Cutaneous Manifestations in Diabetes

Klaus Fritz • George-Sorin Tiplica
Editors

Cutaneous Manifestations in Diabetes

Springer

Editors
Klaus Fritz
Dermatology and Laser Consulting
Landau, Germany

George-Sorin Tiplica
Dermatological Clinic, Carol Davila, UMP
Colentina Clinical Hosp, 2nd
Bucharest, Romania

ISBN 978-3-031-65299-8 ISBN 978-3-031-65300-1 (eBook)
https://doi.org/10.1007/978-3-031-65300-1

This Springer imprint is published by the registered company Springer Nature Switzerland AG
The registered company address is: Gewerbestrasse 11, 6330 Cham, Switzerland

Preface

Diabetes as well as skin disorders are among the most common ailments, but in the highly specialized environment of medical professions, the specialty groups that treat patients affected by diabetes often have less experience with skin conditions. On the other hand, dermatologists only marginally deal with the treatment of diabetes.

Our aim as editors was to highlight the connections between both conditions, and present the most important skin diseases that can be triggered or worsened by diabetes, to help practitioners in differential diagnosis and in the choice of the best therapeutic options. Surprisingly, there are only a few focused and comprehensive works available on this topic, and for that reason this timely work appears as quite unique in Springer's portfolio of clinical medicine books.

To fill this gap and to build the contents of this volume, we primarily thought of colleagues who, while treating diabetes in their everyday practice, suddenly encounter skin changes. In medical care, these interactions are very telling and of growing importance. Diabetes mellitus is a persistent metabolic disorder characterized by elevated blood glucose levels, leading to progressive damage in various tissues and organs, including the skin and nerves. The predominant form is type 2 diabetes, typically occurring in adults, resulting from a combination of insulin resistance and insufficient pancreatic beta cell function. Within a decade from the first appearance of the condition, approximately 50% of patients may require insulin therapy.

On the other side, type 1 diabetes, more prevalent among children and adolescents, is an autoimmune condition marked by chronic inflammation and the destruction of beta cells by autoreactive T lymphocytes. Patients suffering from diabetes have up to a 2.6 times higher risk of premature death, and their life expectancy is about 5–6 years lower than the expectancy of a person without diabetes. The global incidence of diabetes is on the rise, largely attributed to the widespread obesity epidemic, and this escalating trend poses a significant global health challenge.

Between 30% and 70% of all diabetes patients experience temporary as well as long-term dermatological symptoms. Skin problems in diabetes can be an initial warning sign or indicating inadequate therapy, a life-threatening emergency, or undetected type 2 diabetes. In cases of persistent itching and mycoses, dermatological consultation should always be sought, as diabetes can be responsible for—or at least more prevalent in—other skin changes. Skin changes occur in both manifest diabetes and the pre-diabetic stage. Skin changes in diabetes mellitus can be categorized into five groups of diseases: skin infections, skin diseases with a frequent association with diabetes mellitus, due to diabetic complications, due to diabetogenic organ diseases and their secondary effects on the skin, as well as reactions to antidiabetic treatments.

Before examining specific presentations of the skin in diabetic patients, our collective endeavor dwells on epidemiologic considerations, evaluates socio-economic consequences of diabetes, and offers insights to quality-of-life issues in patients. Specific chapters are dedicated to infections of the skin, the issues of reduced circulation including leg ulcers, wound, and skin care. Topics include complications and imaging, dermatoses, and auto-inflammatory skin disorders.

While preserving clarity of style, we looked for an interdisciplinary approach, with authors representing clinical practice in Germany and Romania, but also in Finland, Spain, and Brazil, to cite a few. All contributions were prepared by expert colleagues with sound experience and, in some cases, decades of work in clinical research and practice.

Their participation allowed us to finalize this volume, that will help in navigating diagnostic challenges, and a valued guide for clinical dermatologists, general practitioners, nursing personnel, and health care professionals involved in the care of diabetic patients, enabling early detection and safe treatment.

Landau, Germany — Klaus Fritz
Bucharest, Romania — George-Sorin Tiplica

Contents

Part I
Diabetes Impact on Skin Structure and Functions

Chapter 1
Importance of Diabetes and Skin-Related Conditions in Health Care: Social and Economic Impact

Matthias Augustin

Abstract

- Skin diseases are frequent, burdensome and economically relevant.
- Diabetes is a frequent comorbidity of many chronic inflammatory, vascular and autoimmune skin diseases.
- The disease burden of diabetes adds to the disease burden of the associated skin diseases.
- In Europe there are large socio-economic variations, including access to care, in skin conditions and diabetes, leading to large variations of costs and burden.
- High numbers of patients are in need of health care and have to bear substantial personal costs for health care.
- Better access to innovative care will improve the value for money.
- There is a huge economic potential of prevention, both for diabetes and for many chronic skin conditions.

Skin diseases are associated with considerable socio-economic burden. These result both from the frequency of skin diseases and from the individual burden of disease. Skin diseases associated with diabetes have both the disease burden of the skin disease and the additional burden of diabetes.

The following chapter systematically deals with the epidemiological and health economic aspects of skin diseases associated with diabetes.

M. Augustin (✉)
Institute for Health Services Research in Dermatology and Nursing (IVDP), University Medical Center Hamburg-Eppendorf (UKE), Hamburg, Germany
e-mail: m.augustin@uke.de

K. Fritz, G.-S. Tiplica (eds.), *Cutaneous Manifestations in Diabetes*,
https://doi.org/10.1007/978-3-031-65300-1_1

1.1 Background: Epidemiology as a Determinant of Disease Burden

Skin diseases are among the most common causes of treatment in general medicine. In Western countries, around 25% of people suffer from a skin disease requiring treatment each year [1], while the number of people with skin diseases worldwide is estimated at around 2 billion. Diabetes is also a common metabolic disease positioned by the World Health Organization WHO as one of the most relevant noncommunicable diseases [2]. According to the Organisation for Economic Co-operation and Development (OECD) sources and the report of the International Diabetes Federation (IDF), it affects between 4 and 15% of people, depending on the region and population groups and more than 500 mio. persons worldwide [3, 4]. It shows a general increase in prevalence since several decades [5]. Genetic factors as well as diet and lifestyle contribute to the increased incidence of diabetes.

The most common skin diseases in Western countries are chronic inflammatory conditions, such as eczema, including atopic dermatitis, psoriasis and acne, but also pathogen-related skin diseases such as mycoses, viral warts, herpes and the large group of bacterial skin diseases. In many countries, parasites and infestations also play a role—scabies, for example, is a major health challenge worldwide [6]. Also diseases of the skin appendices such as hair, glands and nails and diseases of the mucous membranes play an important role. Last but not least, vascular skin diseases of the arteries, veins and venous system are socially and economically very relevant.

A considerable number of the aforementioned diseases occur more frequently with diabetes and/or take a particularly severe course in combination with diabetes, imposing additional disease burden and costs. For example, as a consequence of diabetes-related vascular diseases, chronic wounds can result [7]. Also skin sensations such as pruritus are significantly more frequent in persons with diabetes compared to persons without [8, 9]. Vice versa, persons with diabetes suffer more frequently from pruritus than persons without [10].

Remarkably, diabetes can be a causal factor, just as certain skin diseases can lead to an increased risk of diabetes due to a systemic inflammatory process. It is not uncommon for skin and diabetes diseases to be intertwined via obesity and vascular inflammation.

The aforementioned findings are of great importance for the socio-economic assessment of both diseases, as the costs for combinations of diabetes and skin disease are generally higher than for the respective individual diseases.

1.2 Essentials About Economic Burden

From an economic perspective, the total disease burden of skin diseases and diabetes results from the combination of direct costs, indirect costs and intangible costs (Fig. 1.1). The direct costs relate to immediate medical treatment and are mainly

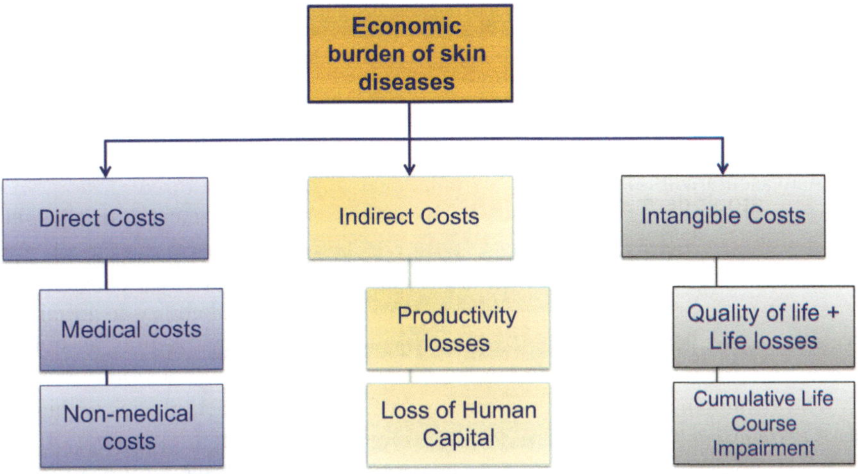

Fig. 1.1 Costs to be considered in the economic characterization of diabetes and skin conditions

borne by payers (health insurers, national healthcare systems) and patients, with the latter being referred to as out-of-pocket costs.

Indirect costs result from loss of productivity, retraining measures and other indirect factors, all of which can be measured in monetary terms. Intangible costs are those associated with the humanitarian burden of disease, which reflect the suffering of those affected. These cannot be measured in monetary units and are therefore referred to as intangibles. However, the loss of quality of life, the loss of well-being and the accumulation of burdens in the sense of cumulative lifetime burdens can be measured indirectly.

A special method for determining the global burden of disease is the global burden of disease method [11]. This method adds up years of life lost and years of life impaired by disability as a function of population size. The losses of quality of life from disease are assessed using a method that determines disease weights in the public. Diabetes ranges number 14 and skin diseases number 18 in the global list of burdensome conditions. In the area of skin diseases, this approach has led to a considerable underestimation of the global burden of disease [12], because the disease weights for skin diseases were assessed as extremely low—an expression of the lack of understanding of skin diseases in the general population.

1.3 Social Burden of Diabetes and Skin Diseases

From an economic point of view, it is therefore more reliable and valid if the humanistic burden of disease is determined using quality of life methods.

Here, people with diabetes already show significant average losses in quality of life compared to the normal population (Fig. 1.2), while people with skin diseases

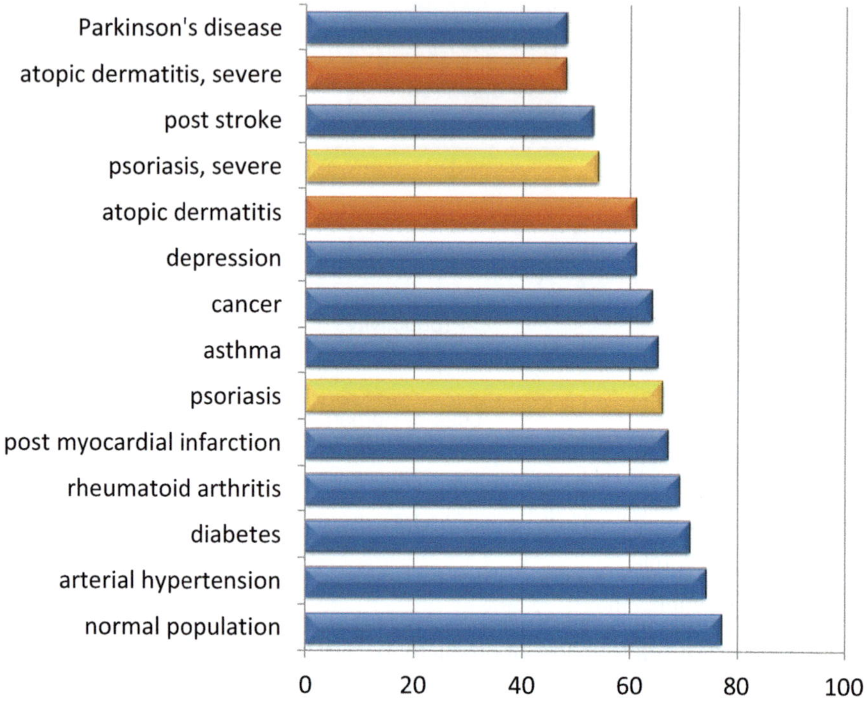

Fig. 1.2 Quality of life impairment in diabetes and in several skin conditions measured by EQ-5D scores. Data from German routine care ($N = 14{,}321$)

such as psoriasis and atopic dermatitis show even greater average losses in quality of life [13, 14]. This is due not only to the heavy physical burden of the disease caused by itching and pain but also to the psychological stress and social burdens such as stigmatization. Comparable burdens are generally not found in diabetes alone.

In the combination of chronic skin disease and diabetes, however, components of the disease can interact additively or even more strongly.

The socio-economic burden of disease includes the phenomenon of cumulative life course impairment (CLCI). This means that physical, psychological and social stresses can accumulate over time and are sometimes irreversible. Such irreversible events can happen at work and in social life but also biological events, such as the loss of extremities due to severe diabetic skin conditions. The term CLCI was introduced to describe the risk of chronic stress during the course of the disease. This indicates that in the case of both skin diseases and diabetes, an essential measure is to avert cumulative damage for the person concerned and to limit the cumulative curve (Fig. 1.3).

The timing of intervention is of great importance both in the early treatment of diabetes and in the timely intervention of skin diseases. If the intervention takes place early, an escalation of both diseases with major damage can be averted, while

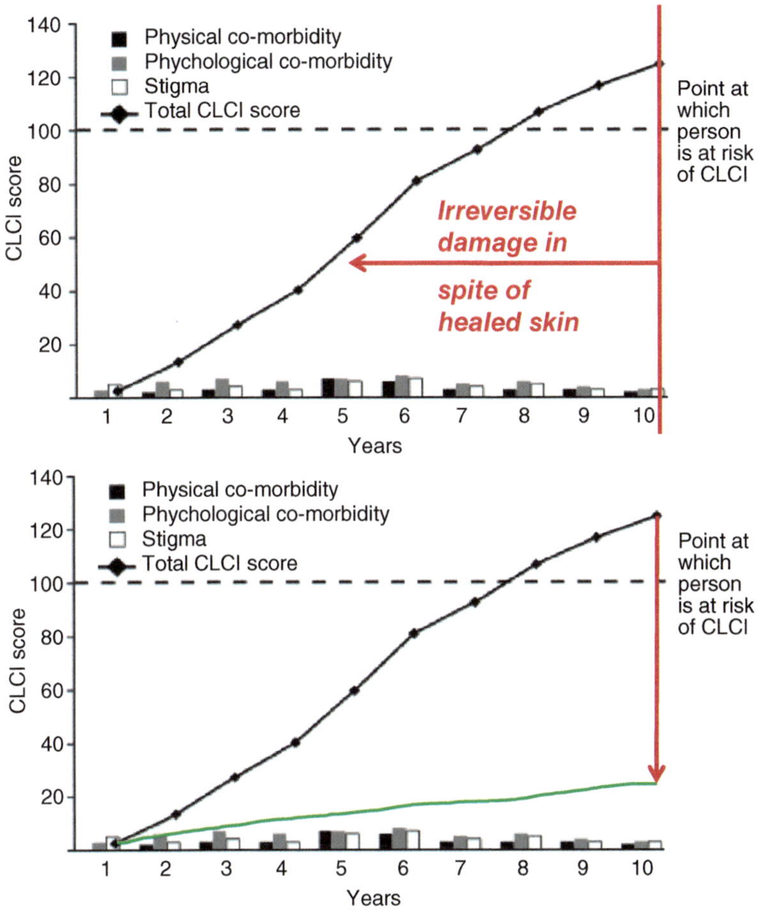

Fig. 1.3 Scheme on the indirect disease burden of skin diseases and diabetes reflected by cumulative life course impairment (left); treatment goal is to "flatten the curve" (right)

late interventions and failure to make timely diagnoses lead to a corridor of burdens over time. These burdens can accumulate and be irreversible, which is referred to as cumulative life course impairment (CLCI) which has also been described for chronic skin wounds including diabetes [15, 16].

Avoiding CLCI in skin diseases and diabetes means promoting early intervention for both. In line with this, controlled studies have shown that early detection of diabetes on a population basis leads to better health economic results [17]. Besides reducing costs, early intervention also leads to reduction of risks for physical damage, morbidity, CLCI and possibly even mortality (Fig. 1.4).

From an economic perspective, the principle of necessary early intervention also means that higher initial treatment costs may be required, for example, through intensified diagnostics, secondary preventive measures or sustainable interventions.

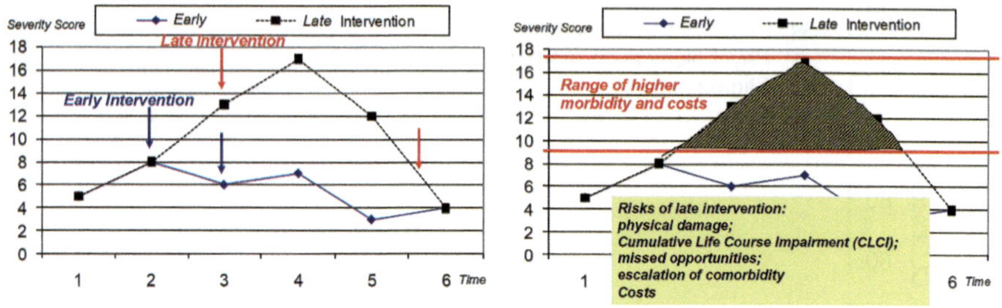

Fig. 1.4 Scheme depicting the importance of early intervention in diabetes and skin diseases for the prevention of disease progression and consecutive damage

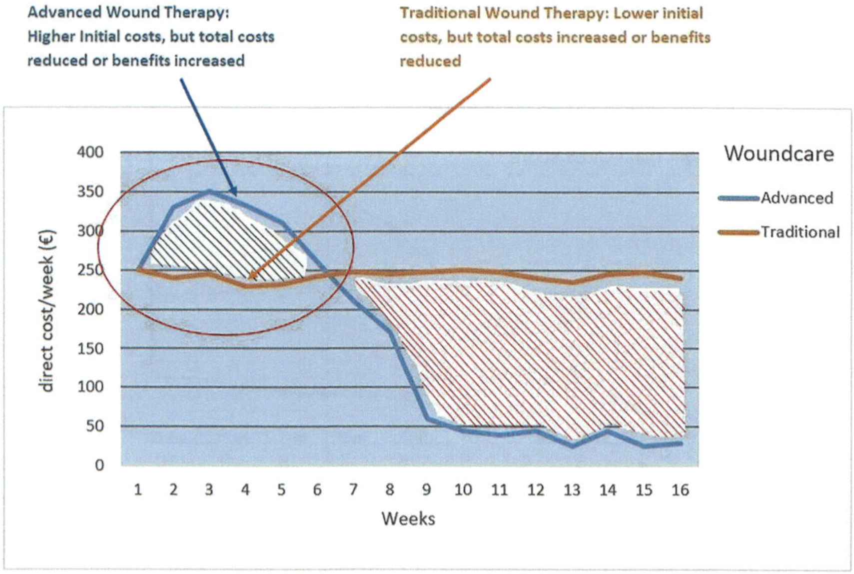

Fig. 1.5 Schematic presentation of the return on investment from advanced wound therapies in chronic wounds including diabetic wounds. Early higher costs can be compensated with greater long-term economic and social benefits

The "return on investment" can then be expected over time [18], so that the overall balance of even expensive and costly therapies is often better (Fig. 1.5).

1.4 Economic Burden of Skin Diseases Related to Diabetes

There are numerous individual studies on the total costs of skin diseases in Germany that focus on specific diseases. For example, the average cost of psoriasis vulgaris is €8000 and that of chronic wounds is €15,000. The costs of many diseases have not been determined in detail. In the case of diabetes, it is assumed that the total cost per affected person in most countries is around €8000–30,000 per year. Depending on the prevalence and the population group, the total costs for the individual healthcare systems therefore vary considerably and amount to around €3 billion in Germany and €15 billion in the USA.

Chronic skin wounds related to diabetes are particularly expensive, as shown in studies for the UK [19], the US [20] and Germany [21].

Diabetes per se is a global political, social and economic challenge with rising costs expected on an annual level [22]. In a recent study from the USA, the total annual cost of diabetes in 2022 was $412.9 billion, which of $306.6 billion derived from direct medical costs and $106.3 billion from indirect costs [23]. People with diagnosed diabetes account for 1 of every 4 healthcare dollars spent in the USA.

A major cost driver of health care for skin disease and diabetes is the patient adherence, both in prevention and treatment [24]. In diabetes, randomized studies have shown that this adherence can be increased using structured interventions [25]. Additionally, patients who felt diabetes and/or skin treatment more burdensome experienced worse diabetes results, measured by HbA1C [26].

Costs of diabetes have been shown to directly being triggered by several skin conditions, such as erysipelas and other skin infections. Increased costs were also found in patients who use insulin pumps and/or glucose sensors but did not apply proper skin care [27].

1.5 Cost-Effectiveness of Interventions for Chronic Skin Conditions and for Associated Diabetes

The economic consequence of the high disease burden of diabetes and skin diseases is to implement sustainable and cost-effective interventions. This involves the use of cost-benefit calculation methods that ideally go beyond a pure cost-cost analysis and also compare the costs with an outcome benefit or, even better, a value benefit (Fig. 1.6).

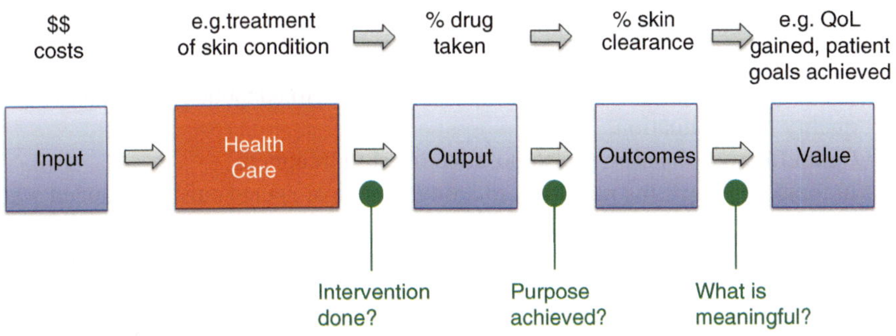

Fig. 1.6 The value chain: the ultimate benefits if interventions for skin conditions and for diabetes need to be measured by the extent of value generated

For these interventions, it is advisable to take into account both the costs of treatment in the main area and those of diabetes and also to apply the benefits to both disease areas or even further comorbidity.

1.6 Recommendations for Practice

For medical practice, the following facts may be considered:

- The disease burden of skin diseases and diabetes is considerable and should be considered in health care.
- From the patient's point of view, the greatest burden is the suffering caused by the skin and the consequences of diabetes; early and consistent intervention is therefore necessary here.
- More efficiency in care in reducing subjective illness is gained if this is systematically measured using validated questionnaires and treatment goals.
- In practice, the Questionnaire on quality of life with chronic wounds (WoundQoL) has proven to be a validated and suitable instrument for measuring quality of life in the wound sector, which should be supplemented by pain measurements.
- This questionnaire can be used to formulate therapy goals which are strongly recommended in diabetes and skin care.
- "Treatment goals" means (a) the definition of goals (ideally shared with the patient), (b) the time to follow-up and (c) the check of achievement.
- Greater efficiency is achieved by setting therapy goals and measuring goal achievement.
- When selecting therapies, those procedures should be used with which the therapy goal can be achieved with the least economic effort.
- However, if more expensive procedures are necessary to achieve the therapy goals, these may still be more efficient in the long term, and the principle of benefit before cost applies anyway.
- The most important predictors of costs for both diabetes and associated skin diseases are inpatient treatments; the duration of these should be shortened or even avoided by suitable outpatient measures.
- Other important cost predictors are the wound dressings; here it is important to use only those that are immediately necessary and to adapt both the quantity and quality to the situation.
- Cost-effective planning is also possible for skin treatment.
- In topical therapy, the necessary quantity of topical agents must be planned well in advance; the fingertip units help here.
- For prudent, psychosocially optimized care, the involvement of family caregivers and other professions is of great importance. Here too, the cost of coordinating measures is usually low compared to the added benefit achieved through better coordinated measures.

- The objective in the care of diabetes and associated skin diseases must therefore be early intervention, careful diagnosis and individualized therapy within the scope of what is necessary.
- This principle is based on the PCHC of the WHO.

References

1. Augustin M, Herberger K, Hintzen S, Heigel H, Franzke N, Schaefer I. Prevalence of skin lesions and need for treatment in a cohort of 90,880 workers. Br J Dermatol. 2011;165(4):865–73.
2. https://www.who.int/news-room/fact-sheets/detail/noncommunicable-diseases. Accessed 6 Jan 2024.
3. OECD. Health at a glance, 2023. https://www.oecd.org/health/health-at-a-glance/.
4. IDF—International Diabetes Federation. IDF diabetes atlas. 10 ed. Brussels: International Diabetes Federation; 2021.
5. NCD Risk Factor Collaboration. Worldwide trends in diabetes since 1980: a pooled analysis of 751 population-based studies with 4.4 million participants. Lancet. 2016;387:1513–30. https://doi.org/10.1016/S0140-6736(16)00618-8.
6. Cox V, Fuller LC, Engelman D, Steer A, Hay RJ. Estimating the global burden of scabies: what else do we need? Br J Dermatol. 2021;184(2):237–42.
7. Heyer K, Herberger K, Protz K, Glaeske G, Augustin M. Epidemiology of chronic wounds in Germany: analysis of statutory health insurance data. Wound Repair Regen. 2016;24(2):434–42.
8. Ständer S, Schaefer I, Phan NQ, Blome C, Herberger K, Heigel H, Augustin M. Prevalence of chronic pruritus in Germany: results of a cross-sectional study in a sample working population of 11,730. Dermatology. 2010;221(3):229–35.
9. Ständer S, Garbe C, Hagenström K, Petersen J, Zeidler C, Augustin M. Healthcare utilization and treatment patterns in patients with chronic Prurigo and chronic pruritus in Germany. Dermatology. 2022;238(4):753–61.
10. Augustin M, Garbe C, Hagenström K, Petersen J, Pereira MP, Ständer S. Prevalence, incidence, and presence of comorbidities in patients with Prurigo and pruritus in Germany: a population-based claims data analysis. J Eur Acad Dermatol Venereol. 2021;35(11):2270–6.
11. GBD 2013 Mortality and Causes of Death Collaborators. Global, regional, and national age-sex specific all-cause and cause-specific mortality for 240 causes of death, 1990–2013: a systematic analysis for the Global Burden of Disease Study 2013. Lancet. 2015;385(9963):117–71.
12. Hay RJ, Johns NE, Williams HC, Bolliger IW, Dellavalle RP, Margolis DJ, Marks R, Naldi L, Weinstock MA, Wulf SK, Michaud C, Murray JLC, Naghavi M. The global burden of skin disease in 2010: an analysis of the prevalence and impact of skin conditions. J Invest Dermatol. 2014;134(6):1527–34.
13. Koenig HH, et al. Z Gesundheitswesen. 2005;67:173–82.
14. Beikert FC, Langenbruch AK, Radtke MA, Kornek T, Purwins S, Augustin M. Willingness to pay and quality of life in patients with atopic dermatitis. Arch Dermatol Res. 2014;306(3):279–86.
15. Augustin M, Mayer A, Goepel LM, Baade K, Heyer K, Herberger K. Cumulative life course impairment (CLCI): a new concept to characterize persistent patient burden in chronic wounds. Wound Med. 2013;1:2–6.
16. Augustin M. Cumulative life course impairment in chronic wounds. In: Kimball AB, Linder MD, Itin P, Jemec G, editors. Dermatological diseases and cumulative life course impairment. Current problems in dermatology, vol. 44. Basel: Karger Verlag; 2013. p. 125–9.
17. Einarson TR, Bereza BG, Acs A, Jensen R. Systematic literature review of the health economic implications of early detection by screening populations at risk for type 2 diabetes. Curr Med Res Opin. 2017;33(2):331–58.

18. Augustin M, Vanscheidt W. Chronic venous leg ulcers: the future of cell-based therapies. Lancet. 2012;380(9846):953–5.
19. Guest JF, Ayoub N, McIlwraith T, Uchegbu I, Gerrish A, Weidlich D, Vowden K, Vowden P. Health economic burden that wounds impose on the National Health Service in the UK. BMJ Open. 2015;5(12):e009283.
20. US costs.
21. Heyer K, Debus ES, Mayerhoff L, Augustin M. Prevalence and regional distribution of lower limb amputations from 2006 to 2012 in Germany: a population based study. Eur J Vasc Endovasc Surg. 2015;50(6):761–6.
22. Bommer C, Sagalova V, Heesemann E, Manne-Goehler J, Atun R, Bärnighausen T, Davies J, Vollmer S. Global economic burden of diabetes in adults: projections from 2015 to 2030. Diabetes Care. 2018;41(5):963–70.
23. Parker ED, Lin J, Mahoney T, Ume N, Yang G, Gabbay RA, ElSayed NA, Bannuru RR. Economic costs of diabetes in the U.S. in 2022. Diabetes Care. 2024;47(1):26–43.
24. Hagenström K, Protz K, Petersen J, Augustin M. Development of a model to predict closure of chronic wounds in Germany: claims data analysis. Int Wound J. 2022;19(1):76–85.
25. Joshi R, Joshi D, Cheriyath P. Improving adherence and outcomes in diabetic patients. Patient Prefer Adherence. 2017;11:271–5. https://doi.org/10.2147/PPA.S122490.
26. Vijan S, Sussman JB, Yudkin JS, Hayward RA. Effect of patients' risks and preferences on health gains with plasma glucose level lowering in type 2 diabetes mellitus. JAMA Intern Med. 2014;174(8):1227–34.
27. Berg AK, Thorsen SU, Thyssen JP, Zachariae C, Keiding H, Svensson J. Cost of treating skin problems in patients with diabetes who use insulin pumps and/or glucose sensors. Diabetes Technol Ther. 2020;22(9):658–65.

Chapter 2
The Types of Diabetes

Alexandra Mirica and Diana Loreta Paun

Abstract Diabetes mellitus is a complex condition with specific diagnostic and treatment features depending on the type of diabetes identified. In this chapter we will summarize the types of diabetes and the clinical management features for each. Diabetes mellitus is a chronic disease affecting all the body's metabolism, with a complex etiopathogenesis, characterized by elevated blood glucose levels.

The etiopathogenic classification of diabetes was proposed in 1997 by the American Diabetes Association (ADA) and accepted 2 years later by the World Health Organization (WHO). It comprises four categories, namely:

- **Type 1 diabetes mellitus**, which can include latent autoimmune diabetes of adults, resulting from the autoimmune destruction of pancreatic beta cells leading to an absolute insulin deficiency.
- **Type 2 diabetes mellitus** characterized by progressive non-autoimmune decrease of insulin secretion due to insulin resistance and metabolic syndrome.
- **Specific types of diabetes** due to other causes or conditions (diseases of the exocrine pancreas, drug- or chemical-induced diabetes and monogenic diabetes syndromes).
- **Gestational diabetes** (diabetes that was not obviously evident before pregnancy but was discovered in the second or third trimester of the pregnancy) [1].

Traditionally, diabetes is divided into two categories: type 2 diabetes, which makes up around 90% of cases, and type 1 diabetes, which makes up the remaining 5–10% of instances. Diabetes type 1 and type 2 are diverse diseases with widely varying clinical presentations and forms of disease development. Although classification is crucial for choosing a course of treatment, differentiating between type 1 and unusual type 2 diabetes presentations has becoming more challenging. Since both diseases affect people of all ages, the outdated stereotypes that type 2 diabetes exclusively affects adults and type 1 diabetes only affects children are no longer valid [2].

A. Mirica (✉) · D. L. Paun
University of Medicine and Pharmacy "Carol Davila" Bucharest, Bucharest, Romania
e-mail: alexandra.mirica@umfcd.ro; diana-loreta.paun@umfcd.ro

K. Fritz, G.-S. Tiplica (eds.), *Cutaneous Manifestations in Diabetes*,
https://doi.org/10.1007/978-3-031-65300-1_2

2.1 Type 1 Diabetes

About 5–10% of all instances of diabetes are type 1 diabetes mellitus, which comes in two forms: idiopathic and immune-mediated. The majority of individuals with type 1 diabetes have markers of beta cell destruction, such as antibodies against islet cell antibodies (ICA), antibodies against insulin, antibodies against tyrosine phosphatases, insulinoma-associated protein 2 antibodies (IA-2 and IA-2 beta), antibodies against zinc transporter 8 (ZnT8), and glutamic acid decarboxylase 65 (GAD65) antibodies. The ADA classification system subclassifies type 1 diabetes into A and B forms. "Type 1A" diabetes includes patients in whom autoantibodies are identified in the serum and is synonymous with autoimmune type 1 diabetes, especially if two or more autoantibodies are positive. And the term "idiopathic" or "type 1B" diabetes is used to include patients with type 1 diabetes without identifiable autoantibodies in serum and patients who have no other known cause for beta cell destruction [3]. Interestingly, new research suggests that individuals with type 1 diabetes may also exhibit insulin resistance and other characteristics of type 2 diabetes, particularly if they have a family history of the condition [4]. It is important to note that intense insulin treatment may extend beta cell activity in the early stages of type 1 diabetes [5]. Diabetic ketoacidosis (DKA) can be the initial presentation in approximately 25% of adults with newly diagnosed type 1 diabetes.

2.1.1 Latent Autoimmune Diabetes in Adults (LADA)

Latent autoimmune diabetes in adults (LADA) is a kind of type 1 diabetes that progresses more slowly in terms of insulin absolute deficiency. An adult patient with this diagnosis will have at least one diabetes autoantibody but will show longer preservation of insulin secretion and a more gradual onset of clinical diabetes than usual type 1 diabetes diagnosed in children and adolescents. Although insulin medication may not be necessary at the time of diagnosis for adults with LADA, insulin dependency usually develops after several years. Regarding LADA, studies indicated that patients have the body mass index (BMI) lower, an earlier age of diabetes onset, and antibody titers higher, especially high glutamic acid decarboxylase antibody titers $\geq$10 U/mL [6, 7].

2.2 Type 2 Diabetes

Type 2 diabetes accounts for approximately 90% of all diabetes cases. The significant increase in type 2 diabetes cases can be justified by the intensification of the urbanization process [according to the International Diabetes Federation (IDF), two thirds of patients come from the urban environment], changes in eating habits, reduction of physical activity, and the general aging of the population. Type 2 diabetes is the most common phenotypic form of diabetes in adults and is characterized by hyperglycemia and varying degrees of insulin resistance and initial relative insulin deficiency. Its prevalence is increasing considerably with the rise in obesity, a pandemic condition in recent years. Environmental or genetic factors may contribute to insulin insufficiency and resistance. In addition, hyperglycemia itself can damage pancreatic beta cell function and increase insulin resistance, through a process termed "glucotoxicity" [4].

Recent research has also identified subtypes of type 2 diabetes, depending on proinsulin levels and the presence of insulin resistance, associated with features of obesity, lipodystrophy, or abnormal liver lipid metabolism [8].

Clinicians should consider islet autoantibody testing, at least two autoantibodies, in all patients who do not exhibit a classic phenotype of overweight-associated type 2 diabetes, given the overlap between type 1 and type 2 diabetes [1].

Individuals who test positive for two or more autoantibodies are likely to develop type 1 diabetes, which should be treated with insulin replacement treatment right at once because these individuals don't react well to diet and oral hypoglycemic medication therapy [1].

2.3 Specific Types of Diabetes

The subclass of specific types of diabetes associated with other causes or conditions represents approximately 1–2% of all diabetes cases. In some situations, the etiopathogenic relationship is known, i.e., diabetes mellitus secondary to pancreatic and endocrine disorders or the administration of drug therapies such as synthetic glucocorticoids. In other situations, the relationship is described due to the frequent association of the condition with specific syndromes.

The summary of the main specific causes of diabetes consists of the following, synthesized in Table 2.1.

1. **Genetic abnormalities of pancreatic beta cell function** [mitochondrial diabetes secondary to mutations in deoxyribonucleic acid (DNA), maturity-onset diabetes of the young (MODY), neonatal diabetes]
2. **Genetic abnormalities in the action of insulin**
3. **Diseases of the exocrine pancreas** (pancreatectomy, pancreatitis, pancreatic carcinoma, cystic fibrosis, hemochromatosis)
4. **Endocrine disorders**
5. **Diabetes induced by medication or generated by chemical substances**
6. **Infections**
7. **Genetic syndromes**
8. **Rare forms** generated by immunologically mediated mechanisms

Table 2.1 Specific types of diabetes

1. Genetic defects of beta cell function	2. Genetic defects in insulin action	3. Diseases of the exocrine pancreas	4. Endocrine disorders	5. Drug or chemical induced	6. Infections	7. Genetic syndromes	8. Rare forms
Chromosome 20, HNF-4-alpha (MODY1)	Leprechaunism	Pancreatitis	Cushing's syndrome	Thyroid hormones	Congenital rubella	Down syndrome	"Stiff man" syndrome
Chromosome 7, glucokinase (MODY2)	Type A insulin resistance	Trauma/ pancreatectomy	Acromegaly	Glucocorticoids	Cytomegalovirus	Klinefelter syndrome	Anti-insulin receptor antibodies
Chromosome 12, HNF-1-alpha (MODY3)	Rabson–Mendenhall syndrome	Cystic fibrosis	Aldosteronoma	Vacor		Turner syndrome	
Chromosome 13, insulin promoter factor-1 (IPF-1; MODY4)	Lipoatrophic diabetes	Neoplasia	Glucagonoma	Pentamidine		Prader–Willi syndrome	
Chromosome 17, HNF-1-beta (MODY5)		Hemochromatosis	Pheochromocytoma	Alpha interferon		Wolfram syndrome	
Chromosome 2, NeuroD1 (MODY6)		Fibrocalculous pancreatopathy	Hyperthyroidism Somatostatinoma	Atypical antipsychotics		Friedreich's ataxia	
Mitochondrial DNA				Thiazides		Huntington's chorea	
Neonatal diabetes				Nicotinic acid		Laurence–Moon–Biedl syndrome	
				Diazoxide		Myotonic dystrophy	
				Beta-adrenergic agonists		Huntington's chorea	

1. **The genetic disorders of pancreatic beta cell function** comprises deoxyribonucleic acid DNA mutations causing mitochondrial diabetes, MODY or maturity-onset diabetes of the young, and neonatal diabetes.

   Mitochondrial diabetes develops secondary to DNA mutations, associated with deafness and moderately elevated blood glucose values [9, 10].

   Monogenic diabetes [formerly called maturity-onset diabetes of the young (MODY)] is a clinically heterogeneous autosomal dominant disease characterized by diabetes diagnosed at a young age (<25 years) with lack of autoantibodies. MODY-type diabetes includes moderately elevated blood glucose values that are mostly asymptomatic, absence of obesity, but a family history of diabetes of three or more generations [11]. Mutant genes are expressed both in pancreatic beta cells and also in other tissues such as liver and kidneys and cause also other organic dysfunctions [12]. The genetic defects and chromosomes involved are shown in Table 2.2. The increased attention given to this form of diabetes through the numerous published studies allowed genetic testing, highlighting the monogenic transmission of the diabetogenic defect, pointing to a much more precise approach to the genetics of type 2 diabetes in which the transmission is polygenic. Published evidence shows that 1/3 of MODY patients are treated with diet, 1/3 with oral therapy, and 1/3 with insulin [13, 14].

Table 2.2 Types of monogenic diabetes

Type MODY	Genetic defect	Frequency	Pancreatic cell defect	Clinical picture	Treatment
1	Chromosome 20, hepatocyte nuclear factor-4-alpha	<10%	Diminished insulin secretory response to glucose	Normal renal threshold for glucose	Sulfonylureas
2	Chromosome 7, glucokinase	15–31%	Defective glucokinase	Mild, stable, fasting hyperglycemia	**Diet**
3	Chromosome 12, HNF-1-alpha	**52–65%**	Abnormal insulin secretion, low renal threshold for glucose	Low renal threshold for glucose, with glycosuria	Sulfonylureas
4	Chromosome 13, insulin promoter factor-1	**Rare**	Reduced binding to the insulin gene promoter, reduced activation of insulin gene in response to hyperglycemia	Rare, pancreatic agenesis in homozygotes, less severe mutations resulting in mild diabetes	
5	Chromosome 17, HNF-1-beta	**Rare**		Pancreatic atrophy, renal dysplasia, renal cysts, renal insufficiency, hypomagnesemia	**Insulin**
6	Chromosome 2, NeuroD1	**Rare**	Pancreatic development		**Insulin**

Differentiating monogenic diabetes from type 1 and type 2 diabetes is crucial because the underlying genetic abnormality affects the best outcome of therapy and the likelihood of complications from the disease.

If any of the following are present, a high suspicion for monogenic diabetes can be suspected and genetic testing should be done [15–17].

- Diabetes with a multigenerational family history (i.e., ≥3 generations or history in one parent and at least one additional first-degree relative of that parent) along with other clinical traits (age below 25 years old, normal weight, low risk of diabetic ketoacidosis) and negative autoantibodies against zinc transporter (ZnT8), insulinoma-associated protein 2 (IA-2), and glutamic acid decarboxylase 65 (GAD65).
- Using the MODY Clinical Risk Calculator available online, clinicians can calculate whether there is a high probability of monogenic diabetes.
- Preserved fasting C-peptide (>0.6 ng/mL when glucose is >72 mg/dL) in people with assumed type 1 diabetes, 3–5 years after diagnosis.

In addition, a mutation in a single gene that impacts pancreatic beta cell activity is often the cause of **neonatal diabetes mellitus** (NDM), which is defined by the emergence of persistent hyperglycemia within the first 6 months of life as a result of reduced insulin action. One of the more than 30 known genetic mutations causes NDM. Depending on the particular gene mutation, NDM can manifest as one of several clinical subtypes, such as transient diabetes, diabetes that responds to oral sulfonylurea, isolated permanent diabetes requiring lifelong insulin therapy, or NDM associated with genetic syndromes that also require lifelong insulin therapy [18, 19].

2. **Genetic abnormalities in insulin action include** [20]:

   - Insulin resistance type A, characterized by significant insulin resistance, the presence of ovarian cysts, hirsutism or virilization, as well as acanthosis nigricans.
   - Leprechaunism associated with marked insulin resistance and craniocerebral changes.
   - Rabson–Mendenhall syndrome presenting severe insulin resistance, hyperplasia of the pineal gland, as well as dental and nail abnormalities.
   - Lipoatrophic diabetes characterized by marked reduction of adipose tissue, insulin resistance, hepatomegaly, and xanthomas [1].

3. **Exocrine pancreatic diseases**

   Following pancreatectomy surgery consisting in the surgical removal of over half to three quarters of the pancreas (for pancreatic neoplasia, congenital hyperinsulinism, other pancreatic diseases), insulin-requiring diabetes can develop. Diseases of the exocrine pancreas that can be associated with diabetes are represented by chronic pancreatitis, carcinoma of the pancreas, cystic fibrosis, and hemochromatosis. Inflammation and fibrosis of pancreatic tissue impair both endocrine and exocrine function, leading to insulin or glucagon deficiency and pancreatic enzyme deficiencies. Moreover, patients with pancreatic disease typically require insulin treatment. There is a greater chance of hypoglycemia because the alpha cells that produce glucagon are also affected [21, 22].

Furthermore, reduced insulin production and insulin resistance are two characteristics of type 1 and type 2 diabetes that are shared by the distinct processes of diabetes associated with cystic fibrosis. The most prevalent comorbidity in individuals with cystic fibrosis is cystic fibrosis-related diabetes, which affects 20% of adolescents and 40–50% of adults. The ADA presents several recommendations regarding cystic fibrosis-related diabetes, as follows [2]:

- Diabetes screening must be initiated at the age of 10 in patients diagnosed with this condition.
- The oral glucose tolerance test is recommended, and HbA1C is not recommended for diagnosis of diabetes in children with cystic fibrosis or symptoms suggestive of acute onset of type 1 diabetes.
- Patients diagnosed with diabetes benefit from insulin therapy in order to attain individualized glycemic goals.
- After 5 years from the diagnosis, the annual screening of complications specific to diabetes is required.
- In addition, individuals with hereditary hemochromatosis frequently have diabetes; in fact, up to 50% of symptomatic individuals had diabetes at the time of diagnosis [23].

Moreover, tropical pancreatitis is the cause of fibrocalculous pancreatic diabetes, an uncommon sort of diabetes that is common in various parts of the world (like southern India). The fatality rate from this condition is further increased by complications from pancreatic cancer and chronic pancreatitis, as well as macro- and microvascular issues that are frequently connected to diabetes [24].

4. **Endocrine disorders**

Regarding the endocrinopathies associated with diabetes, it is known that numerous hormones such as epinephrine, glucagon, cortisol, and growth hormone antagonize the physiological actions of insulin on glucose metabolism, so that the secretion of these hormones constitutes the counter-regulatory protective response to hypoglycemia. On the other hand, the primary oversecretion of these hormones in the context of endocrine disorders can lead to altered glucose tolerance or clinically manifest diabetes. Endocrine conditions that can generate diabetes are mainly represented by acromegaly, hyperthyroidism, Cushing's syndrome, primary hyperaldosteronism, pheochromocytoma, glucagonoma, and somatostatinoma [1].

Acromegaly is a condition caused by a chronic excess of growth hormone (GH) and insulin-like growth factor 1 (IGF-1), in most cases caused by a GH-secreting pituitary tumor. This pathology is associated with severe comorbidities (cardiovascular, metabolic, respiratory, neoplastic, and musculoskeletal), which have a negative impact on the patients' quality of life. Excess GH decreases insulin sensitivity and favors gluconeogenesis, these changes resulting in altered glucose metabolism. In addition, excess GH determines increased insulin resistance due to excessive lipolysis and altered fat distribution and dysfunctional adipose tissue. Thus, an increased number of patients diagnosed with acromegaly have altered glucose tolerance or secondary diabetes. Moreover, the drug treatment used to control the disease can determine, as an adverse effect, the alteration of carbohydrate metabolism, independent of the acromegaly status [25].

Furthermore, diabetes mellitus and thyroid dysfunction are strongly related conditions. Numerous research investigations have reported that individuals with diabetes mellitus are more likely to have thyroid disorders, associated with both hyperfunction and thyroid hypofunction. Patients with diabetes who have untreated thyroid dysfunction may have impaired metabolic regulation, and this correlation may have significant effects on the course of both conditions [26].

Thus, in hyperthyroidism, an increase in blood sugar occurs through several mechanisms [26]:

- Increasing food intake
- Increasing the absorption of glucose at the intestinal level
- Increase in hepatic gluconeogenesis
- Increased secretion of insulin and proinsulin
- Hepatic resistance to the action of insulin
- Increased glucose utilization in muscle and adipose tissue but with the development of peripheral insulin resistance
- On the other hand, in hypothyroidism there is an alteration of blood sugar, with a tendency to hypoglycemia, through [27]:
- Decrease in the intestinal absorption of glucose.
- Decrease in hepatic gluconeogenesis.
- Reduction of glycogenolysis at liver and muscle level.
- Decreased use of glucose at the peripheral level, with the development of insulin resistance [28].

In addition, by encouraging the growth of thyroid tissue and enlarging thyroid nodules, hyperinsulinemia can alter the shape of the thyroid gland. Metformin can provide advantages in both endocrinopathies, but other antidiabetics, such as sulfonylureas, can negatively impair thyroid function [27].

In addition, patients with Cushing's syndrome, due to pituitary or adrenal disease or to exogenous glucocorticoid administration, frequently develop numerous metabolic and systemic complications, such as insulin resistance, prediabetes and diabetes mellitus, dyslipidemia, hypertension, and hypercoagulability [29]. It should be noted that the most important metabolic effects of excess glucocorticoids occur postprandially and a large proportion of patients with hypercorticism have normal fasting blood glucose. Thus, oral glucose tolerance test is considered a gold standard in the diagnosis of abnormalities of carbohydrate metabolism in this category of patients [30–32].

In the case of catecholamine excess in pheochromocytoma, the hypersecretion of catecholamines occurs, and hyperglycemia can develop through the activation of the sympathetic system. Thus, both altered glucose tolerance and overt clinical diabetes can be found as an associated clinical picture [29, 33–35].

A very uncommon pancreatic α-islet cell tumor, glucagonoma frequently presents with a number of clinical signs, such as necrotizing migratory erythema, diabetes, anemia, and weight loss. It can be associated with an association of other clinical features, including skin rash and thromboembolic problems [36].

In addition, somatostatin-secreting tumors (somatostatinomas) typically are associated with the triad of diabetes mellitus, cholelithiasis, and diarrhea with steatorrhea [37].

5. **Diabetes induced by medication or generated by chemical substances**

   Furthermore, drug-induced or chemical-induced diabetes is a subclass caused by drugs that can alter the secretion or action of insulin, can increase hepatic glucose production, or can cause resistance to the action of insulin [38, 39]. The main ones are shown in Table 2.3.

In addition, glucocorticoid therapy is increasingly used today. In pharmacological doses, they can generate the alteration of the glycemic homeostasis by stimulating gluconeogenesis, inducing insulin resistance, altering the function of pancreatic beta cells, and initiating autoimmune insulitis. The management of steroid-induced diabetes presents difficulties due to the vast variations in postprandial hyperglycemia and the absence of well-defined therapeutic guidelines. Insulin therapy administered at mealtimes is the cornerstone of treatment [40].

6. **Infections**

   Furthermore, some viruses (including Coxsackie virus, mumps, and SARS-CoV-2) can cause diabetes directly by destroying beta cells or by triggering an autoimmune reaction [41]. There are studies that indicate the association between diabetes and chronic hepatitis C virus infection. In individuals with or without a

Table 2.3 Drugs or chemicals associated with diabetes

Main drugs or chemicals
Glucocorticoids
Statins
Lithium
β-Adrenergic blockers
Thyroid hormones
Calcium channel blockers
Testosterone
Nicotinic acid
Atypical antipsychotics
Rifampicin
Indomethacin Isoniazid
Cimetidine
Phenothiazides
Thiazide diuretics
Ciclosporin
Alpha interferon

history of diabetes, SARS-CoV-2 (COVID-19) seems to trigger severe diabetes symptoms, such as hyperosmolar hyperglycemic state, diabetic ketoacidosis, and severe insulin resistance [42].

7. **Genetic syndromes associated with diabetes**

   The Wolfram or DIDMOAD (abbreviation for arginine vasopressin deficiency previously named diabetes insipidus, diabetes mellitus, optic atrophy, and deafness) syndrome is another instance of a rare genetic illness linked to diabetes. This condition, encompassing two syndromic subforms, type 1 and type 2, has incomplete penetrance, with autosomal recessive mode of transmission, with distinct genes responsible for the conditions but similar clinical manifestations [43].

   The main syndromes associated with diabetes and their principal characteristic are summarized in Table 2.4.

8. **Rare forms of diabetes**

   Rare forms of diabetes are generated by immunologically mediated mechanisms and include stiff man syndrome, which is generated by the production of anti-insulin receptor antibodies. Clinical manifestations include stiffness of axial

Table 2.4 Main genetic and clinical features of genetic syndromes associated with diabetes

Genetic syndromes associated with diabetes mellitus	Genetic and clinical features
Down syndrome	Presence of an extra chromosome 21, moderate mental retardation, obesity, thyroid disorders [44]
Klinefelter syndrome	Presence of an extra X chromosome, lack of sexual development at puberty, obesity, infertility, micropenis, osteoporosis, cardiovascular disease [45]
Turner syndrome	Complete or partial absence of the X chromosome, lack of development of sexual characteristics at puberty, infertility, cardiovascular disease, autoimmune disorders [46]
Wolfram/DIDMOAD syndrome	Autosomal recessive inherited condition, associated with diabetes insipidus, type 1 diabetes mellitus, optic nerve atrophy, hypoacusis, mental and neurological manifestations [47]
Friedreich's ataxia	FXN gene mutation located on chromosome 9, balance disorders, reduced muscle coordination, dysarthria, hypertrophic cardiomyopathy [48]
Huntington's chorea	Mutation at the HTT gene, motor symptoms, cognitive and psychiatric disorders [49]
Laurence-Moon Biedl syndrome	Autosomal recessive inherited disorder, retinitis pigmentosa, polydactyly, mental retardation, renal dysplasia, obesity [50]
Myotonic dystrophy	Mutations of the DMPK gene present on chromosome 19, respiratory failure, persistent arrhythmias, cognitive impairment [51]
Prader-Willi syndrome	Loss of paternally inherited imprinted genes at 15q11.2-q13, short stature, cardiovascular problems, hypothalamic dysfunction, severe hypotonia, hypogonadism, central hypothyroidism [52]

muscles and painful spasms; it may be associated with other autoimmune conditions such as systemic lupus erythematosus. The condition is characterized by elevated anti-GAD antibody titers [53].

2.4 Gestational Diabetes

Gestational diabetes is defined as any degree of glucose intolerance with onset or first diagnosis during pregnancy [1].

A woman develops gestational diabetes when her body cannot produce enough insulin to combat the increased fuel consumption required to support her growing body and developing fetus, as well as the insulin resistance caused by the anti-insulin hormones secreted by the placenta during pregnancy (such as prolactin, estrogen, human placental lactogen, cortisol, and progesterone). It is thought to affect 2.1% of pregnant women [1, 54].

In addition, a rising corpus of research has shown additional lifetime consequences beyond type 2 diabetes for mothers in recent decades, such as an increased chance of eventually acquiring cardiovascular disease [55].

References

1. American Diabetes Association Professional Practice Committee. Diagnosis and classification of diabetes: standards of care in diabetes-2024. Diabetes Care. 2024;47:S20.
2. American Diabetes Association (ADA). Standards of care in diabetes—2023. Diabetes J. 2023;46(1):1–298. https://diabetesjournals.org/care
3. Chiang JL, Kirkman MS, Laffel LMB, Peters AL. Type 1 diabetes through the life span: a position statement of the American Diabetes Association. Diabetes Care. 2014;37(7):2034–54. https://doi.org/10.2337/dc14-1140.
4. Purnell JQ, Dev RK, Steffes MW, Cleary PA, Palmer JP, Hirsch IB, Hokanson JE, Brunzell JD. Relationship of family history of type 2 diabetes, hypoglycemia, and autoantibodies to weight gain and lipids with intensive and conventional therapy in the diabetes control and complications trial. Diabetes Care. 2003;52(10):2623–9. https://www.ncbi.nlm.nih.gov/pmc/articles/PMC3624763/pdf/nihms412728.pdf.
5. Lachter J. Effect of intensive therapy on residual 0-cell function in patients with type 1 diabetes in the diabetes control and complications trial. Ann Intern Med. 1998;128(7):517–23. https://doi.org/10.7326/L23-0065.
6. Maruyama T, Nakagawa T, Kasuga A, Murata M. Heterogeneity among patients with latent autoimmune diabetes in adults. Diabetes Metab Res Rev. 2011;27(30):971–4. https://doi.org/10.1002/dmrr.
7. Zhu Y, Qian L, Liu Q, et al. Glutamic acid decarboxylase autoantibody detection by electrochemiluminescence assay identifies latent autoimmune diabetes in adults with poor islet function. Diabetes Metab J. 2020;44(2):260–6. https://doi.org/10.4093/DMJ.2019.0007.
8. Udler MS, Kim J, von Grotthuss M, et al. Type 2 diabetes genetic loci informed by multi-trait associations point to disease mechanisms and subtypes: a soft clustering analysis. PLoS Med. 2018;15(9):1–23. https://doi.org/10.1371/journal.pmed.1002654.

9. Low HC, Chilian WM, Ratnam W, et al. Changes in mitochondrial epigenome in type 2 diabetes mellitus. Br J Biomed Sci. 2023;80:1–10. https://doi.org/10.3389/bjbs.2023.10884.
10. Schapira AHV. Mitochondrial diseases. Lancet. 2012;379(9828):1825–34. https://doi.org/10.1016/S0140-6736(11)61305-6.
11. Harris AG, Letourneau LR, Greeley SAW. Monogenic diabetes: the impact of making the right diagnosis. Curr Opin Pediatr. 2018;30(4):558–67. https://doi.org/10.1097/MOP.0000000000000643.
12. Gupta RK, Vatamaniuk MZ, Lee CS, et al. The MODY1 gene HNF-4α regulates selected genes involved in insulin secretion. J Clin Invest. 2005;115(4):1006–15. https://doi.org/10.1172/JCI200522365.
13. Thanabalasingham G, Owen KR. Diagnosis and management of maturity onset diabetes of the young (MODY). BMJ. 2011;343(7828):1–9. https://doi.org/10.1136/bmj.d6044.
14. Shields BM, Hicks S, Shepherd MH, Colclough K, Hattersley AT, Ellard S. Maturity-onset diabetes of the young (MODY): how many cases are we missing? Diabetologia. 2010;53(12):2504–8. https://doi.org/10.1007/s00125-010-1799-4.
15. Greeley SAW, Polak M, Njølstad PR, et al. ISPAD Clinical Practice Consensus Guidelines 2022: the diagnosis and management of monogenic diabetes in children and adolescents. Pediatr Diabetes. 2022;23(8):1188–211. https://doi.org/10.1111/pedi.13426.
16. Broome DT, Pantalone KM, Kashyap SR, Philipson LH. Approach to the patient with MODY-monogenic diabetes. J Clin Endocrinol Metab. 2021;106(1):1052. https://doi.org/10.1080/00498254.2020.1737890.
17. Maloney KA, Mizerik E, King RH, McGinnis EM, Perkowitz S, Diamonstein CJ, Schmanski AA, Saliganan S, Shipper AG, Udler MS, Guan Y. Genetic counseling in diabetes mellitus: a practice resource of the National Society of Genetic Counselors. J Genet Couns. 2023;33(3):493–505.
18. Rubio-Cabezas O, Ellard S. Diabetes mellitus in neonates and infants: genetic heterogeneity, clinical approach to diagnosis, and therapeutic options. Horm Res Paediatr. 2013;80(3):137–46. https://doi.org/10.1159/000354219.
19. Nayak S, Sarangi AN, Sahoo SK, et al. Neonatal diabetes mellitus: novel mutations. Indian J Pediatr. 2021;88(8):785–92. https://doi.org/10.1007/s12098-020-03567-7.
20. Challis BG, Semple RK. Genetic disorders of insulin action: far more than diabetes. Curr Obes Rep. 2013;2(4):293–300. https://doi.org/10.1007/s13679-013-0075-6.
21. Richardson A, Park WG. Acute pancreatitis and diabetes mellitus: a review. Korean J Intern Med. 2021;36(1):15–24. https://doi.org/10.3904/kjim.2020.505.
22. Hart PA, Conwell DL. Chronic pancreatitis: managing a difficult disease. Am J Gastroenterol. 2020;115(1):49–55. https://doi.org/10.14309/ajg.0000000000000421.
23. Utzschneider KM, Kowdley KV. Hereditary hemochromatosis and diabetes mellitus: implications for clinical practice. Nat Rev Endocrinol. 2010;6(1):26–33. https://doi.org/10.1038/nrendo.2009.241.
24. Kumaran S, Unnikrishnan AG. Fibrocalculous pancreatic diabetes. J Diabetes Complicat. 2021;35(1):107627. https://doi.org/10.1016/j.jdiacomp.2020.107627.
25. Moustaki M, Paschou SA, Xekouki P, et al. Secondary diabetes mellitus in acromegaly. Endocrine. 2023;81(1):1–15. https://doi.org/10.1007/s12020-023-03339-1.
26. Biondi B, Kahaly GJ, Robertson RP. Thyroid dysfunction and diabetes mellitus: two closely associated disorders. Endocr Rev. 2018;40:789. https://doi.org/10.1210/er.2018-00163.
27. Grigoriadis G, Koufakis T, Kotsa K. Epidemiological, pathophysiological, and clinical considerations on the interplay between thyroid disorders and type 2 diabetes mellitus. Medicina. 2023;59(11):1–12. https://doi.org/10.3390/medicina59112013.
28. Eom YS, Wilson JR, Bernet VJ. Links between thyroid disorders and glucose homeostasis. Diabetes Metab J. 2022;46(2):239–56. https://doi.org/10.4093/dmj.2022.0013.
29. Adlan MA, Bondugulapati LN, Premawardhana LD. Glucose intolerance and diabetes mellitus in endocrine disorders—two case reports and a review. Curr Diabetes Rev. 2010;6(5):266.

30. Szychlińska M, Baranowska-Jurkun A, Matuszewski W, Wołos-Kłosowicz K, Bandurska-Stankiewicz E. Markers of subclinical cardiovascular disease in patients with adrenal incidentaloma. Medicina. 2020;56(2):69. https://doi.org/10.3390/medicina56020069.
31. Kelsall A, Iqbal A, Newell-Price J. Adrenal incidentaloma: cardiovascular and metabolic effects of mild cortisol excess. Gland Surg. 2020;9(1):94–104. https://doi.org/10.21037/gs.2019.11.19.
32. Paun DL, Vija L, Stan E, et al. Cushing syndrome secondary to ectopic adrenocorticotropic hormone secretion from a Meckel diverticulum neuroendocrine tumor: case report. BMC Endocr Disord. 2015;15(1):34–6. https://doi.org/10.1186/s12902-015-0070-x.
33. Kvasnička J, Zelinka T, Petrák O, et al. Catecholamines induce left ventricular subclinical systolic dysfunction: a speckle-tracking echocardiography study. Cancers (Basel). 2019;11(3):318. https://doi.org/10.3390/cancers11030318.
34. Pang Y, Liu Y, Pacak K, Yang C. Pheochromocytomas and paragangliomas: from genetic diversity to targeted therapies. Cancers (Basel). 2019;11(4):1–16. https://doi.org/10.3390/cancers11040436.
35. Păun DL, Mirica A. Pheochromocytomas and paragangliomas: genotype–phenotype correlations. IntechOpen; 2021. p. 13–24. https://doi.org/10.5772/intechopen.95888.
36. Song X, Zheng S, Yang G, et al. Glucagonoma and the glucagonoma syndrome (review). Oncol Lett. 2018;15(3):2749–55. https://doi.org/10.3892/ol.2017.7703.
37. Bevere M, Gkountakos A, Martelli FM, Scarpa A, Luchini C, Simbolo M. An insight on functioning pancreatic neuroendocrine neoplasms. Biomedicines. 2023;11(2):1–23. https://doi.org/10.3390/biomedicines11020303.
38. Jain V, Patel RK, Kapadia Z, Galiveeti S, Banerji M, Hope L. Drugs and hyperglycemia: a practical guide. Maturitas. 2017;104:80–3. https://doi.org/10.1016/j.maturitas.2017.08.006.
39. Anyanwagu U, Idris I, Donnelly R. Drug-induced diabetes mellitus: evidence for statins and other drugs affecting glucose metabolism. Clin Pharmacol Ther. 2016;99(4):390–400. https://doi.org/10.1002/cpt.274.
40. Arlt W, Lang K, Sitch AJ, et al. Steroid metabolome analysis reveals prevalent glucocorticoid excess in primary aldosteronism. JCI Insight. 2017;2(8):1–14. https://doi.org/10.1172/JCI.INSIGHT.93136.
41. Dotta F, Censini S, Van Halteren AGS, et al. Coxsackie B4 virus infection of β cells and natural killer cell insulitis in recent-onset type 1 diabetic patients. Proc Natl Acad Sci USA. 2007;104(12):5115–20. https://doi.org/10.1073/pnas.0700442104.
42. Bode B, Garrett V, Messler J, et al. Glycemic characteristics and clinical outcomes of COVID-19 patients hospitalized in the United States. J Diabetes Sci Technol. 2020;14(4):813–21. https://doi.org/10.1177/1932296820924469.
43. Barrett T, Bundey SE, Macleod AF. (DIDMOAD) syndrome UK nationwide study of Wolfram. Lancet. 1995;346:1458–63.
44. Aslam AA, Baksh RA, Pape SE, Strydom A, Gulliford MC, Chan LF. Diabetes and obesity in down syndrome across the lifespan: a retrospective cohort study using U.K. electronic health records. Diabetes Care. 2022;45(12):2892–9. https://doi.org/10.2337/dc22-0482.
45. Liu S, Yuan T, Song S, et al. Glucose metabolic disorder in Klinefelter syndrome: a retrospective analysis in a single Chinese hospital and literature review. BMC Endocr Disord. 2021;21(1):1–10. https://doi.org/10.1186/s12902-021-00893-5.
46. Mitsch C, Alexandrou E, Norris AW, Pinnaro CT. Hyperglycemia in turner syndrome: impact, mechanisms, and areas for future research. Front Endocrinol (Lausanne). 2023;14:1–12. https://doi.org/10.3389/fendo.2023.1116889.
47. Urano F. Wolfram syndrome: diagnosis, management, and treatment. Curr Diab Rep. 2016;16(1):1–8. https://doi.org/10.1007/s11892-015-0702-6.
48. Cnop M, Mulder H, Igoillo-Esteve M. Diabetes in Friedreich ataxia. J Neurochem. 2013;126(SUPPL.1):94–102. https://doi.org/10.1111/jnc.12216.

49. Lee CY, Ro JS, Jung H, Kim M, Jeon B, Lee JY. Increased 10-year prevalence of Huntington's disease in South Korea: an analysis of medical expenditure through the National Healthcare System. J Clin Neurol. 2023;19(2):147–55. https://doi.org/10.3988/jcn.2022.0212.
50. Dhakchinamoorthi KK, Palathingal JT, Sreenivasan S. Laurence–Moon–Bardet–Biedl syndrome with maturity onset diabetes of the young (Mody)—case report. J Young Pharm. 2018;11(1):114–6. https://doi.org/10.5530/jyp.2019.11.25.
51. Takeshima K, Ariyasu H, Ishibashi T, et al. Myotonic dystrophy type 1 with diabetes mellitus, mixed hypogonadism and adrenal insufficiency. Endocrinol Diabetes Metab Case Rep. 2018;2018:1–6. https://doi.org/10.1530/edm-17-0143.
52. Clerc A, Coupaye M, Mosbah H, et al. Diabetes mellitus in Prader–Willi syndrome: natural history during the transition from childhood to adulthood in a cohort of 39 patients. J Clin Med. 2021;10(22):1–14. https://doi.org/10.3390/jcm10225310.
53. Rathbun JT, Imber J. Stiff person syndrome and type 1 diabetes mellitus: a case of the chicken or the egg? J Gen Intern Med. 2019;34(6):1053–7. https://doi.org/10.1007/s11606-019-04835-9.
54. Coţofană I, Roşca R, Mirică A, Coţofană M, Păduraru DN, Mirică R, Beuran M, Păun S, Păun DL. Clinical and surgical attitude in a MEN2 syndrome case with medullary thyroid carcinoma recurrence during pregnancy. J Surg Sci. 2015;2(4):189–93.
55. Wicklow B, Retnakaran R. Gestational diabetes mellitus and its implications across the life span. Diabetes Metab J. 2023;47(3):333–44. https://doi.org/10.4093/dmj.2022.0348.

Chapter 3
Metabolism and Pathophysiology of Diabetes and Skin Involvement

Petra Staubach and Charlotte Staubach

Abstract Diabetes mellitus is a widespread increasing systemic disorder with a high impact on health systems worldwide. Skin disorders with diabetes can be found in about one third of all people with diabetes and frequently occur before the diagnosis, thus playing an important role in the initial recognition of underlying disease.

Due to increased serum glucose level, different cell types like keratinocytes and fibroblasts but also endothelial cells, and neurons, are damaged. Thus different causalities like diabetic angiopathy and neuropathy skin manifestations may appear. The physiological changes cause skin reactions more often like xerosis and pruritus but also skin infections like mycoses or erysipelas. Necrobiosis lipoidica, scleredema adultorum of Buschke, and granuloma annulare are examples of frequent noninfectious skin diseases.

3.1 The Impact of Diabetes on Skin Structure and Functions

3.1.1 Importance of Diabetes and Skin-Related Conditions in Health Care: Social and Economic Impact

The term diabetes mellitus refers to a group of diseases that are diagnosed by an increase in blood glucose concentrations. The disease occurs in all age groups and affects all ethnicities. Worldwide, the prevalence of diabetes mellitus in adults up to the age of 79 was estimated at 537 million in 2021. In 2024, 783 million people are expected to be affected worldwide. In 2024 around the world, with approximately 642 million people predicted. Approximately 30% of all diabetics develop skin changes, which are divided into different groups according to Perez [1–3].

P. Staubach (✉) · C. Staubach
Department of Dermatology, University Medical Center Mainz, Mainz, Germany
e-mail: petra.staubach@unimedizin-mainz.de

K. Fritz, G.-S. Tiplica (eds.), *Cutaneous Manifestations in Diabetes*,
https://doi.org/10.1007/978-3-031-65300-1_3

3.1.2 QoL in Skin-Induced Conditions in the Diabetic Patient

In principle, the impact on the quality of life of chronic, partially itchy skin symptoms with or without an underlying diseases is considerable. The results of examinations, primarily of type II diabetes, distinguish between four categories: skin changes caused by diabetes mellitus, by infections, as a consequence of complications or comorbidity, and by the therapy. A particularly high impact on quality of life was found in the group with skin changes due to diabetes [3, 4].

3.1.3 The Types of Diabetes

Diabetes mellitus is a metabolic disorder associated with hyperglycemia. Defects in insulin secretion or insulin action or both cause disorders of carbohydrate, fat, and protein metabolism in particular. In the long term, damage, dysfunction, and failure of various organs may occur. On the one hand, small blood vessels (microangiopathy) with diseases of the eyes (retinopathy) can occur, and kidneys (nephropathy) and nerves (neuropathy) are affected. On the other hand, processes in the large vessels in the form of arteriosclerosis can be accelerated by diabetes (macroangiopathy).

3.1.4 Type I (T1D)

Autoimmune-related diabetes mellitus usually begins in childhood or adolescence due to autoimmunological destruction of the pancreatic β-cells, which leads to a relative and later absolute insulin deficiency. Diabetes-specific autoantibodies are often conspicuous in the serum of patients; in less than 10% of cases, these are not found (idiopathic). Type I diabetes rarely occurs with absolute insulin deficiency due to destruction of the pancreatic cells (latent autoimmune diabetes in adults). Titer level and age at autoantibody detection are associated with the progression of type I diabetes. Type I diabetes occurs in 7–10% of all diabetics.

3.1.5 Type II (T2D)

Eighty percent of all diabetics have type II diabetes. Due to the reduction in insulin action (insulin resistance), the loss of beta cell function progresses, and a relative insulin deficiency with disruption of glucose-dependent insulin secretion occurs.

The disorders are often already present long before the diagnosis is made. This also increases subsequent damage such as macrovascular consequences or association with other diseases such as metabolic syndrome. Further subclassifications of T2D depending on the extent of insulin resistance and subsequent damage/complications are planned in the future [5].

3.1.6 Gestational Diabetes

In gestational diabetes a glucose tolerance disorder occurs for the first time during the second or third trimester. Seven percent of all pregnant women are affected by it. Every fourth woman with gestational diabetes develop T2D after pregnancy [6].

3.1.7 Other Types of Diabetes

Diabetes mellitus can be caused by pathology of the exocrine pancreas and associated insufficiency such as pancreatitis, mucoviscidosis, or hemochromatosis or diseases of other endocrine organs, e.g., Cushing's syndrome, glucagonoma syndrome, or pheochromocytoma, or infections such as congenital rubella.

Further causes of other types of diabetes are drugs such as systemic glucocorticoids, genetic defects in insulin action or beta cell function, as well as genetic syndromes [5].

3.1.8 Metabolism and Pathophysiology of Diabetes Mellitus and Skin Involvement

Fundamentally, the process that leads to skin involvement in diabetes mellitus is multifactorial, and the skin symptoms are often associated with other diabetes complications. Skin changes occur predominantly in uncontrolled diabetes mellitus and usually regress as soon as the diabetes is controlled.

It is assumed that hyperglycemia induces oxidative stress. This leads to a reduction in the immune response, which in turn leads to the formation of advanced glycation end products (AGEs). This is caused by excess tissue glucose, which reacts with macromolecules such as lipids, proteins, or nucleic acids and leads to an irreversible change in these macromolecules and their functions. Such pathologies also occur in old age or as a result of smoking and are greatly accelerated by other factors such as DM [7–9].

3.1.9 Histology of the Skin in Diabetes Mellitus

The pathogenesis of skin changes in diabetes mellitus can be explained by the accumulation of glycated proteins and amino acids. This leads to a disturbance of the intracellular signals in the skin. As a result, keratinocytes and fibroblasts are restricted in terms of proliferation, differentiation, and migration. This in turn causes a disrupted and thus weakened barrier function of the skin, which is noticeable, for example, in delayed wound healing. If other factors such as comorbidity, skin ageing, and increased skin stress are added, the already weakened skin barrier is significantly weakened and shows pathological signs [10].

3.1.10 II Diabetes-Related Skin Conditions: Vascular Damage

Diabetic microangiopathy can lead to stenoses and even occlusion of end-stream vessels. Here too, the accumulation of AGEs plays a decisive role in causing damage to the vascular endothelium. Microangiopathy occurs predominantly in the renal glomeruli and retinal vessels. Macroangiopathy is also caused by the glycation and oxidation of LDL and the lack of inhibition of lipolysis due to insulin deficiency, which leads to atherosclerotic vascular wall deposits in the peripheral arteries (PAOD), the coronary arteries (CHD), and the central vessels, resulting, for example, in carotid stenosis [7, 8].

3.1.11 Diabetic Foot Syndrome (DFS) [11, 12]

The pathogenesis of diabetic foot syndrome is complex. Additional symptoms like trigger finger, Dupuytren's disease, carpal tunnel syndrome, cubital tunnel syndrome and osteoarthritis of the first carpometacarpal joint occur significantly more frequently in patients with diabetes mellitus type one or two. In addition to a possible circulatory disorder, which is present in at least 50% of cases, neuropathy plays a key role. Sensorimotor polyneuropathy is found in at least 90% of cases. Overlaps between the two clinical pictures are common. Sensory polyneuropathy leads to a loss of protective perception and a lack of pain sensation. Motor polyneuropathy causes foot deformities due to a muscular imbalance. People with diabetes also suffer from a disorder of depth sensitivity with a change in gait pattern and consecutive incorrect loading. Autonomic neuropathy leads to dry, less resistant skin. The smallest injuries, bleeding, or blistering can lead to ulcerations on the foot. Diabetic foot syndrome is divided into different stages:

Armstrong stage

A, without ischemia or infection

B, with infection
C, with ischemia
D, with infection and ischemia
Wagner grade
0, pre- or postulcerative foot
1, superficial wound
2, wound up to the level of tendons or capsule
3, wound up to the level of bones and joints
4, necrosis of parts of the foot
5, necrosis of the entire foot

3.1.12 *Diabetic Dermopathy*

This skin condition occurs in one in ten diabetics. Brownish to reddish, roundish atrophic areas are conspicuous, predominantly on the extensor sides of the lower leg. Diabetic microangiopathy and/or microtraumas are suspected to be the cause. An early necrobiosis lipoidica is discussed as a differential diagnosis. The skin changes are regressive due to the cessation of the underlying disease.

3.1.13 *Wet Gangrene (Foot)*

Gangrene, usually in the area of the feet, occurs more frequently in diabetics due to the angiopathies described but also due to the weakened skin barrier and additionally the increased tendency to infection, usually beginning with a trivial injury. A distinction is made between dry gangrene (mummified gangrene) and moist gangrene in diabetes patients, which is often greasy due to superinfection.

3.2 Erysipelas-Like Erythema

3.2.1 *III Diabetes-Related Skin Conditions: Infections*

Due to the impaired skin barrier, the reduced immune system, and the increased glucose concentration in the epidermis, mycoses and bacterial infections can develop more frequently and spread more quickly. Every second diabetic suffers from skin infections. Twenty-five percent show clinical signs of candidiasis.

3.2.2 *Mycoses in the Diabetic Patient*

Of the dermatomycoses, yeast infection, candidiasis, is the most common fungal infection of the skin diagnosed in diabetics, occurring predominantly in the intertriginous area. In women, vulvovaginitis caused by *Candida* is known to be an early sign of diabetes mellitus [12].

Dermatophytes, mainly *Trichophyton rubrum*, but also molds play a common role. Dermatophytes in the area of the feet including nails are also observed more frequently than in the normal population due to the angiopathy-related undersupply. Early treatment is essential here to prevent microtraumas in the course of the disease, which in turn can lead to serious consequences such as diabetic foot syndrome or gangrene [3, 4].

A very rare but very dangerous rhinocerebral mucormycosis can occur in the otorhinolaryngological tract, caused by a special class of fungi named Zygomycetes, like *Rhizopus*, *Rhizomucor*, and *Absidia*. The first symptoms are clinically, it starts with a sinusitis combined with facial erythema edemarsh fever like cellulitis. Over time complications can accur like damage of nerves or vessels up to sphenoid sinus or cavernous sinus. The gold standard therapy is intravenous amphotericin B with surgical debridement of necrosis [13].

3.2.3 *Bacterial Infections in the Diabetic Patient*

Pronounced and/or recurrent folliculitis, abscesses, erysipelas, erythrasma, and impetigo can be an early sign of diabetes mellitus alongside mycoses or indicate that diabetes mellitus is present or not well controlled. Due to the disturbed metabolic situation, these are often mixed infections, which must be taken into account when choosing the appropriate therapeutic agent. Topical antibiotics are obsolete due to the tendency of infections to recur and the development of multiresistant germs [3, 4].

In diabetics, very pronounced infections such as necrotizing fasciitis or the special form of Fournier's gangrene in the area of the external genitals and perineum are more common than in the normal population, which can occur predominantly in men [14].

3.3 Skin Infestations in the Diabetic Patient

3.3.1 *Diabetes-Related Skin Conditions: Neurological Damage*

In addition to angiopathy with its circulatory disorders, neurological disorders play a decisive role in the pathomechanisms of individual diseases such as the diabetic foot. In addition to sensorimotor polyneuropathy, which occurs due to the loss of protective pain sensation, there is a parallel motor polyneuropathy, which leads to foot shape deformities due to muscular disharmonies and thus to incorrect loading. The third form of neuropathy is autonomic neuropathy, which leads to a dry and weakened skin barrier. The smallest injuries lead to bleeding, blistering, and even serious ulceration.

3.3.2 *The Diabetic Foot*

The pathogenesis is caused by angiopathy with circulatory disorders and neuropathy. The overlap of both pathologies is frequent.

3.4 Diabetes-Related Skin Conditions: Various Associated Symptoms

3.4.1 *Common Skin Manifestations Related to Obesity*

Type II diabetes mellitus in particular is associated with obesity and frequently also with metabolic syndrome. Similar to diabetes, obesity favors infections mainly in the intertriginous area such as candidiasis. Furthermore, chronic venous insufficiency with varicose veins up to ulcerations, lymphedema, or diabetic foot syndrome occurs more frequently [2, 7, 15].

3.4.2 *Eruptive Xanthomas*

These are papules that are grouped in a pale reddish color and occur predominantly in uncontrolled diabetes mellitus but also in triglyceridemia. Therapeutically, the aim is to control the underlying disease. They can be easily removed surgically (excision, curettage) or by laser therapy [15].

3.4.3 *Acanthosis Nigricans Benigna*

Characterisitc skin skigns of acanthosis nigricans are hyperpigment plaques in intertriginous areas are characteristics of acanthosis nigricans, in diabetic patients often axillary and nuchal. Histopathological findings are keratinocyte hyperproliferation, with papillomatosis, acanthosis, and a hyperpigmented epidermis. Females with polycystic ovary syndrome and obesity develop acanthosis nigricans often. It is discussed that the hyperinsulinism starts the keratinocyte hyperproliferation due to the binding of insulin to insulin-like growth factor receptors. It has to be mentioned that acanthosis nigricans maligna is to be distinguished. This subtype appears in patients with malignome sometimes as a first sign. Different to the benign or pseudoacanthosis nigricans, it appears rapidly [15–17].

3.4.4 *Metabolic Effects on the Skin Produced by Obesity: Hyperandrogenism*

The obesity guidelines refer to obesity-related comorbidities. Metabolic disorders (insulin resistance, dyslipidemia, hyperuricemia, homeostasis disorders) play a decisive role here. As increased fatty tissue also has inflammatory properties, the insulin effect is influenced and the development of atherosclerotic processes is accelerated. Gout is diagnosed in every fourth patient with type II diabetes mellitus, with women being affected more frequently. Hormonal disorders (hyperandrogenemia, polycystic ovary syndrome) as well as lower pregnancy rates and increased complications during pregnancy are known to occur in women with obesity [15, 18].

3.4.5 *Metabolic Effects on the Skin Produced by Obesity: Necrobiosis Lipoidica*

Necrobiosis lipoidica is a common skin sign in patients with diabetes. It starts with erythematous papular efflorescences, which then turn into brownish-yellow and coalesce into non-itching plaques, some of which are atrophic and some of which have telangiectasias. Predilection sites are ventral area of the legs, often symmetrical. Ulcerations are known to occur in every third patient as a complication, sometimes superinfected. The pathomechanism is not yet understood [19].

The chosen treatment is often frustran. The occlusive application of topical high-potency corticosteroids such as clobetasol and/or calcineurin inhibitors such as tacrolimus is recommended.

3.4.6 *Metabolic Effects on the Skin Produced by Obesity: Granuloma Annulare*

Granuloma annulare is a granulomatous annular skin change that occurs predominantly on the distal extremities and in diabetics, so an association is controversially discussed here, as an increased occurrence in infections or other diseases is also known [15].

3.4.7 Pruritus in the Diabetic Patient

Pruritus is a symptom that diabetics complain about. The causes of pruritus are heterogeneous: Increased glucose levels, oxidative stress, xerosis, and hypohidrosis lead to pruritus, but diabetic nephropathy due to microangiopathy and diabetic neuropathy can also cause pruritus. Furthermore, oral antidiabetic drugs such as metformin, glimepiride, or tolbutamide are known to cause the development of pruritus. It is important that the intensity of the pruritus is reduced by good control of the diabetes and adequate skin care/basic therapy [20].

3.4.8 Diabetic Blisters

Blistering, mainly on the back and soles of the feet, occurs in patients with a long history of diabetes. It is striking that no inflammatory reaction occurs. It is suspected that the skin becomes more vulnerable during the long course of the disease [15].

3.4.9 Sclerosis in the Diabetic Patient

The occurrence of thickened, indurated, sometimes erythematous waxy plaques at the predilection sites of the neck and upper back is predominantly seen in type II diabetes and is referred to as scleroedema diabeticorum. Sclerosis type Buschke is known to occur in type I diabetes but also in diseases like gammopathy, which is characterized by thickening of the skin in the hip, shoulder, and neck area [12, 15].

In principle, digital sclerosis can also occur; the thickening significantly restricts mobility, which leads to immense strain and the risk of infection due to microtrauma [12].

3.4.10 Nail Changes in Diabetic Patients

Due to the altered metabolism and micro- and macroangiopathy combined with the elevated infection rates and the reduced skin barrier, nail pathologies are increased mostly in toenails. The color of the nails appears as yellowish or brownish (yellow nails). Dystrophia but also melanonychia striata may occur. Elevated fungal infections with high recurrence occur [12].

3.4.11 *Acne Inversa*

Acne inversa is a severe, previously underdiagnosed systemic disease which, similar to psoriasis, is often associated with concomitant diseases such as diabetes, obesity, lipid metabolism disorders, cardiovascular diseases, chronic inflammatory bowel disease, and spinal diseases due to systemic inflammation and has an immense impact on quality of life [21]. Upcoming publications show a response of antidiabetic therapies such as metformin to the treatment of acne inversa [22].

3.4.12 *Influence of Diabetes on Skin Disease*

3.4.12.1 Psoriasis in Diabetic Patients

The increased incidence in patients with psoriasis is known. It is fact that psoriasis is a systemic disease. Obesity and overall metabolic syndrome and other chronic inflammatory diseases such as chronic inflammatory bowel disease occur two to three times more frequently than in the normal population. Therapeutically, early intervention in psoriasis is necessary in order to reduce the inflammatory burden at an early stage and thus also has a positive effect on comorbidity. Treat smart and early is necessary to influence the cumulative life course impairment [23].

3.4.12.2 Atopic Dermatitis in Diabetic Patients

Since years it is discussed that atopic dermatitis can be diagnosed more often in atopic dermatitis. But a new study on atopic dermatitis and diabetes found no association. The study published in February 2024 showed data of a longitudinal study of parents and children in a British longitudinal birth cohort [24].

3.4.12.3 Vitiligo in Diabetic Patients

Vitiligo is an autoimmune disease that is often associated with other autoimmune diseases such as type I diabetes. In principle, vitiligo occurs more frequently with other diseases such as discoid lupus erythematosus, alopecia areata, Sjögren's syndrome, myasthenia gravis, systemic lupus erythematosus, and rheumatoid arthritis. The non-segmental subform of vitiligo is observed as a particularly chronic and stationary form. Treatment of the concomitant diseases is the treatment of choice. In addition to topical steroids or calcineurin inhibitors, topical therapy with a JAK inhibitor ruxolitinib has been approved for the non-segmental subtype since 2023, provided that the facial area is also affected [25, 26].

3.4.12.4 Acne and Rosacea

Acne vulgaris, rosacea, and hidradenitis suppurativa are diseases that can be provoked by hyperandrogenism, angiogenesis fibrosis, and oxidative stress. They are chronic inflammatory skin diseases, and studies show positive effects in treating patients with metformin, an antidiabetic drug. Discussed are antiandrogenic, antioxidants, antiangiogenic, and anti-fibrotic effects. Syndromes are known, where acne, hirsutismus, and diabetes as well as obesity occur (like Achard–Thiers syndrome). Rosacea is known to be associated with diabetic macular edema, dry eye disease, glaucoma, and cataract development in diabetic patients [12, 22, 27].

3.4.13 Skin Disorders in Pregnancy

Itch is common symptom that can be an early sign of gestational diabetes or worsening of existing diabetes, even if there are no visible skin lesions. In this case, daily basic therapy, with, e.g., urea, should definitely be pointed out. Every chronic inflammatory or autoimmune disorder can be influenced in a negative but also positive way during pregnancy. Therapeutic adjustment and tight monitoring should be considered. Important to notice is that patients with other systemic diseases should be monitored closely. In families with autoimmune skin diseases, it could be shown that there was a higher risk of spontaneous abortions than in control population [28].

3.4.14 Diabetes Mellitus: Disease Associations and Genetic Syndromes

Diabetes mellitus is increasingly associated with rare syndromes (e.g., trisomy 21, Klinefelter syndrome, Ullrich–Turner syndrome) or hereditary neuromuscular diseases (e.g., Friedreich's ataxia, Huntington's chorea).

The DIDMOAD syndrome ("diabetes insipidus, diabetes mellitus, optic atrophy, and deafness syndrome") is characterized by hypogonadism, diabetes insipidus, optic atrophy, and deafness as well as increasing neurological and mental deficits during the third and fourth decade of life.

Patients with Prader–Labhart–Willi syndrome, which is mainly characterized by extreme obesity and later onset of type II diabetes, usually become insulin-dependent.

Wolfram syndrome is an autosomal recessive hereditary disease in which insulin-dependent diabetes occurs in the first decade of life [2, 12].

Diseases with skin complications are:

Cushing's syndrome	Striae, distensae, Ekchymosen, rubeosis faciei
Achard–Thiers syndrome	Hirsutismus, acne
Flynn–Aird syndrome	Skin atrophy
Morgagni syndrome	Hypertrichosis, hirsutismus
Werner syndrome	Skleropoikilodermie, ulcera crurum, canities
Progeria adultorum	Teleangiektasien, cavities
Miescher syndrome II	Acanthosis nigricans benigna, hypertrichose, lingua scrotalis

References

1. Jaacks LM, Siegel KR, Gujral UP, Narayan KM. Type 2 diabetes: a 21st century epidemic. Best Pract Res Clin Endocrinol Metab. 2016;30(3):331–43.
2. International Diabetes Foundation (IDF) Diabetes Atlas [database on the Internet]. 2015. http://www.diabetesatlas.org/. Guidelines. 2023. https://www.idf.org/e-library/guidelines/128-idf-clinical-practice-recommendations-for-managing-type-2-diabetes-in-primary-care.html.
3. Perez MI, Kohn SR. Cutaneous manifestations of diabetes mellitus. J Am Acad Dermatol. 1994;30(4):519–31. quiz 32–4.
4. Kurtalic N, Kurtalic S, Salihbegovic EM. Skin changes in patients with diabetes mellitus type 2 and their impact on quality of life. Mater Sociomed. 2020;32(4):283–6.
5. Danne T, Kordonouri O, Lange K. Diabetes bei Kindern und Jugendlichen. In: Definition, Klassifikation und Epidemiologie des Diabetes bei Kindern und Jugendlichen. Berlin: Springer; 2015.
6. Bellamy L, Casas JP, Hingorani AD, Williams D. Type 2 diabetes mellitus after gestational diabetes: a systematic review and meta-analysis. Lancet. 2009;373(9677):1773–9.
7. Roglic G. Global report on diabetes. Geneva: World Health Organization; 2016. p. 86.
8. Demirseren DD, et al. Relationship between skin diseases and extracutaneous complications of diabetes mellitus: clinical analysis of 750 patients. Am J Clin Dermatol. 2014;15(1):65–70.
9. Hosseini MS, Razavi Z, Bahri RA, Ehsani AH, Firooz A, Aryanian Z, Ehsani A, Sadeghi Y. Is skin autofluorescence a novel non-invasive marker in diabetes? A systematic review and meta-analysis of case-control studies. J Res Med Sci. 2023;28:68.
10. Li M, Zhao Y, Hao H, et al. Mesenchymal stem cell-conditioned medium improves the proliferation and migration of keratinocytes in a diabetes-like microenvironment. Int J Low Extrem Wounds. 2015;4:73–86.
11. Brandl R, Stiegler H. Das diabetische Fußsyndrom. Dtsch Med Wochenschr. 2015;140:593–602.
12. Hautveränderungen bei endokrinologischen Erkrankungen. V. Voigtländer, D. Maaßen in Dermatologie und Innere Medizin 74–81.
13. Prabhu RM, Patel R. Mucormycosis and entomophthoramycosis: a review of the clinical manifestations, diagnosis and treatment. Clin Microbiol Infect. 2004;10(Suppl 1):31–47.
14. Tschachler E, Brockmeyer N, Effendy I, Geiss HK, Harder S, Hartmann M, et al. Streptococcal infections of the skin and mucous membranes. J Dtsch Dermatol Ges. 2007;5(6):527–32.
15. David P, Singh S, Ankar R. A comprehensive overview of skin complications in diabetes and their prevention. Cureus. 2023;15(5):e38961.
16. Kutlubay Z, Engin B, Bairamov O, Tuzun Y. Acanthosis nigricans: a fold (intertriginous) dermatosis. Clin Dermatol. 2015;33(4):466–70.
17. Kutane Paraneoplasien V, Voigtländer D. Maaßen in Dermatologie und Innere Medizin. 155–156.

18. https://register.awmf.org/assets/guidelines/0500011_S3_Adipositas_Praevention_Therapie_2014-11-.pdf.
19. Sibbald C, Reid S, Alavi A. Necrobiosis lipoidica. Dermatol Clin. 2015;33(3):343–60.
20. Ständer S, et al. S2k-Leitlinie zur Diagnostik und Therapie des chronischen Pruritus. https://register.awmf.org/assets/guidelines/013-048l_S2k_Diagnostik-Therapie-des-chronischen-Pruritus_2022-09.pdf.
21. Vişan MA, Căruntu C, Costache RS, Tiplica G, Costache DO. Hidradenitis suppurativa: detangling phenotypes and identifying common denominators. J Eur Acad Dermatol Venereol. 2024;38(1):62–76.
22. Cho M, Woo YR, Cho SH, Lee JD, Kim HS. Metformin: a potential treatment for acne, hidradenitis suppurativa and rosacea. Acta Derm Venereol. 2023;103:adv18392.
23. Augustin J, Wolf S, Stephan B, Augustin M, Andrees V. Psoriasis comorbidities in Germany: a population-based study on spatiotemporal variations. PLoS One. 2022;17(3):e0265741.
24. Kantor J. This month in JAAD international: February 2024: atopic dermatitis and diabetes. J Am Acad Dermatol. 2023;90(2):254.
25. Rosmarin D, et al. Two phase 3, randomized, controlled trials of ruxolitinib cream for vitiligo. N Engl J Med. 2023;387:1445–55.
26. Lee JH, Ju HJ, Seo JM, Almurayshid A, Kim GM, Ezzedine K, Bae JM. Comorbidities in patients with vitiligo: a systematic review and meta-analysis. J Invest Dermatol. 2023;143(5):777–789.e6.
27. Wang FY, Kang EY, Liu CH, Ng CY, Shao SC, Lai EC, Wu WC, Huang YY, Chen KJ, Lai CC, Hwang YS. Diabetic patients with rosacea increase the risks of diabetic macular edema, dry eye disease, glaucoma, and cataract. Asia Pac J Ophthalmol (Phila). 2022;11(6):505–13.
28. Keum H, Bermas B, Patel S, Jacobe HT, Chong BF. Patients with autoimmune skin diseases are at increased risk of adverse pregnancy outcomes. Am J Obstet Gynecol MFM. 2023;6(1):101226.

Chapter 4
Diabetes and Skin Histology

Klaus Fritz, Carmen Salavastru, and George-Sorin Tiplica

Abstract Primary complications associated with diabetes mellitus (DM) encompass the kidneys, retina, and peripheral nerves, with diabetic patients commonly experiencing skin injuries. Consequently, there is a growing interest in understanding the structural and molecular characteristics of non-compromised diabetic skin, i.e., prior to the onset of injuries. The existing insights into this domain have predominantly emerged in recent times and, to some extent, stem from diverse models involving diabetic animals.

Elevated blood sugar levels are the primary cause of skin changes in people with diabetes. The increased blood sugar can trigger various metabolic processes, leading to complex disruptions in skin cells and connective tissue. High levels of blood lipids and uric acid also increase the risk of skin changes, especially in individuals with type 2 diabetes. Maintaining good glucose control can help prevent skin alterations.

The histology of the skin in diabetes reveals changes such as thickening of the reticular dermis, fraying of collagen fibers, lymphohistiocytic infiltrate, and edema of the papillary dermis [1].

It is evident that diabetes mellitus damages elevated pathological glucose concentrations both directly and indirectly through the formation of "advanced glycation end products (AGEs)." AGEs result from a nonenzymatic reaction (glycation)

K. Fritz (✉)
Carol Davila University of Medicine and Pharmacy, Bucharest, Romania

Dermatology and Laser Consulting, Landau, Germany
e-mail: drklausfritz@drklausfritz.com

C. Salavastru
Carol Davila University of Medicine and Pharmacy, Bucharest, Romania

Colentina Clinical Hospital, Bucharest, Romania

Pediatric Dermatology Discipline, Dermato-oncology Research Facility, Bucharest, Romania

G.-S. Tiplica
Carol Davila University of Medicine and Pharmacy, Bucharest, Romania

Colentina Clinical Hospital, Bucharest, Romania

K. Fritz, G.-S. Tiplica (eds.), *Cutaneous Manifestations in Diabetes*,
https://doi.org/10.1007/978-3-031-65300-1_4

between glucose and proteins, lipids, and nucleic acids. They exert detrimental effects on nearly all cell systems. Pathological glucose concentrations, for instance, inhibit the proliferation, migration, and protein synthesis of keratinocytes and fibroblasts. In endothelial cells, they induce apoptosis and inhibit nitric oxide synthase (NOS), thereby suppressing NO synthesis. This, in vivo, leads to reduced vasodilation. Pathological glucose concentrations also suppress the chemotaxis and phagocytosis of cell types involved in the innate immune response.

AGEs interact with a variety of intracellular and extracellular proteins, such as collagen type I, superoxide dismutase 1, or the epidermal growth factor receptor, weakening their biological functions. Additionally, AGEs bind to RAGE (receptor for AGEs), leading to the activation of the NF-κB signaling pathway and the induction of pro-inflammatory cytokines. Both pathological glucose concentrations and AGEs contribute to increased intracellular oxidative stress [formation of reactive oxygen species (ROS)]. This is causally linked to the depletion of antioxidant protective enzymes like glutathione or mitochondrial superoxide dismutase. Furthermore, it results in the induction of ROS-generating enzymes, such as nicotinamide adenine dinucleotide phosphate oxidase [2].

Macrophages play a crucial role in the wound healing process. In the initial phases, they actively promote inflammation and eliminate pathogens, as well as clear wound debris and apoptosed cells. As the repair progresses, they shift toward dampening inflammation and secreting factors that control the proliferation, differentiation, and migration of keratinocytes, fibroblasts, and endothelial cells, facilitating neovascularization and eventual wound closure.

Macrophages in individuals with diabetes undergo alterations, exhibiting heightened responsiveness to inflammatory stimuli and an increased release of pro-inflammatory cytokines. Additionally, their ability to phagocytose pathogens and efferocytose apoptotic cells is reduced. This diminished capability to eliminate pathogens, coupled with the impaired efferocytosis triggering a phenotypic switch, results.

This results in a diminished presence of M2 reparative macrophages within the wound, potentially culminating in the development of diabetic foot ulcers (DFUs). This circumstance heightens the risk of impaired healing, susceptibility to infections, and, in severe cases, the necessity for amputation. Gaining insights into the dysregulation of macrophages in DFUs and exploring potential alterations in these cells, coupled with an understanding of the related inflammatory processes, holds promise for the development of enhanced therapies. Such interventions could complement existing treatments and improve the overall healing rates of DFUs [3].

An examination revealed pathological and physiological alterations in dermal tissue in a rat model of diabetes mellitus (DM). The skin tissue of diabetic rats displayed notable changes, including a reduction in thickness, loss of the multilayer epithelium structure, degeneration of collagen fibers, and an escalation in inflammatory cell infiltration. Additionally, there was a substantial rise in skin glucose and AGEs (advanced glycation end products). Diabetic rats exhibited elevated levels of plasma glycosylated protein (GSP) and malondialdehyde (MDA), along with a decrease in plasma glutathione (GSH).

While the percentage of epidermal cells in the S phase was similar between the two groups of rats, there was a significant decrease in the G2/M phase in Group DM. Furthermore, exposing ECV304 cells to AGE-HSA resulted in a time-dependent and dose-dependent increase in apoptosis. Thus, the heightened glucose levels in skin tissue, coupled with the accumulation of detrimental substances like AGEs, contribute to the dysfunction of dermal cells and/or the matrix. This mechanism may play a crucial role in the early-stage endogenous skin damage induced by diabetes [4].

The elevated quantity of blood vessels reaching the skin, along with the increased numbers and thickness of endothelial cells, could serve as factors contributing to issues associated with the diabetic foot. These problems may manifest as a predisposition to skin ulceration, infection, and impaired wound healing in affected individuals. Additionally, these factors may play a role in the secondary alterations observed in diabetic foot lesions, suggesting a lack of sufficient vascularization in the foot [5].

The evaluation of cutaneous innervation through skin biopsies is increasingly recognized as a valuable approach for both diagnosing and categorizing diabetic neuropathy. Numerous studies have consistently reported a decrease in intraepidermal nerve fiber density in skin biopsies obtained from individuals with diabetes [6].

Small fiber neuropathy constitutes a substantial component of diabetic sensorimotor polyneuropathy (DSPN), an aspect that has been largely overlooked in most recommendations for DSPN diagnosis. These small fibers are predominant in the peripheral nerve, playing essential and clinically significant roles such as pain perception and the regulation of microvascular blood flow. They are pivotal in mediating the mechanisms underlying foot ulceration, adding a crucial dimension to our understanding of diabetic neuropathic complications [7].

Disturbed wound healing, sclerosis, infection, and reduced vascularization can be observed in various diabetes-related skin disorder.

References

1. Quondamatteo F. Skin and diabetes mellitus: what do we know? Cell Tissue Res. 2014;355(1):1–21. https://doi.org/10.1007/s00441-013-1751-2. Epub 2013 Dec 7.
2. Lima AL, et al. Cutaneous manifestations of diabetes mellitus: a review. Am J Clin Dermatol. 2017;18:541–53.
3. Aitcheson SM, Frentiu FD, Hurn SE, Edwards K, Murray RZ. Skin wound healing: normal macrophage function and macrophage dysfunction in diabetic wounds. Molecules. 2021;26(16):4917. https://doi.org/10.3390/molecules26164917. PMID: 34443506; PMCID: PMC8398285.
4. Chen XF, Lin WD, Lu SL, Xie T, Ge K, Shi YQ, Zou JJ, Liu ZM, Liao WQ. Mechanistic study of endogenous skin lesions in diabetic rats. Exp Dermatol. 2010;19(12):1088–95. https://doi.org/10.1111/j.1600-0625.2010.01137.x.
5. Yusof MI, Al-Astani AD, Jaafar H, Rashid FA. Morphometric analysis of skin microvasculature in the diabetic foot. Singap Med J. 2008;49(2):100–4.

6. Beiswenger KK, Calcutt NA, Mizisin AP. Epidermal nerve fiber quantification in the assessment of diabetic neuropathy. Acta Histochem. 2008;110(5):351–62. https://doi.org/10.1016/j.acthis.2007.12.004. Epub 2008 Apr 1. PMID: 18384843; PMCID: PMC2561960.
7. Javed S, Petropoulos IN, Tavakoli M, Malik RA. Clinical and diagnostic features of small fiber damage in diabetic polyneuropathy. Handb Clin Neurol. 2014;126:275–90. https://doi.org/10.1016/B978-0-444-53480-4.00019-9. PMID: 25410229.

Part II
Diabetes-Related Skin Conditions: Vascular Damage

Chapter 5
Diabetes-Related Foot Disease

George-Sorin Tiplica, Constantin Ionescu-Tirgoviste, Maria-Cristina Voicu, Maria Bianca Dragomir, and Lawrence Chukwudi Nwabudike

Abstract Diabetes-related foot disease was redefined in 2023 by the International Working Group on the Diabetic Foot as the disease of the foot of a person suffering from diabetes mellitus that includes one or more of the following: peripheral neuropathy, peripheral artery disease, infection, skin ulcer, neuro-osteoarthropathy, gangrene, and amputation. A multidisciplinary team is necessary for the management of those complex patients including endocrinologists and dermatologists. The dermatologist's role is related to the recognition and prevention of the apparition and development of ulcers that can ultimately necessitate amputation. Screening, clinical evaluations, early referral, and education of the patient and caregivers are pivotal, revealing foot lesions that can evolve dramatically demanding meticulous clinical examination to identify the risk factors. Investigations performed for the evaluation of the patient with diabetes-related foot disease include the 10-g monofilament test, the ankle-brachial index testing, ultrasound examination, and others. The classification of foot ulcers is difficult, but several systems are in use for a more accurate treatment and prognosis: the site, ischemia, neuropathy, bacterial infection, and depth (SINBAD) system, the society for vascular surgery classification system for wound, ischemia, and foot infection (SVS WIfI) classification system, and the IDSA/IWGDF (Infectious Diseases Society of America/International Working Group on the Diabetic Foot) classification. The management of diabetes-related foot disease involves eliminating or mitigating risk factors, treating existing disorders (neuropathy, arteriopathy, and infections), preventing future injuries, treating existing lesions, and educating the patient on proper foot care.

G.-S. Tiplica (✉) · M.-C. Voicu · M. B. Dragomir
Dermatology 2, Colentina Clinical Hospital, "Carol Davila" University of Medicine and Pharmacy, Bucharest, Romania
e-mail: Maria-cristina.voicu@rez.umfcd.ro; maria-bianca.dragomir@rez.umfcd.ro

C. Ionescu-Tirgoviste
Romanian Academy, Bucharest, Romania

L. C. Nwabudike
N. Paulescu National Institute of Diabetes, Bucharest, Romania

K. Fritz, G.-S. Tiplica (eds.), *Cutaneous Manifestations in Diabetes*,
https://doi.org/10.1007/978-3-031-65300-1_5

Diabetes-related foot disease (also known as "diabetic foot" or "diabetic foot syndrome") was redefined in 2023 by the International Working Group on the Diabetic Foot (IWGDF) as the disease of the foot of a person suffering from diabetes mellitus that includes one or more of the following: peripheral neuropathy, peripheral artery disease, infection, skin ulcer, neuro-osteoarthropathy, gangrene, and amputation [1]. Foot disease is frequently associated with diabetes mellitus [2]. Foot ulceration is the most dreaded complication of diabetes, as there is increased risk of amputation and mortality. Patients with diabetes have 34% lifetime risk of developing foot ulcer [2]. Epidemiologic data shows that global diabetic foot ulcer prevalence is 6.3% and 5.1% in Europe, higher in males (4.5%) than in females (3.5%), and higher in type 2 diabetic patients (6.4%) than in type 1 (5.5%) [3]. Every 30 s a lower limb is amputated due to diabetes mellitus [4] and the average annual cost of care for a patient with diabetic foot is US$ 8659 [3].

Diabetes-related foot disease has a complex pathology which is not fully understood, and it is different from other chronic ulcers of the lower limb due to the development of diabetic polyneuropathy in combination with repetitive stress, infection, and peripheral artery disease (PAD). Diabetic polyneuropathy manifests as diminished or altered perception of stimuli, thus decreased pain, pressure, proprioception, and thermal sensitivity. These predispose to alteration in the anatomy of the foot and structure and function of skin (diminished sweating, dry skin, fissuring of skin, calluses, among others), which may increase risk of ulceration. The ulcers may be deep, are prone to infection, and heal with difficulty due to neuropathy and reduced blood flow.

The management of such complex patients requires a multidisciplinary approach that includes endocrinologists, neurologists, vascular surgeons, orthopedics, plastic surgeons, dermatologists, infectious disease specialists, general practitioners, and others. The dermatologist's role in a multidisciplinary team that manages diabetes-related foot disease is related to the recognition and prevention of the occurrence and progression of ulcers that can ultimately necessitate lower extremity amputation. Regular dermatological screening and education of the patient and of the patient's caregivers are essential in diminishing the risk of foot amputation [5]. According to the "IWGDF Risk Stratification System and corresponding foot screening and examination frequency," the examination should be once a year for diabetic patients with no loss of protective sensation and no peripheral artery disease, but the examinations should be once every 1–3 months when those conditions are present [6].

The clinical evaluation of patients with diabetes-related foot disease is recommended to be done in accordance with the existing guidelines of IWGDF [6] and of the American Diabetes Association [7] for the identification of the risk factors that favor the occurrence of ulcers in patients. These factors include poor glycemic management, peripheral neuropathy (loss of protective sensation), PAD, foot deformities (e.g., bunions, hammertoes, Charcot joint), pre-ulcerative corns or calluses, dry skin, fissuring of soles of feet, prior ulceration, prior amputation, smoking, retinopathy, and nephropathy.

The medical history is relevant and can be related to the prevalent pathogenic change. Neuropathy is perceived by the patient as numbness; tingling; pain; cramps; sensation of cold or hot foot, burning, and stabbing; or heavy sensation of the limb. These symptoms worsen at night or in the morning upon waking and at rest, with improvement upon movement. PAD is perceived by the patient as calf pain on walking. Varicose veins can also be present, and the patient reports sensation of heavy legs, tingling, and numbness that can be very similar to those caused by neuropathy, but the symptoms worsen with a reclined sitting position, especially when prolonged.

5.1 The Clinical Examination

Inspection may identify the deformities of the foot (e.g., claw toes, *hallux valgus*, *pes cavus*), accompanied by a change in gait pattern, which may alter the pressure distribution on the plantar level, leading to hyperkeratosis and callus; changes in gait can also be caused by the pain accompanying ulcerative lesions and infections.

Hyperkeratosis (Fig. 5.1), fissures, and plantar calluses (Fig. 5.2) will develop as signs of abnormal pressure and dry skin in the respective area, and they constitute risk factors for the occurrence of ulcers; interdigital spaces will be inspected as calluses at this level can be formed as a consequence of inadequate footwear (a situation commonly encountered); interdigital tinea pedis may also be the first step to formation of an ulcer. The presence of a hematoma under a callus, indicated by red or black discoloration, suggests the existence of an ulcer at this level. Subungual hematoma may occur asymptomatically in patients with diabetic neuropathy. This is a serious sign as it is indicative of trauma (severe enough to cause hematoma), which passed unnoticed by the patient. The skin may be pale or cyanotic, indicating significant vascular damage. The presence of erythema with a cyanotic tinge (a reddish-purple coloration of the skin) suggests the potential for rapid development of gangrene.

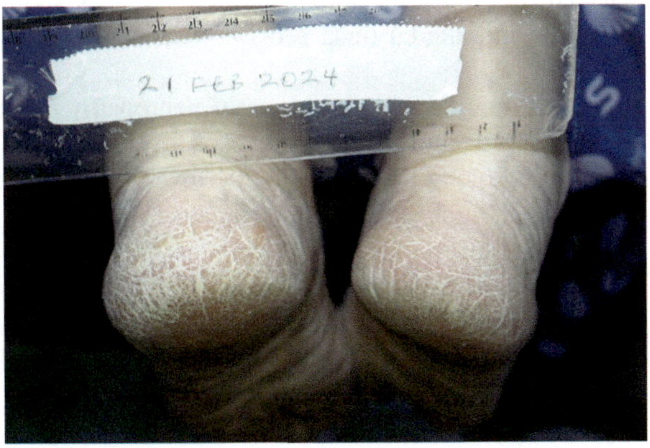

Fig. 5.1 Hyperkeratosis with fissuring of the heels in a patient with diabetes mellitus

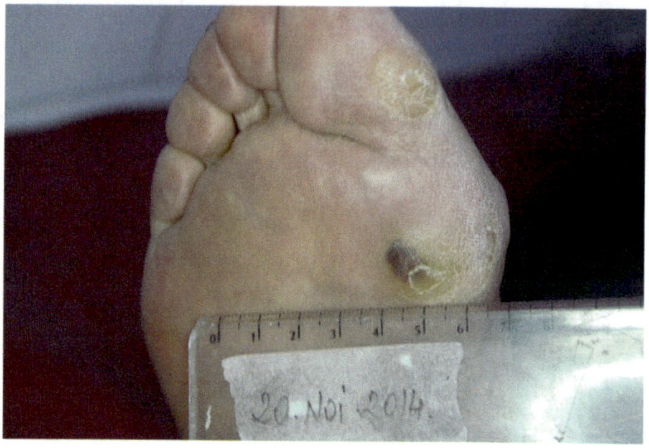

Fig. 5.2 Plantar callus in a patient with diabetes mellitus

Diabetic dermopathy is observed as brown atrophic plaques located on the anterior surface of the shin. The lesions appear following repeated trauma or infection, often unnoticed by the patient due to the presence of neuropathy. Healing of these lesions occurs with slight atrophy due to microangiopathy.

Varicose veins are associated with the presence of brown pigmented macules (ochre dermatitis) followed by more advanced stages by the appearance of an atrophic plaque that may develop a central ulceration. Varicose ulcers are commonly located on the inner side of the leg, especially in the lower third.

Petechiae can indicate significant vascular compromise; they are found on the shin and occur due to the red blood cell extravasation accompanying the varicose veins or the microangiopathy.

Previous amputations should be noted as they constitute risk factors for the appearance of new ulcers, both through the persistence of the causative factors of previous lesions and through the actual modification of foot biomechanics, leading to altered pressure distribution and the occurrence of deformities. Additionally, amputation stumps can be sites for contact eczema, fungal/bacterial infections, pain, and other ulcers.

Tinea pedis and tinea unguium constitute risk factors for ulcers and can be easily detected through inspection; interdigital spaces should be carefully examined to determine interdigital tinea pedis. These can become an entry point for bacterial infections.

Edema may be a consequence of neuropathy (neuropathic edema—associated with increased temperature in the respective lower limb and dilated dorsal veins due to increased blood flow through arteriovenous shunts opened as a consequence of loss of innervation) but can also be caused by chronic venous insufficiency or cardiac or renal insufficiency. Erythematous edema can be caused by infection, neuroarthropathy, or trauma, while varicose veins and cardiac insufficiency produce edema with a slightly bluish or pale discoloration. Diabetic muscle infarction (DMI) may manifest as acute onset of unilateral or bilateral edema and pain, most often in the upper thigh.

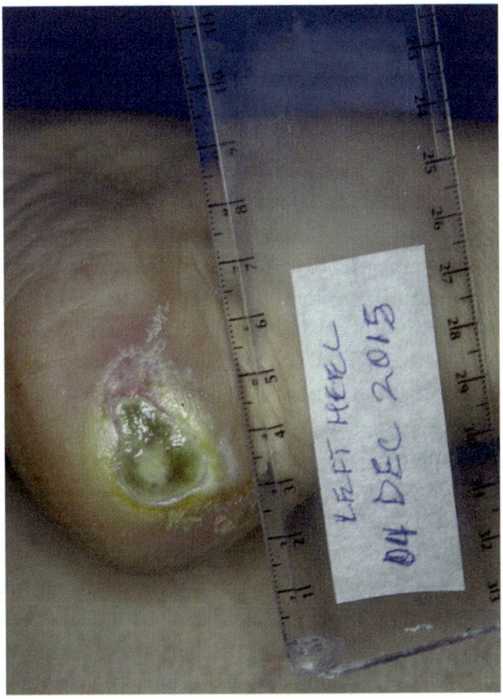

Fig. 5.3 Heel ulcer in a patient with diabetes mellitus

The description of the ulcers (Fig. 5.3) must include the location, dimensions, edges, and the base of the lesion, as well as the condition of the surrounding skin. Neurotrophic ulcers are usually located in high-pressure areas (plantar area of the metatarsal heads, plantar surface of the toes, heel, tip of a hallux valgus), or dorsa of toes. They are usually surrounded by callus, with well-defined margins, and have a pink, granulating base, with no signs of ischemia.

Arteriopathic ulcers are painful and well-defined, lack surrounding callus, and sometimes have an ischemic tinge of the surrounding skin. They may be covered by a black eschar.

Palpation Peripheral pulse should be examined at both the dorsalis pedis and posterior tibial arteries; its presence suggests the absence of significant ischemia.

Temperature of the skin is relevant as a low temperature indicates vascular involvement of the respective lower limb and correlates with changes in skin color; a high temperature is encountered in the acute phase of Charcot arthropathy, infections, and neuropathic edema.

Vascular lesions are differentiated by purpuric lesions by palpation as a slight or moderate pressure leads to the emptying of vascular lesions with their filling up again with the reduction of pressure. Purpuric lesions remain unchanged when pressure is applied. Pain upon palpation confirms the inflammatory nature of the lesions. Diabetic muscle infarction can be detected through palpation as a tender and fluctuant mass within the muscle tissue.

Enlarged regional lymph nodes on palpation may be suggestive of infection.

Neuro-osteoarthropathy (Charcot foot) is observed in patients with diabetic neuropathy or, in endemic areas, it can be a consequence of leprosy. The pathogenesis of this condition is complex, arising from a combination of mechanical and vascular factors resulting from diabetic peripheral and autonomic neuropathy, along with metabolic abnormalities in bone. The neuropathic joint appears to undergo two distinct phases: an initial resorptive phase and followed by a hypertrophic repair phase [8]. Probably, osteopenia associated with diabetes and silent traumas (sensory neuropathy) lead to repeated fractures. Diabetic peripheral neuropathy increases susceptibility to joint damage by causing loss of proprioception and autonomic neuropathy. Diminished and loss of proprioception may lead to minor trauma that harms the joint and bones of the foot, expanding the range of joint movement and causing instability and ligament laxity. Changes to joint and foot architecture further alter the mechanical axis of the foot, making the patient more prone to additional joint damage. Autonomic neuropathy can induce vasomotor changes and the formation of arteriovenous shunts. Despite normal foot pulses, these changes reduce blood flow to the skin and bone, hindering the ability to repair damaged bone and joints. The damaged joint is replaced with abnormal bone and cartilage, often resulting in ankylosis. The altered joint anatomy places stress on the plantar fascia and surrounding tendons, making the joint more susceptible to additional damage [9]. The preferred location of Charcot-type lesions is at the tarsometatarsal and tarsal joints. Metatarsophalangeal joints are also frequently affected.

In the acute phase, the foot is swollen, local temperature is elevated, and erythema is present. Radiological examination identifies fractures (resulting from minor traumatic events often unnoticed by the patient), areas of osteolysis, bone fragmentation, joint subluxations, bone sclerosis, and erosions. In the chronic phase, Charcot arthropathy leads to the appearance of the "rocker bottom foot" by displacing the tarsometatarsal joint or shifting the talonavicular joint (convex protrusion of the foot in the plantar area—the so-called rocker bottom deformity). This deformity becomes a significant risk factor for the development of ulcers in newly emerged high-pressure areas.

5.2 Investigations Performed for the Evaluation of the Patient with Diabetes-Related Foot Disease

The evaluation of the loss of protective sensation is usually done by the 10-g Semmes-Weinstein monofilament test together with one of the following: pinprick, temperature perception, ankle reflexes, and vibratory perception with a 128-Hz tuning fork. The absence of the monofilament sensation together with an abnormal result from one of the other tests confirms the existence of the neuropathy. The monofilament test evaluates the sensation at 12 of the most frequent foot sites of ulcer formation (Fig. 5.4).

Fig. 5.4 10-g monofilament test sites

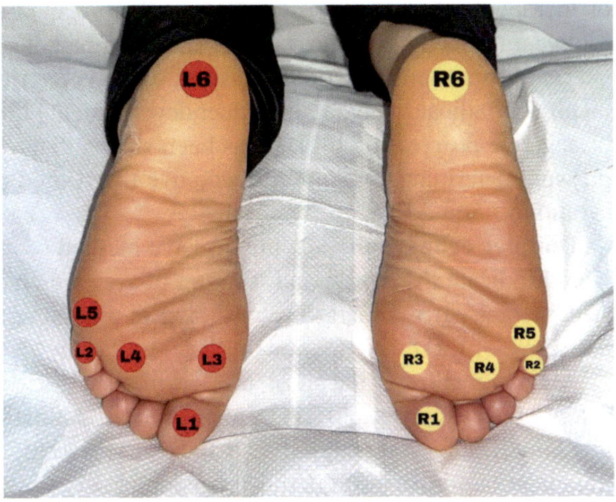

The evaluation of PAD is based on the history of the patient, the clinical examination, and the ankle-brachial index (ABI) testing. History can reveal no symptoms at the beginning of the disease, but, with the arterial narrowing, symptoms will be present, and their intensity increases with the degree of narrowing and with the number of affected arteries. Patients will report pain in the muscle groups of the lower limb during physical activities, initially with cessation of the pain at rest (intermittent claudication), and when the disease progresses, patients will report atypical pain or pain at rest (including acute pain that wakens the patient from sleep). The pain is reduced by a dependent position of the leg (e.g., patient sleeps sitting in a chair). Physical examination will assess pedal, popliteal, and femoral pulses. Skin color may be indicative of ischemic disease. There may be absence of hair on the skin of the leg and feet. The diminished or absent pulses are highly suggestive for PAD, and ABI testing will be necessary to confirm the clinical suspicion of lower extremity arterial stenosis or occlusion [10]. ABI is calculated by dividing the higher value of the systolic blood pressure at the ankle to the higher systolic brachial pressure. ABI normal values are in the interval 1.00–1.29 and 0.91–0.99 is considered equivocal. ABI values of 0.41–0.90 are considered mild-to-moderate PAD and 0.00–0.40 are suggestive for severe PAD (with a 5-year mortality of 50% [11]). Patients with extensive vascular calcification and noncompressible arteries have ABI over 1.30. Without a foot ulcer, it is challenging to predict the risk of foot ulceration in a patient with a low ankle-brachial index (ABI) [12]. However, if a patient has both a low ABI and a foot ulcer, the prognosis can be enhanced through reconstructive vascular surgery.

Optical pedobarography is a computerized method for measuring pressures on the plantar level, allowing the creation of a true "map" of pressures at this level. This method has demonstrated a strong relationship between increased pressure and the incidence of ulcers. In addition to identifying at-risk areas and areas with increased pressure, information obtained through this method can be used for the manufacture of therapeutic footwear (providing complete ulcer pressure relief) and protective footwear (reducing pressure below the ulcer threshold) for each patient.

Transcutaneous partial pressure of oxygen determination values below 30 mmHg indicate a high risk of ulcer development [13] and an increased likelihood of negative progression [14]. It has been shown that transcutaneous oxygen partial pressure determination is more predictive than blood pressure in forecasting ulcer evolution.

Doppler echography is a noninvasive method of assessing the vascular bed. It would indicate the degree and location of stenotic changes in large- and medium-sized vessels. It is usually the next step in assessing the vascular limb, if ABI is indicative of PAD.

Arteriography is the most precise method for determining the location and extent of occlusive lesions. It is a mandatory investigation for patients scheduled for revascularization intervention. Hypersensitivity to the contrast substance is a contraindication for performing this procedure.

Magnetic resonance imaging allows confirmation of the nature of a lesion in diabetic muscle infarction, as this pathology has characteristic features. It may also be indicative of the degree of damage to the foot in Charcot arthropathy especially in incipient stages.

Mycological examination enables the identification of mycelial filaments, and their culture allows the identification of the fungal species, thus facilitating the selection of the appropriate therapeutic agent. Usually, detecting these mycelial filaments is sufficient to treat the patient appropriately.

Gram staining, culture, and antibiotic sensitivity testing are laboratory investigations used in the assessment of an infected ulcer. After collecting microbiological samples, empirical antibiotic treatment can be initiated, with the choice of antibiotics based on the most commonly encountered microorganisms. After obtaining culture and antibiotic testing sensitivity results, antimicrobial therapy can be readjusted, which may not be necessary if the clinical course is favorable.

Skin biopsy is indicated, especially in the case of painless and long-standing ulcers, to exclude potential neoplastic causes. Biopsy is also useful in determining the nature of other lesions, such as non-mycotic onychodystrophy.

5.3 The Classification of Foot Ulcers

The authors recommend the use of the risk stratification system developed by IWGDF [15] in order to characterize foot ulcers in people with diabetes for routine clinical practice.

There is no system available for predicting the outcome of an ulcer in a specific individual.

The SINBAD system [16] is recommended for communication among healthcare professionals and for the audit of outcome(s) of populations. It is simple to use and requires no specialist equipment to allow for triage by a specialist team. This scoring system has been validated in multiple studies for several foot ulcer-related clinical outcomes (including healing, amputation, hospitalization, death, etc.).

The SVS WIfI classification system [17] (the Society for Vascular Surgery Lower Extremity Threatened Limb Classification System) is recommended for communication among specialists dedicated to wound healing. It can also be used for the characterization of infected wounds. The SVS WIfI classification system is intended to a more precise stratification of the patients according to their initial disease burden. It cannot dictate the therapy.

The IDSA/IWGDF (Infectious Diseases Society of America/International Working Group on the Diabetic Foot) classification [18] is recommended for infected ulcers, mainly to identify which patients require hospital admission.

5.4 Therapeutic Approach in Diabetes-Related Foot Disease

The management of diabetes-related foot disease involves eliminating or mitigating risk factors, treating existing disorders (neuropathy, arteriopathy, and infections), preventing future injuries, treating existing lesions, and educating the patient on proper foot care.

Elimination and Mitigation of Risk Factors Calluses and plantar hyperkeratosis should be carefully removed. It is crucial to prohibit patients from using sharp tools. Their use under conditions of neuropathic impairment, reduced visual acuity, or impaired joint mobility or by unqualified personnel poses a significant risk of causing injuries with subsequent unfavorable outcomes. Preferably, surgical removal using a scalpel or a mechanical abrasion device should be performed in specialized clinics under the supervision of a specialist. It should be noted that in approximately 50% of cases, corns are accompanied by underlying ulcers. For long-term treatment, the use of mild keratolytic is preferable. These have the advantage of inducing keratolysis with an almost nonexistent risk of injuries or chemical burns. Additionally, this approach avoids the need for multiple visits associated with surgical methods. Moisturizing creams also alleviate the itching associated with dryness of the skin on the feet and calves, thereby reducing the incidence of scratching-related injuries. Wearing appropriate shoes cannot be underestimated. Offloading should not be ignored, and pressure relief should be assured using casting techniques (total contact casting), custom-made or industrially manufactured orthesis, or therapeutic footwear [19]. Footwear for mobile patients should be designed based on the presence or absence of deformities and alterations in plantar pressure distribution. Shoes should be soft, devoid of rigidity, with a broad and covered toe, possibly with a rounded toe in the case of "claw toes." It is recommended to use insoles and heel cups tailored to the foot's specific conformation. Socks should be without elastic on their upper part, thus avoiding excessive pressure on the toes and calves. When choosing shoes, the patient should ensure that the footwear, with the use of insoles or heel cups, allows enough space for the foot. Selecting shoes is a challenging issue for patients with neuropathy.

Peripheral neuropathy necessitates good glycemic control. Antioxidants can be administered, preferably alpha-lipoic acid, considered a pathogenetic treatment. However, vitamin E can be useful from the same perspective, especially in cases where financial resources are limited [20]. Some patients experience more intense symptoms and signs in one of the lower limbs, indicating vascular involvement. In fact, in cases with asymmetrical neuropathy and symptoms, vascular impairment seems to be more significant. Both neuropathy and arteriopathy will be treated. Acupuncture has proven useful not only for symptomatic treatment but also for bringing certain parameters, such as nerve conduction velocity and vibratory sensitivity threshold, back to normal limits. It is also highly beneficial in treating mononeuropathy [21]. Acupuncture acts by stimulating the endogenous production of endorphins, but this mechanism inadequately explains its multiple observed beneficial effects in medical practice. Side effects are practically nonexistent for experienced hands. Amitriptyline and gabapentin can be used in cases of resistant painful neuropathy and can be helpful in combination with topical NSAIDs. The patient will be educated about choosing appropriate footwear and socks.

Arteriopathy may be treated with vasodilators and antiplatelet agents. The authors have experience with *Ginkgo biloba* extracts which increase collagen concentration in the vascular wall and has an antioxidant effect by reducing the number of circulating endothelial cells. Sulodexide can be also used in the treatment of vascular impairment in diabetes as it increases the basement membrane's filtration capacity by enhancing the vascular wall's negative ion load. Pentoxifylline also has a good effect in arteriopathies but is not effective in severe cases. A more detailed discussion on the pharmacological therapy of arteriopathy is found in Chapter "Gangrene." Walking has proven to be effective in the treatment of symptomatic arteriopathy, increasing the maximum walking distance without symptoms by up to 88% [22]. Angioplasty significantly increases transcutaneous oxygen partial pressure both immediately after the procedure and in the weeks following [23]. Bypass surgery should be considered when arteriopathy is severe, especially if an ulcer is present under these conditions and is not healing, posing a risk of degenerating into gangrene.

Fungal infections should be treated with antifungals, with topical agents being the first choice, reserving systemic treatment for severe cases. For onychomycosis, the use of keratolytic ointments with 40–60% urea or antifungal nail lacquers is recommended. In selected cases, where hepatic conditions do not contraindicate itraconazole, fluconazole or terbinafine systemic treatment can be prescribed [24]. Surgical removal of nails should be avoided since healing is often challenging and serious complications may arise.

Bacterial Infections generally respond to synthetic penicillin or cephalosporins. If anaerobic infection is suspected, metronidazole, clindamycin, or imipenem should be used. To establish specific treatment, cultures can be performed, with antimicrobial therapy adjustment after obtaining antibiogram results. In cases of ulcers, culture with antibiogram can be helpful for more specific antibiotic treatment. In cases of necrotizing fasciitis, aggressive antibiotic therapy is combined with the removal of affected tissues. Sometimes amputation is necessary to remove affected areas and save the patient's life.

References

1. van Netten JJ, Bus SA, Apelqvist J, Chen P, Chuter V, Fitridge R, et al. Definitions and criteria for diabetes-related foot disease (IWGDF 2023 update). Diabetes Metab Res Rev. 2023;40:e3654.
2. Armstrong DG, Boulton AJM, Bus SA. Diabetic foot ulcers and their recurrence. N Engl J Med. 2017;376(24):2367–75.
3. Zhang P, Lu J, Jing Y, Tang S, Zhu D, Bi Y. Global epidemiology of diabetic foot ulceration: a systematic review and meta-analysis. Ann Med. 2017;49(2):106–16.
4. Boulton AJ, Vileikyte L, Ragnarson-Tennvall G, Apelqvist J. The global burden of diabetic foot disease. Lancet. 2005;366(9498):1719–24.
5. Wexler DJ, Nathan DM, Rubinow K, editors. Evaluation of the diabetic foot. Waltham: UpToDate Inc.; 2019.
6. Schaper NC, van Netten JJ, Apelqvist J, et al. Practical guidelines on the prevention and management of diabetes-related foot disease (IWGDF 2023 update). Diabetes Metab Res Rev. 2024;40:e3657.
7. American Diabetes Association Professional Practice Committee. 12. Retinopathy, neuropathy, and foot care: standards of care in diabetes—2024. Diabetes Care. 2023;47(Supplement _1):S231–43.
8. Sequeira W. The neuropathic joint. Clin Exp Rheumatol. 1994;12(3):325–37.
9. Rosenbaum AJ, DiPreta JA. Classifications in brief: Eichenholtz classification of Charcot arthropathy. Clin Orthop. 2015;473(3):1168–71.
10. Hirsch AT, Haskal ZJ, Hertzer NR, Bakal CW, Creager MA, Halperin JL, et al. ACC/AHA 2005 practice guidelines for the Management of Patients with Peripheral Arterial Disease (lower extremity, renal, mesenteric, and abdominal aortic): a collaborative report from the American Association for Vascular Surgery/Society for Vascular Surgery,* Society for Cardiovascular Angiography and Interventions, Society for Vascular Medicine and Biology, Society of Interventional Radiology, and the ACC/AHA task force on practice guidelines (writing committee to develop guidelines for the Management of Patients with Peripheral Arterial Disease): endorsed by the American Association of Cardiovascular and Pulmonary Rehabilitation; National Heart, Lung, and Blood Institute; Society for Vascular Nursing; TransAtlantic intersociety consensus; and vascular disease foundation. Circulation. 2006;113(11):1474. https://doi.org/10.1161/CIRCULATIONAHA.106.174526.
11. McKenna M, Wolfson S, Kuller L. The ratio of ankle and arm arterial pressure as an independent predictor of mortality. Atherosclerosis. 1991;87:119–28.
12. Mcneely MJ, Boyko EJ, Ahroni JH, Stensel VL, Reiber GE, Smith DG, et al. The independent contributions of diabetic neuropathy and vasculopathy in foot ulceration. Diabetes Care. 1995;18(2):216.
13. Sumpio BE. Foot ulcers. N Engl J Med. 2000;343:787–93.
14. Kalani M, Brismar K, Fagrell B, Ostergren J, Jörneskog G. Transcutaneous oxygen tension and toe blood pressure as predictors for outcome of diabetic foot ulcers. Diabetes Care. 1999;22(1):147–51.
15. Monteiro-Soares M, Hamilton EJ, Russell DA, Srisawasdi G, Boyko EJ, Mills JL, et al. Guidelines on the classification of foot ulcers in people with diabetes (IWGDF 2023 update). Diabetes Metab Res Rev. 202;40:e3648.
16. Ince P, Abbas ZG, Lutale JK, Basit A, Ali SM, Chohan F, et al. Use of the SINBAD classification system and score in comparing outcome of foot ulcer management on three continents. Diabetes Care. 2008;31(5):964–7.
17. Mills JL, Conte MS, Armstrong DG, Pomposelli FB, Schanzer A, Sidawy AN, et al. The Society for Vascular Surgery Lower Extremity Threatened Limb Classification System: risk stratification based on wound, ischemia, and foot infection (WIfI). J Vasc Surg. 2014;59(1):220–234.e2.
18. Schaper NC. Diabetic foot ulcer classification system for research purposes: a progress report on criteria for including patients in research studies. Diabetes Metab Res Rev. 2004;20(S1):S90–5.

19. Stephan M, Gerhard R. Disease patterns in diabetes mellitus. In: Chronic wounds. 1st ed. Elsevier; 2021.
20. Tütüncü NB, Bayraktar M, Varli K. Reversal of defective nerve conduction with vitamin E supplementation in type 2 diabetes: a preliminary study. Diabetes Care. 1998;21(11):1915–8.
21. Nwabudike L, Ionescu-Tirgoviste C, Anghel V, Buligescu S. Acupuncture in the treatment of diabetic mononeuropathy: a case presentation. Roman J Diabetes. 1999;7:70–1.
22. Ubels FL, Links TP, Sluiter WJ, Reitsma WD, Smit AJ. Walking training for intermittent claudication in diabetes. Diabetes Care. 1999;22(2):198–201.
23. Wagner HJ, Schmitz R, Alfke H, Klose KJ. Influence of percutaneous transluminal angioplasty on transcutaneous oxygen pressure in patients with peripheral arterial occlusive disease. Radiology. 2003;226(3):791–7.
24. Gupta AK, Stec N, Summerbell RC, Shear NH, Piguet V, Tosti A, et al. Onychomycosis: a review. J Eur Acad Dermatol Venereol. 2020;34(9):1972–90.

Chapter 6
Diabetic Dermopathy (Diabetic Shin Spots)

Lawrence Chukwudi Nwabudike

Abstract Diabetic dermopathy is a common cutaneous manifestation of diabetes mellitus. It was first described by the Swede, Dr. Hans Melin in 1964. The prevalence varies from 0.2 to 35%, and may be more common in type 2 diabetes. There is no apparent sex or racial predisposition. Although it has often been classified as a microangiopathic disorder, studies suggest that other factors such as hyperglycaemia, neuropathy and possibly immune disorders may play a role. Diabetic dermopathy presents with asymptomatic, atrophic, round or roundish, well-defined lesions, located asymmetrically on the shins. They have rarely involved the abdomen and other anatomic sites. Histopathologic features include atrophy of the rete ridges, hyperkeratosis, papillary oedema and telangiectasis, with mucopolysaccharide infiltration of the vessel walls. Therapy is not necessary, as not only is the disorder benign and an incidental finding but it is also spontaneously remitting. Nevertheless, data suggests that laser therapy may help remit lesions.

6.1 Definition

Diabetic dermopathy is a cutaneous manifestation presenting as atrophic, well-defined, bilateral plaques located asymmetrically, usually on the anterior legs of patients with diabetes mellitus.

L. C. Nwabudike (✉)
N. Paulescu National Institute of Diabetes, Nutrition and Metabolic Diseases, Bucharest, Romania

K. Fritz, G.-S. Tiplica (eds.), *Cutaneous Manifestations in Diabetes*, https://doi.org/10.1007/978-3-031-65300-1_6

6.2 History

Diabetic dermopathy, also known as diabetic shin spots, is a common disorder associated with diabetes mellitus. It was first described in 1964 by Hans Melin of Sweden [1]. This work was part of his doctoral thesis and his paper suggested his findings were the result of several years of careful observation. Melin also noted the presence of deposits of gamma globulins in the skin lesions of patients with diabetic dermopathy and lupus erythematosus [2], which were not seen in the skins of control subjects. These deposits were located primarily immediately beneath the basal layer and in the vessel walls in the dermis [2]. Binkley [3] of the USA first coined the term "dermopathy" in 1966 and advanced the view that the disorder is a manifestation of microangiopathy in patients with diabetes mellitus.

6.3 Epidemiology

The prevalence of diabetic dermopathy varies. This variation depends largely on the study size and methodology. Some authors noted 12.5% of their cohort ($n = 457$) [4]. Their diabetic dermopathy patients were seen in the non-insulin dependent diabetes mellitus (NIDDM) subgroup ($n = 393$); thus, this proportion is probably lower as a percentage of the total. A Turkish study ($n = 151$), of type 2 diabetic patients, observed diabetic dermopathy in 11.2% of their study group, with no sex prevalence [5]. An Argentinian study found 35% of their cohort ($n = 125$, 88% type 2 diabetes) had diabetic dermopathy [6]. Most of their cases of diabetic dermopathy (40/44, 90.9%) were type 2 diabetic patients, as in the Turkish cohort. An Indian cohort ($n = 680$) found 9.4% with diabetic dermopathy [7], mostly in patients with type 2 diabetes. In spite of this apparent bias towards type 2 diabetes, a study of patients with type 1 diabetes ($n = 500$) showed 29 (5.8%) of patients with diabetic dermopathy, with no apparent sex difference [8]. Notably, although this cohort had a short average duration of diabetes (4.43 years), it nonetheless had poor average metabolic control (HbA1c = 9.72%) [8], suggesting that metabolic control might be an important pathogenic factor in production of diabetic dermopathy, at least in type 1 diabetes. A group from India found a prevalence of 6.3% of a cohort of 294 patients [9]. A very low prevalence of diabetic dermopathy was found in another Indian cohort ($n = 500$, 494 type 2) [10]. The study authors found only one case of diabetic dermopathy (0.2%). While it has been hypothesised that this may be due to the skin complexion of Indians, the other studies show much higher prevalence of diabetic dermopathy, albeit lower than studies from populations with lighter skin.

There has been no consistent predilection of lesions based on sex seen in these patients. It appears to be commoner in older patients, with longer duration of diabetes.

One may summarise that the prevalence of diabetic dermopathy is of the order of 0.2–35%, with a greater tendency to occur in type 2 diabetes than in type 1 and without apparent sex or racial predilection.

6.4 Pathogenesis

Melin [1] initially thought diabetic dermopathy might be caused by trauma, which passed unobserved. He reported negative results in attempting to replicate the lesions of diabetic dermopathy by applying trauma using a rubber hammer to the shins of his patients. Diabetic dermopathy is often classified as a microangiopathic complication of diabetes mellitus. In newly diagnosed type 2 diabetes, there is already a 13% prevalence of microangiopathy [11] and a cumulative 24.3% incidence of neuropathy in the prediabetic state [12]. The prevalence of neuropathy in Europe is of the order of 28–51% [13, 14]. Thus, one may expect an association between diabetic dermopathy, microvascular disease and neurological disease due to the frequency of the latter two complications.

Skin blood flow has been found to be significantly increased at sites of dermopathy lesions compared with contiguous skin, and to standard sites, in spite of decreased responsiveness of the cutaneous microvasculature generally of these patients to thermal stimuli [15, 16]. This would suggest that, although cutaneous blood flow is affected generally in these patients, the microvasculature may not be the critical aetiological factor for production of diabetic dermopathy that it has been thought to be. Yet there still may be a case for microangiopathy as an aetiological factor, since data from a study suggests that dermopathy is much commoner in patients with retinopathy than without [17]. It should be noted that the patients in this study also had significantly longer duration of diabetes, thus greater risk of having complications [17], again suggesting the argument of potential pathogenic association by virtue of high frequency.

Another study showed that patients with diabetic dermopathy and neuropathy have significantly smaller compound muscle action potentials, slower nerve conduction velocities and longer mean distal latencies than patients with neuropathy alone. This study was carried out only in male patients. The authors concluded that diabetic dermopathy could be a marker of severe neuropathy [18]. A further study with only female subjects found significantly reduced mean distal latencies of the ulnar nerve in patients with diabetic dermopathy as compared to those without [19]. There is therefore an argument for neuropathy as a potential aetiopathogenic factor for diabetic dermopathy.

Melin [2] found gamma globulin (immunoglobulin) deposition in lesional and perilesional skin of patients with diabetic dermopathy and patients with lupus erythematosus, but not in normal controls. This suggests that diabetic dermopathy might have an immunologic pathogenic component. However, other studies would be necessary to confirm this finding.

6.5 Clinical Features

Diabetic dermopathy is primarily a clinical diagnosis. The lesions are only very rarely biopsied, as the diagnosis is benign and there is the potential for significant morbidity following a biopsy in a patient with diabetes. Patients with this disorder rarely report antecedent trauma or cutaneous infection and the lesions are often an incidental clinical finding.

Lesions of diabetic dermopathy are asymptomatic. The initial lesions have not been established, although there is some speculation of trauma due to some patients recalling some preceding minor ulcerations [1]. They are classically atrophic, round or roundish, well-defined lesions with variable degrees of pigmentation, located on the anterior shins in an asymmetrical manner (Fig. 6.1). Some authors have noted initial red/purple papules with central vesiculation, which tend towards the atrophic lesions that are classically seen [20]. The lighter lesions tend to be less atrophic than the older lesions, may have a light overlying scale and are between 1 and 2.5 cm in diameter [1, 20–22] (Fig. 6.2). Within a span of 18–24 months, the lesions may fade and new ones appear [1]. A rare case with atrophic reddish-brown patches on the thighs and abdomen of a female patient with type 2 diabetes was histopathologically confirmed to be diabetic dermopathy [23].

Some authors carried out a dermoscopic study in a patient whose diagnosis was apparently confirmed with histopathology [24]. Although their work was limited to one patient, their study showed dermoscopic findings of one or more whitish, central areas surrounded by a brown rim containing ring-like globular structures. The central areas had linear vessels separated by dusky, blurred greyish-white streaks [24]. The authors speculated that the whitish central areas may be areas of increased collagen deposition, the ring-like structures areas of hemosiderin deposition and the telangiectases vessels in the papillary dermis seen through atrophic skin.

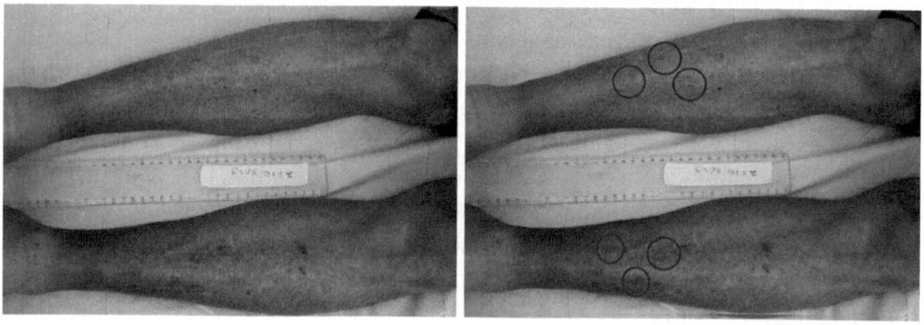

Fig. 6.1 Asymmetrically distributed hyperpigmented, atrophic patches, some with some hypopigmentation surrounded by a ring of hyperpigmentation (blue circles)

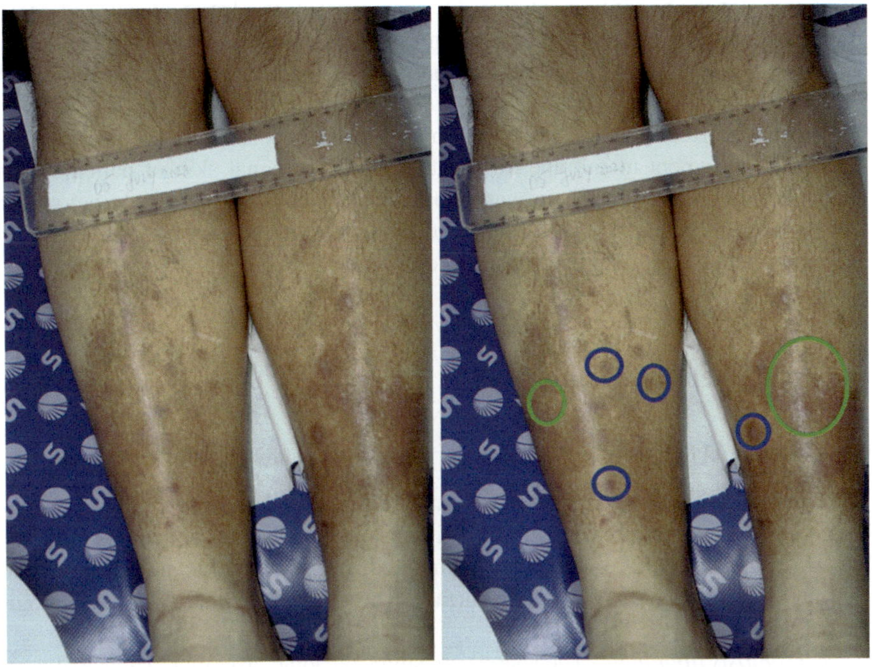

Fig. 6.2 Multiple, hypopigmented, atrophic patches on the legs (green circles) on a background of stasis hyperpigmentation, possibly illustrating why diabetic dermopathy may be harder to detect on dark skin. Blue circles illustrated as in Fig. 6.1

6.6 Histopathologic Features

Epidermal changes include atrophy of the rete ridges, with moderate hyperkeratosis and variable basal pigmentation [20–22]. There are oedema, fibroblastic proliferation and telangiectasia of the papillary dermis [20–22]. There are hemosiderin deposition and mucopolysaccharide infiltration of the vessel walls, the latter shown by periodic acid-schiff (PAS) staining [22]. There is some PAS-positive thickening of the blood vessels in the skin [1, 25]. There is a perivascular infiltrate of lymphoid, histiocytic and plasma cells [23]. Some workers [22] felt that this in itself would be a marker for diabetic dermopathy histologically in the appropriate setting, but others' findings failed to confirm this [25]. The latter [25] comprised a histopathological study of autopsy samples, which the study authors believed might have contributed to the paucity of plasma cells. Other suggested histologic markers of this disorder include hemosiderin and melanin deposition [25], which might appear to account for the hyperpigmentation. Of note, sepsis was a frequent cause of death in the subjects from whom post-mortem samples were obtained, and the study authors noted this [25] as a potential cofounding factor in assessing the significance of the hemosiderin deposits.

Others reported the presence of gamma globulin deposition in the vessel walls and at the basement membrane in affected and perilesional skin of patients with diabetic dermopathy [2]. There was also a similar deposit immediately below the basement membrane [2]. This fluorescent deposition was also seen in subjects with lupus erythematosus, but not in normal controls [2].

6.7 Differential Diagnosis

The differential diagnoses of diabetic dermopathy include the following:

- *Superficial fungal infection*—In the early stages of diabetic dermopathy, but fungal infections may present with more intense itch and active, squamous margins.
- *Neurotic excoriations*—Scars are pigmented, slightly atrophic and irregular and may occur anywhere on the skin surface. There may be a history of psychological disorder.
- *Necrobiosis lipoidica*—The lesions are shiny, atrophic, irregular, patches of variable size, which are initially reddish and then progress to yellow colour.
- *Papulonecrotic tuberculids*—The scars would usually be smaller, more numerous in a younger age group and a history of prior ulceration or excoriation would be present. There may be a history of prior tuberculosis.
- *Stasis dermatitis*—Hyperpigmentation, usually most intense over medial leg. There may be associated induration and lipodermatosclerosis.
- *Schamberg disease (progressive pigmented purpura)*—Red-brown patches, appearing anywhere on the skin.
- *Simple post-traumatic scars*—Usually one or several, of varying size and shape. Preceding history of a traumatic lesion is present.
- *Drug-induced pigmentation*—This may occur following ingestion of minocycline or quinolines.

6.8 Therapy

Treatment is usually not necessary, as the condition is benign and often diagnosed incidentally. Also, lesions may go into remission spontaneously with time [1].

Nonetheless, attempts have been made to find therapeutic solutions for this disorder. In one such attempt, low-level laser therapy using a helium–neon, non-heating laser was compared with placebo in a cohort ($n = 12$) [26]. The laser was applied to both limbs of the same patient but turned off on the placebo side. Lesional and perilesional skin blood flow as well as size of the lesions were measured. The authors found that there was significant improvement in diabetic dermopathy lesions for both treated and placebo areas, but increase in cutaneous blood flow was only significant for the treated areas [26]. The authors proffered no explanation for the improvement seen in the placebo arm. There were no side effects recorded and the study authors considered this a safe and effective modality of treatment, worthy of further study [26].

A topically applied combination of glycerine and modified collagen in a lotion reportedly helped improve the appearance of diabetic dermopathy lesions [21].

Most practitioners do not treat the patients' lesions for the reasons stated above. Nonetheless, the presence of lesions of diabetic dermopathy may be considered an indication to aggressively investigate and treat affected patients for microvascular and neuropathic complications of diabetes mellitus.

6.9 Conclusions

Diabetic dermopathy is a common, benign, acquired dermatosis associated with diabetes mellitus. Its prevalence ranges from 0.2 to 35%, with a predilection for type 2 diabetes. There is no apparent sex or racial predilection for this disorder. Data suggests that diabetic dermopathy may be specific to diabetes. The cause of this disorder is unknown, but there is evidence that implicates microangiopathy, neuropathy and perhaps some immune mechanisms. Diabetic dermopathy is asymptomatic and often an incidental clinical finding. It is usually located on the anterior legs, but lesions have rarely been found on other sites.

There is no specific therapy for this disorder, it is benign, and lesions have been documented as remitting spontaneously over 18–24 months. Laser therapy showed some beneficial effect in a blinded, placebo-controlled study and is worthy of further study, though costs of this form of therapy may be a factor limiting access.

The presence of lesions of diabetic dermopathy in a patient should be an indication to aggressively investigate for systemic manifestations of diabetic microangiopathy and neuropathy.

References

1. Melin H. An atrophic circumscribed skin lesion in the lower extremities of diabetics. Acta Med Scand. 1964;176:1–75.
2. Larsson O, Melin H. Chapter IX: an investigation with the fluorescent antibody technique on the occurrence of gammaglobulin in skin from the lower extremities of diabetics. Acta Med Scand. 1964;176:56–8. https://doi.org/10.1111/J.0954-6820.1964.Tb06340.X.
3. Binkley GW. Dermopathy in the diabetic syndrome. Arch Dermatol. 1965;92(6):625–34. https://doi.org/10.1001/archderm.1965.01600180017003.

4. Romano G, Moretti G, Di Benedetto A, Giofrè C, Di Cesare E, Russo G, et al. Skin lesions in diabetes mellitus: prevalence and clinical correlations. Diabetes Res Clin Pract. 1998;39(2):101–6. https://doi.org/10.1016/s0168-8227(97)00119-8.
5. Sasmaz S, Buyukbese M, Cetinkaya A, Celik M, Arican O. The prevalence of skin disorders in type-2 diabetic patients. Int J Dermatol. 2004;3(1):1–4.
6. Galdeano F, Zaccaria S, Parra V, Giannini ME, Salomón S. Cutaneous manifestations of diabetes mellitus: clinical meaning. Dermatol Argent. 2013;16:117–21. http://www.dermatolarg.org.ar/index.php/dermatolarg/article/view/1093
7. Chatterjee N, Chattopadhyay C, Sengupta N, Das C, Sarma N, Pal SK. An observational study of cutaneous manifestations in diabetes mellitus in a tertiary care Hospital of Eastern India. Indian J Endocrinol Metab. 2014;18(2):217–20. https://doi.org/10.4103/2230-8210.129115.
8. Sawatkar GU, Kanwar AJ, Dogra S, Bhadada SK, Dayal D. Spectrum of cutaneous manifestations of type 1 diabetes mellitus in 500 South Asian patients. Br J Dermatol. 2014;171:1402–6. https://doi.org/10.1111/bjd.13077.
9. Timshina DK, Thappa DM, Agrawal A. A clinical study of dermatoses in diabetes to establish its markers. Indian J Dermatol. 2012;57(1):20–5. https://doi.org/10.4103/0019-5154.92671.
10. Ragunatha S, Anitha B, Inamadar AC, Palit A, Devarmani SS. Cutaneous disorders in 500 diabetic patients attending diabetic clinic. Indian J Dermatol. 2011;56(2):160–4. https://doi.org/10.4103/0019-5154.80409.
11. Ponto KA, Koenig J, Peto T, Lamparter J, Raum P, Wild PS, et al. Prevalence of diabetic retinopathy in screening-detected diabetes mellitus: results from the Gutenberg Health Study (GHS). Diabetologia. 2016;59(9):1913–9. https://doi.org/10.1007/s00125-016-4013-5.
12. Ziegler D, Rathmann W, Dickhaus T, Meisinger C, Mielck A, KORA Study Group. Prevalence of polyneuropathy in pre-diabetes and diabetes is associated with abdominal obesity and macroangiopathy: the MONICA/KORA Augsburg Surveys S2 and S3. Diabetes Care. 2008;31(3):464–9. https://doi.org/10.2337/dc07-1796.
13. Tesfaye S, Stevens LK, Stephenson JM, Fuller JH, Plater M, Ionescu-Tirgoviste C, et al. Prevalence of diabetic peripheral neuropathy and its relation to glycaemic control and potential risk factors: the EURODIAB IDDM complications study. Diabetologia. 1996;39(11):1377–84. https://doi.org/10.1007/s001250050586.
14. Hicks CW, Selvin E. Epidemiology of peripheral neuropathy and lower extremity disease in diabetes. Curr Diab Rep. 2019;19:86. https://doi.org/10.1007/s11892-019-1212-8.
15. Wigington G, Ngo B, Rendell M. Skin blood flow in diabetic dermopathy. Arch Dermatol. 2004;140(10):1248–50. https://doi.org/10.1001/archderm.140.10.1248.
16. Brugler A, Thompson S, Turner S, Ngo B, Rendell M. Skin blood flow abnormalities in diabetic dermopathy. J Am Acad Dermatol. 2011;65(3):559–63. https://doi.org/10.1016/j.jaad.2010.06.010.
17. Abdollahi A, Daneshpazhooh M, Amirchaghmaghi E, Sheikhi S, Eshrati B, Bastanhagh MH. Dermopathy and retinopathy in diabetes: is there an association? Dermatology. 2007;214(2):133–6. https://doi.org/10.1159/000098572.
18. Kiziltan ME, Benbir G, Akalin MA. Is diabetic dermopathy a sign for severe neuropathy in patients with diabetes mellitus? Nerve conduction studies and symptom analysis. Clin Neurophysiol. 2006;117(8):1862–9. https://doi.org/10.1016/j.clinph.2006.05.007.
19. Kiziltan ME, Benbir G. Clinical and nerve conduction studies in female patients with diabetic dermopathy. Acta Diabetol. 2008;45(2):97–105. https://doi.org/10.1007/s00592-008-0031-1.
20. Morgan AJ, Schwartz RA. Diabetic dermopathy: a subtle sign with grave implications. J Am Acad Dermatol. 2008;58(3):447–51. https://doi.org/10.1016/j.jaad.2007.11.013.
21. George SMC, Walton S. Diabetic dermopathy. Br J Diabetes. 2014;14:95–7. https://doi.org/10.15277/bjdvd.2014.027.
22. Naik PP, Farrukh SN. Clinical significance of diabetic dermatopathy. Diabetes Metab Syndr Obes. 2020;13:4823–7. https://doi.org/10.2147/DMSO.S286887.
23. Minelli L, Gon ADS, De Medeiros RA. Case for diagnosis. An Bras Dermatol. 2008;83(5):480–1. https://doi.org/10.1590/S0365-05962008000500015.

24. Navarro-Gilo M, Alberti-Masalleras N, de Gea-Fernández M, Domingo A, Sagristà M. Dermoscopy of diabetic dermopathy. Dermatol Pract Concept. 2022;12(4):e2022185. https://doi.org/10.5826/dpc.1204a185.
25. McCash S, Emanuel PO. Defining diabetic dermopathy. J Dermatol. 2011;38:988–92. https://doi.org/10.1111/j.1346-8138.2011.01251.x.
26. Abdelhalim NM, Abdelbasset WK, Alqahtani BA, Samhan AF. Low-level laser therapy for diabetic dermopathy in patients with type 2 diabetes: a placebo-controlled pilot study. J Lasers Med Sci. 2020;11(4):481–5. https://doi.org/10.34172/JLMS.2020.75.

Chapter 7
Foot Gangrene in Diabetes

Lawrence Chukwudi Nwabudike

Abstract Gangrene is a consequence of localised tissue necrosis or tissue death, often due to compromised blood circulation to the affected tissue. Three main types of lower extremity gangrene are seen in patients with diabetes—dry, wet and gas gangrene. Dry gangrene is consequent on ischaemia, wet gangrene has associated infection and oedema on the backdrop of ischaemia, and gas gangrene is myonecrosis from bacterial exotoxins, classically from *Clostridium* species. Prevalence rates of gangrene vary from 4.1 to 41.4%, with a male-female ratio of 3:1. Dry gangrene manifests as an area of black, dry, shrunken tissue that is well-delineated from the surrounding area, wet gangrene shows associated oedema, oozing and sometimes has malodour, and there is less delineation, while with gas gangrene there is a then blue-black discolouration of the skin, with associated bullae and systemic symptoms such as high fever. Pathology shows coagulative necrosis in dry gangrene and liquefactive necrosis in wet, with myonecrosis and presence of bacteria in clostridial gas gangrene. Therapy depends on the clinical scenario. It may be general, medical and surgical and include smoking cessation, exercise, antibiotics, vasoactive agents to improve circulation, hyperbaric oxygen therapy and revascularisation procedures.

7.1 Introduction

Gangrene may be defined as localised tissue death or tissue necrosis. Often, this is due to compromised blood supply to the involved tissue. This work will be limited to diabetic lower extremity gangrene of which there are three main types—dry, wet and gas gangrene [1].

Dry gangrene is usually consequent on ischaemia, without bacterial infection, leaving behind dry, mummified, necrotic tissue. *Wet gangrene* is associated with

L. C. Nwabudike (✉)
N. Paulescu National Institute of Diabetes, Nutrition and Metabolic Diseases, Bucharest, Romania

K. Fritz, G.-S. Tiplica (eds.), *Cutaneous Manifestations in Diabetes*, https://doi.org/10.1007/978-3-031-65300-1_7

infections, often on the backdrop of ischaemia and oedema. *Gas gangrene* can be clostridial, with infection by *Clostridium perfringens* and other *Clostridium* species, which leads to myonecrosis [1] and non-clostridial [2], due to other organisms such as *Escherichia coli*, *Proteus* species, *Pseudomonas aeruginosa*, *Klebsiella pneumoniae*, *Enterococcus* species and *Bacteroides* species.

Therapy may be conservative or radical, depending on the extent of pathology. *Fournier gangrene* will not be discussed here.

7.2 Epidemiology

Gangrene is the final stage of a process and is an indication for amputation to preserve health. In an Iranian cohort ($n = 217$ patients, 81 female; mean age 54.25 years), the commonest indication for amputation was diabetic gangrene (41.47%), and below knee amputations were the commonest level of amputation (48.29%) [3]. A Chinese study ($n = 971$, 360 female; mean age 65.1 years) showed a 32.5% prevalence of gangrene [4], with most cases not being amputated; their fate was unclear from this study. Amputation levels were not indicated in this study. Another Chinese study ($n = 3181$, 45.8–42.9% female; average age 65.3–66.3 years) showed between 14.7 and 11.3% decreasing prevalence over an 8-year period [5]. A 4.1% prevalence rate of gangrene was found in an Australian study [6] ($n = 3035$). This study, in contrast to other studies, suggested a 3:1 male–female ratio regarding prevalence of diabetic gangrene. Data from another study ($n = 100$) suggests that patients with gangrene had higher postprandial glycaemia, inflammatory markers (C-reactive protein, fibrinogen and white blood cell), arteriosclerosis and vessel inflammation than patients with intermittent claudication [7], indicating that inflammation and poor glycaemic control may be integral to the process of tissue death.

7.3 Pathogenesis

Dry gangrene is a condition of tissue necrosis following total or almost total ischaemia [1]. Peripheral arteriosclerosis, diabetes and smoking are risk factors for dry/ischaemic gangrene [1, 7]. Peripheral artery disease affects more than 200 million people worldwide and leads to amputation in 3–4% of cases [8]. Dry gangrene occurs in diabetes when tissue needs are no longer met by almost completely compromised circulation. Peripheral artery disease is asymptomatic in up to 50% of patients [8, 9]. Only about 10% of sufferers show classic symptoms [9]. There is a 15–22% 1-year rate of limb amputation in patients with chronic limb-threatening ischaemia [10, 11]. Microvascular disease accounts for 18% of lower extremity amputations. The combination of peripheral artery disease and microvascular disease accounts for 45% of lower extremity amputations according to one study [12]. The authors postulated that microvascular disease could lead to impaired wound healing and therefore to tissue death. In patients with diabetes mellitus, microvascular and macrovascular disease are present and play prominent roles in dry gangrene.

Wet gangrene occurs when tissue compromised by poor venous or arterial flow is affected by infection with associated oedema [1]. Of 194 patients with dry gangrene, who underwent revascularisation [13], 15 (7.7%) converted to wet gangrene over an average 13.5 days, suggesting that there is a greater level of ischaemia needed to produce dry, as opposed to wet, gangrene. The increased blood flow following revascularisation presumably converts dry to wet gangrene by inflow of fluids to the already desiccated area. Wet gangrene is responsible for 29% of cases (total cohort = 100) [14] of infected diabetic foot ulcers, with 42% of this cohort having monomicrobial infections with *Staphylococcus aureus* (31.3%), methicillin-resistant *Staphylococcus aureus* [MRSA] (16.7%) and *Pseudomonas aeruginosa* (16.7%) being the most common species for monomicrobial infections in one cohort [14]. Polymicrobial infections comprised 52% of this cohort, with *Staphylococcus aureus* (48.1%), *Bacteroides fragilis* (46.2%) and *Pseudomonas aeruginosa* (34.6%) as the most common organisms detected [14]. Thus, initial antibiotic therapy covering these organisms, prior to obtaining specific microbiology results, is probably acceptable and may be more indicated for wet, than dry, gangrene.

Gas gangrene is a myonecrosis, which is classically associated with *Clostridium* infections [1, 15]. Post-traumatic gas gangrene is most frequently associated with *Clostridium perfringens*, while *Clostridium septicum* is the most frequent culprit in non-traumatic gas gangrene [16]. While clostridial gas gangrene is the classic form of this disorder, case series suggest that other organisms may be at work, including *Staphylococcus aureus* and *Peptostreptococcus* [17, 18], with infrequent *Clostridium* or no *Clostridium* grown [17]. The mechanism of necrosis in gas gangrene is tissue destruction from bacterial exotoxin production as opposed to ischaemia in dry and wet gangrene [1, 15]. It is a clinical scenario that can rapidly become lethal.

7.4 Clinical Features

Dry gangrene usually manifests as an area of shrunken, black, dry tissue [1, 18]. There may be associated dependent limb rubor, with reduced capillary refill [1]. Associated hair loss over the affected area, with anaesthesia, may be observed, and the affected area is often sharply delineated from the surrounding tissue, especially at the level of the toes [18]. This may be preceded by pallor and diminished function or paralysis of the limb. Violaceous or grey areas with ulceration and blistering at the distal ends of the toes may be seen. Ankle pulses are usually not palpable (Fig. 7.1 dry gangrene).

Wet gangrene, as opposed to dry gangrene, is associated with oedema, oozing, drainage and malodour, which may occur in some cases. Pain and tenderness of the foot may be observed, the latter suggestive of a deep abscess [1] (Fig. 7.2 wet gangrene).

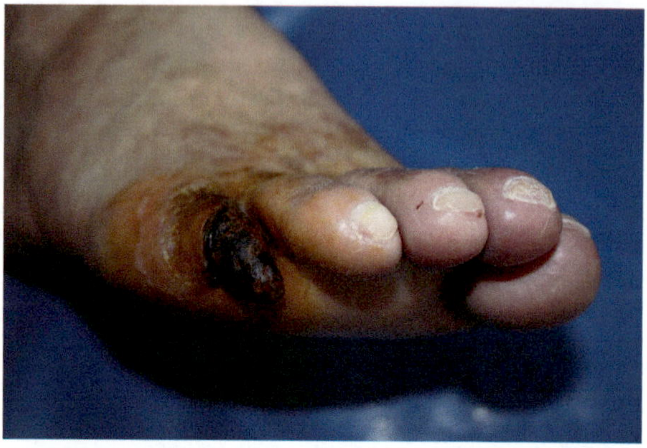

Fig. 7.1 Dry gangrene of right fifth toe. Note shrunken appearance of toe with clear limitation from neighbouring tissue

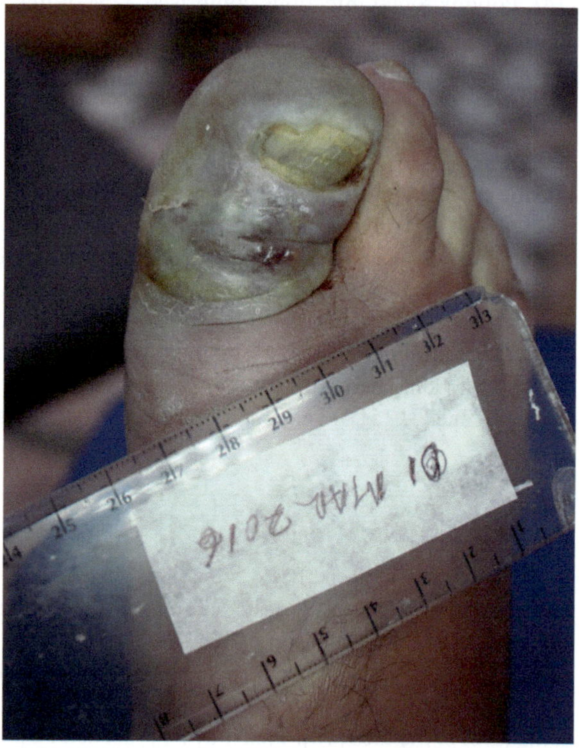

Fig. 7.2 Wet gangrene of right first toe. Note denudation of overlying skin, partly from underlying wet necrosis

Gas gangrene often begins with acute onset of pain in the affected extremity. The skin turns bronze, then blue-black, with haemorrhagic bullae. There may be associated fever and chills, non-pitting oedema and crepitus. The oedema may occasionally mask the crepitus. There may be rapid deterioration to sepsis [15] (Fig. 7.3 gas gangrene).

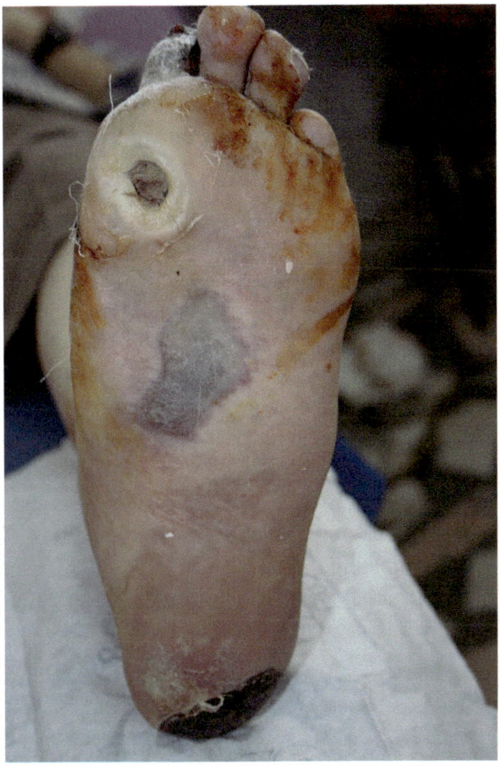

Fig. 7.3 Gas gangrene of left foot. Note bullae with liquid and gas in mid plantar area. There are toe gangrene, heel necrosis and an anterior foot ulcer

7.5 Pathology

Necrosis is cell death, and it is almost invariably a consequence of a pathological process, unlike apoptosis, which may be physiological. Two main kinds of necrosis are involved in the process of gangrene [19]—coagulative and liquefactive necrosis. Liquefactive necrosis relies on autophagy and heterophagy from enzymes within and outside (from bacteria) the cell. The cells do not maintain their architecture and a viscous mass is the result [19]. In coagulative necrosis, cellular enzymes are destroyed due to the ischaemic process, while the desiccation makes it difficult for bacteria to survive, thereby delaying the process of cellular degeneration and progression to liquefactive necrosis. Histopathologically, the cells in coagulative necrosis maintain their architecture for much longer than in liquefactive necrosis. In gas gangrene, the histopathologic image is one of widespread myonecrosis with paucity of leucocytes and large, Gram-positive rods on Gram stain, when *Clostridium* is involved.

7.6 Differential Diagnosis

While the diagnosis is usually fairly clear from a clinical standpoint, possible differential diagnoses for gangrene include the following:

- Gangrenous ergotism—There may be a history of consumption of grains, which may have been contaminated by fungi.
- Frostbite—A history of cold exposure would be elicited.
- Raynaud phenomenon—There may be a history of autoimmune disease and cold exposure, with the classical symptoms and return to normal tissue colour being seen.
- Calciphylaxis—There is usually a history of renal failure, though a significant number of patients are non-uremic.
- Compartment syndrome—A history of trauma, especially fractures, may be present.
- Septic shock—Fever, tachycardia, leucocytosis and tachypnoea may be present, in contrast to the localised manifestations of foot gangrene; sepsis may, in itself, complicate gangrene.
- Toxic shock—This is an acute, life-threatening, toxin-mediated disorder, which may be associated with wounds.

7.7 Therapeutic Approaches

The therapeutic approach to gangrene is aimed at mitigating tissue loss. Aetiological factors such as ischaemia and infection need to be addressed, while non-viable tissue should be eliminated.

Therapy is medical and surgical.

Medical therapy includes the following:

1. *Agents to improve blood flow*

   (a) *Antiplatelet agents* such as clopidogrel, rivaroxaban and aspirin are useful.

   (b) *Pentoxifylline* is a synthetic methylxanthine useful for the therapy of occlusive peripheral artery disease and intermittent claudication [20]. Pentoxifylline improves microcirculation, increases red cell deformability and diminishes platelet aggregation and plasma viscosity [20]. It also improves leucocyte deformability and chemotaxis, while diminishing their sensitivity to cytokines [20, 21], as well as cytokine production, including tumour necrosis factor-α [21]. It increases walking distance and improves symptoms of claudication [20]. Nausea, vomiting, bloating, dizziness, hypotension and flushing are potential side effects.

   (c) *Cilostazol* is a quinolone derivative. Initial claudication distance is significantly greater with cilostazol compared with placebo, with no significant difference compared with pentoxifylline [22]. Cilostazol is a phosphodiesterase

III inhibitor that brings about increased intracellular levels of cyclic adenosine monophosphate; as a result, inhibition of platelet aggregation, anti-inflammatory effects and vasodilation occur [22]. Side effects of cilostazol include headaches, diarrhoea, palpitations, dizziness and pains [23].

(d) *Naftidrofuryl* is a selective serotonin 5-HT_2 (5-HTR) receptor inhibitor. This prevents 5-hydroxy serotonin-induced release by the endothelium and platelets in consequence of hypoxia and atherogenesis. Naftidrofuryl also inhibits platelet aggregation caused by serotonin. The result is an inhibition of vasoconstriction, rather than a production of vasodilation [24]. Naftidrofuryl increases pain-free walking distance and maximum walking distance, albeit moderately [25]. Nausea, vomiting, rash and nephrolithiasis are possible side effects.

(e) *Sulodexide* is a glycosaminoglycan, which is a large family of naturally occurring substances in the body, including heparin [26]. It is comprised of a fast-moving heparin (80%) and dermatan sulphate (20%) [26]. Sulodexide improves pain-free and maximal walking distances in patients with peripheral occlusive artery disease, as well as accelerates healing of trophic ulcers [27]. It has a good safety profile, with gastrointestinal symptoms including nausea, dyspepsia and potential bleeding as possible side effects.

(f) *Prostanoids* are prostaglandin analogues with potent vasodilatory and platelet inhibitory activity [28]. They also increase erythrocyte deformability while inhibiting proliferation of cells in the vessel wall [28]. A Cochrane review concluded that there is some benefit of prostanoids on ischaemic rest pain and ulcer healing compared to placebo, with no apparent impact on incidence of amputations [29]. Potential side effects include nausea, diarrhoea, headaches, flushing and hypotension.

(g) *Hyperbaric oxygen therapy* is the utilisation of 100% oxygen at greater than atmospheric pressure [30]. It stimulates angiogenesis and diminishes inflammation [31]. It is indicated in the therapy of gas gangrene, Fournier gangrene and wound healing in diabetes [31]. Barotrauma, usually to the middle ear and sinuses, acute oxygen neurotoxicity and seizures as well as pulmonary oxygen toxicity are potential side effects.

(h) *Antibiotics* should be initiated where infection is suspected, especially with gas gangrene. Vancomycin, tazobactam, ceftriaxone, penicillin, clindamycin and metronidazole are frequently recommended [15].

2. *General measures*

(a) *Smoking cessation* is important, as smoking is a strong independent risk factor for peripheral artery disease [32].

(b) *Metabolic control* should be strictly maintained as chronic hyperglycaemia is an independent risk factor for cardiovascular events and mortality amongst diabetic patients [33].

(c) *Exercise* improves pain-free walking distance in patients with diabetes but appears to have no effect on ankle brachial pressure indices [34].

3. *Surgery*

   (a) *Endovascular revascularisation* is achieved by balloon angioplasty with stenting as its mainstay. It has the advantage of being less risky than open surgery [35]. Bleeding, stent crush, wire perforation of vessels and stent thrombosis are potential side effects [36].
   (b) *Transcatheter arterialisation* of deep veins creates an arteriovenous connection, with a view to delivering oxygenated blood to distal ischaemic tissue [37]. It appears to have a 66% amputation avoidance rate at 6 months [37].
   (c) *Open surgical revascularisation* is utilised when endovascular interventions may not be feasible [37]. It is sometimes used in a hybrid manner with endovascular interventions. There is a greater risk of morbidity and mortality than the endovascular group.
   (d) *Surgical* debridement is often recommended in the early stages of gas gangrene to limit spread of infection, tissue damage and sepsis [15]. It is also useful for eliminating areas of localised tissue necrosis that may not have gas gangrene as a component.
   (e) *Amputation* may be minor (toe, transmetatarsal) or major (leg or above-knee may be required to limit the process of tissue loss) [36]. Minor amputations do not limit functional independence but may sometimes require prosthesis or orthesis to prevent future ulcerations. Major amputations require prosthesis and full mobility is regained in only 20% of above-knee versus below-knee amputees [36]. Autoamputation sometimes occurs in dry gangrene, usually involving a part or whole toe.

7.8 Conclusions

Gangrene is an end-stage process of tissue loss which may be a consequence of limb ischaemia, infection or both. Diabetes mellitus is a major risk and aetiological factor for gangrene. Gangrene is thrice as common in males than females. Three forms of diabetic foot gangrene are considered in this chapter—dry, wet and gas gangrene. Limb loss is a severe consequence of gangrene. Clinically, dry gangrene manifests as a black, shrunken area of tissue, which is sharply delineated from the neighbouring tissue; wet gangrene is a black area of tissue with oedema and oozing in which malodour may be present; and gas gangrene is a bronze and then blue-black area of skin and subcutaneous tissue, associated with bullae containing liquid and gas. Liquefactive and coagulative necrosis are histopathologic features. Therapy for gangrene may be divided into medical (pharmacological agents), general strategies (exercise, lifestyle changes) and surgery (vascular surgery and amputation).

Since gangrene is preventable, aggressive approaches to the underlying risk factors and causes, especially glycaemic control, are recommended.

References

1. Buttolph A, Gangrene SA. StatPearls [Internet]. Treasure Island (FL): StatPearls Publishing; 2023. https://www.ncbi.nlm.nih.gov/books/NBK560552/.
2. Yang Z, Hu J, Qu Y, Sun F, Leng X, Li H, et al. Interventions for treating gas gangrene. Cochrane Database Syst Rev. 2015;2015(12):CD010577. https://doi.org/10.1002/14651858.CD010577.
3. Saaiq M. Epidemiology and outcome of nontraumatic lower limb amputations. Med J Islam Repub Iran. 2023;37:18. https://doi.org/10.47176/mjiri.37.18.
4. Gong H, Ren Y, Li Z, Zha P, Bista R, Li Y, et al. Clinical characteristics and risk factors of lower extremity amputation in the diabetic inpatients with foot ulcers. Front Endocrinol (Lausanne). 2023;14:1144806. https://doi.org/10.3389/fendo.2023.1144806.
5. Lin CW, Armstrong DG, Lin CH, Liu PH, Hung SY, Lee SR, et al. Nationwide trends in the epidemiology of diabetic foot complications and lower-extremity amputation over an 8-year period. BMJ Open Diabetes Res Care. 2019;7(1):e000795. https://doi.org/10.1136/bmjdrc-2019-000795.
6. Ahmed MU, Tannous WK, Agho KE, Henshaw F, Turner D, Simmons D. Prevalence and burden of diabetes-related foot disease in New South Wales, Australia: evidence from the 45 and up study survey data linked with health services data. Int J Environ Res Public Health. 2021;18:11528. https://doi.org/10.3390/ijerph182111528.
7. Jing DQ, Ma XY, Yin SN, Hu JS, Bai H, Sun Y. Risk factors for diabetic foot gangrene: a clinical analysis of 100 cases of type 2 diabetic foot for 15 years. Chin J Clin Rehabil. 2006;10(36):24–6.
8. Shamaki GR, Markson F, Soji-Ayoade D, Agwuegbo CC, Bamgbose MO, Tamunoinemi BM. Peripheral artery disease: a comprehensive updated review. Curr Probl Cardiol. 2022;47(11):101082. https://doi.org/10.1016/j.cpcardiol.2021.101082.
9. Medical Advisory Secretariat. Stenting for peripheral artery disease of the lower extremities: an evidence-based analysis. Ont Health Technol Assess Ser. 2010;10(18):1–88.
10. Duff S, Mafilios MS, Bhounsule P, Hasegawa JT. The burden of critical limb ischemia: a review of recent literature. Vasc Health Risk Manag. 2019;15:187–208. https://doi.org/10.2147/VHRM.S209241.
11. Abu Dabrh AM, Steffen MW, Undavalli C, Asi N, Wang Z, Elamin MB, et al. The natural history of untreated severe or critical limb ischemia. J Vasc Surg. 2015;62(6):1642–51.e3. https://doi.org/10.1016/j.jvs.2015.07.065.
12. Behroozian A, Beckman JA. Microvascular disease increases amputation in patients with peripheral artery disease. Arterioscler Thromb Vasc Biol. 2020;40(3):534–40. https://doi.org/10.1161/ATVBAHA.119.312859.
13. Latz CA, Deluca E, Lella S, Waller HD, DeCarlo C, Dua A. Rates of conversion from dry to wet gangrene following lower extremity revascularization. Ann Vasc Surg. 2002;83:20–5. https://doi.org/10.1016/j.avsg.2022.01.005.
14. Aziz Z, Lin WK, Nather A, Huak CY. Predictive factors for lower extremity amputations in diabetic foot infections. Diabet Foot Ankle. 2011;2:2. https://doi.org/10.3402/dfa.v2i0.7463.
15. Buboltz JB, Murphy-Lavoie HM. Gas gangzrene. In: StatPearls [Internet]. Treasure Island (FL): StatPearls Publishing; 2023. https://www.ncbi.nlm.nih.gov/books/NBK537030/.
16. Stevens DL, Bisno AL, Chambers HF, Dellinger EP, Goldstein EJ, Gorbach SL, et al. Practice guidelines for the diagnosis and management of skin and soft tissue infections: 2014 update by the Infectious Diseases Society of America. Clin Infect Dis. 2014;59(2):147–59. https://doi.org/10.1093/cid/ciu296.
17. Brucato MP, Patel K, Mgbako O. Diagnosis of gas gangrene: does a discrepancy exist between the published data and practice. J Foot Ankle Surg. 2014;53(2):137–40. https://doi.org/10.1053/j.jfas.2013.10.009.
18. Al Wahabi A. Autoamputation of diabetic toe with dry gangrene: a myth or a fact? Diabetes Metab Syndr Obes. 2018;11:255–64. https://doi.org/10.2147/DMSO.S164199.

19. Adigun R, Basit H, Murray J. Cell liquefactive necrosis. In: StatPearls [Internet]. Treasure Island (FL): StatPearls Publishing; 2023. https://www.ncbi.nlm.nih.gov/books/NBK430935/.
20. Zhang M, Xu YJ, Mengi SA, Arneja AS, Dhalla NS. Therapeutic potentials of pentoxifylline for treatment of cardiovascular diseases. Exp Clin Cardiol. 2004;9(2):103–11.
21. Fossat C, Fabre D, Alimi Y, Bienvenu J, Aillaud MF, Lenoble M, et al. Leukocyte activation study during occlusive arterial disease of the lower limb: effect of pentoxifylline infusion. J Cardiovasc Pharmacol. 1995;25(Suppl 2):S96–100. https://doi.org/10.1097/00005344-199500252-00021.
22. Brown T, Forster RB, Cleanthis M, Mikhailidis DP, Stansby G, Stewart M. Cilostazol for intermittent claudication. Cochrane Database Syst Rev. 2021;30(6):CD003748. https://doi.org/10.1002/14651858.CD003748.pub5.
23. Asal NJ, Wojciak KA. Effect of cilostazol in treating diabetes-associated microvascular complications. Endocrine. 2017;56(2):240–4. https://doi.org/10.1007/s12020-017-1279-4.
24. Parakramawansha R, Fisher M, McKay G. Naftidrofuryl. Pract Diabetes. 2014;31:129–30. https://doi.org/10.1002/pdi.1848.
25. de Backer TL, Vander Stichele R, Lehert P, Van Bortel L. Naftidrofuryl for intermittent claudication. Cochrane Database Syst Rev. 2012;12(12):CD001368. https://doi.org/10.1002/14651858.CD001368.pub4.
26. Lauver DA, Lucchesi BR. Sulodexide: a renewed interest in this glycosaminoglycan. Cardiovasc Drug Rev. 2006;24(3–4):214–26. https://doi.org/10.1111/j.1527-3466.2006.00214.x.
27. Bignamini AA, Chebil A, Gambaro G, Matuška J. Sulodexide for diabetic-induced disabilities: a systematic review and meta-analysis. Adv Ther. 2021;38(3):1483–513. https://doi.org/10.1007/s12325-021-01620-1.
28. Rai KM, Maudar KK. Prostanoids in the management of limb ischemia. Med J Armed Forces India. 1997;53(1):66–7. https://doi.org/10.1016/S0377-1237(17)30651-2.
29. Vietto V, Franco JV, Saenz V, Cytryn D, Chas J, Ciapponi A. Prostanoids for critical limb ischaemia. Cochrane Database Syst Rev. 2018;1(1):CD006544. https://doi.org/10.1002/14651858.CD006544.pub3.
30. Bhutani S, Vishwanath G. Hyperbaric oxygen and wound healing. Indian J Plast Surg. 2012;45(2):316–24. https://doi.org/10.4103/0970-0358.101309.
31. Ortega MA, Fraile-Martinez O, García-Montero C, Callejón-Peláez E, Sáez MA, Álvarez-Mon MA, et al. A general overview on the hyperbaric oxygen therapy: applications, mechanisms and translational opportunities. Medicina (Kaunas). 2021;57(9):864. https://doi.org/10.3390/medicina57090864.
32. Krishna SM, Moxon JV, Golledge J. A review of the pathophysiology and potential biomarkers for peripheral artery disease. Int J Mol Sci. 2015;16(5):11294–322. https://doi.org/10.3390/ijms160511294.
33. Zhang Y, Hu G, Yuan Z, Chen L. Glycosylated hemoglobin in relationship to cardiovascular outcomes and death in patients with type 2 diabetes: a systematic review and meta-analysis. PLoS One. 2012;7(8):e42551. https://doi.org/10.1371/journal.pone.0042551.
34. Lane R, Harwood A, Watson L, Leng GC. Exercise for intermittent claudication. Cochrane Database Syst Rev. 2017;12(12):CD000990. https://doi.org/10.1002/14651858.CD000990.pub4.
35. Thukkani AK, Kinlay S. Endovascular intervention for peripheral artery disease. Circ Res. 2015;116(9):1599–613. https://doi.org/10.1161/CIRCRESAHA.116.303503.
36. Kinlay S. Management of critical limb ischemia. Circ Cardiovasc Interv. 2016;9(2):e001946. https://doi.org/10.1161/CIRCINTERVENTIONS.115.001946.
37. Shishehbor MH, Powell RJ, Montero-Baker MF, Dua A, Martínez-Trabal JL, Bunte MC, PROMISE II Investigators, et al. Transcatheter arterialization of deep veins in chronic limb-threatening ischemia. N Engl J Med. 2023;388(13):1171–80. https://doi.org/10.1056/NEJMoa2212754.

Chapter 8
Mycoses in Diabetic Patients and Treatment of Cutaneous Fungal Infections in Diabetic Patients

Pietro Nenoff

Abstract Previous studies have shown that people with diabetes have a significantly higher risk of bacterial and fungal infections. In particular, diabetes mellitus is a risk factor for tinea pedis or onychomycosis. Previous studies had found that people with diabetes and onychomycosis have a higher risk of diabetic foot ulcers, but no such significant connection could be demonstrated in recent studies. However, a significant connection was found between onychomycosis and diabetic neuropathy as well as an increased HbA1c value. The most common fungal skin infections in patients with diabetes affect the feet and toenails. Tinea pedis is a dermatophytosis that primarily affects the spaces between the toes and can then spread to the plantar area and ultimately the entire foot. Spread of the fungi to other parts of the body like groins, trunk, even the face, and the scalp is possible. Onychomycosis affects the nail plate and nail bed. Yellow stripes in the longitudinal direction are an indication of matrix involvement in onychomycosis, the maximum form of the fungal nail infection. Dermatophytes are the main pathogens of dermatomycosis and onychomycosis. *Trichophyton rubrum* and *Trichophyton interdigitale* are the most frequently isolated causative agent, followed by yeasts (*Candida albicans*), and sometimes mold fungi like *Scopulariopsis brevicaulis* or *Aspergillus* species. Dermatomycological diagnostics are based on microscopic and cultural detection of pathogens. Polymerase chain reaction (PCR) is able to improve sensitivity and specificity of mycological diagnostics. Nail fungal infection is treated with topical and systemic (orally applied) antimycotics. Mild or moderate infections of the nails can be successfully treated with topical antifungals in the form of nail polish. According to the current German S1 Guideline onychomycosis, it is recommended to treat severe onychomycosis by oral terbinafine, fluconazole, or itraconazole. The best therapeutic results in onychomycosis can be achieved when combined topical and systemic antifungal treatment is used.

P. Nenoff (✉)
Labopart, Laboratory Leipzig-Mölbis (Labor Leipzig-Mölbis), Leipzig, Germany
e-mail: p.nenoff@labopart.de

K. Fritz, G.-S. Tiplica (eds.), *Cutaneous Manifestations in Diabetes*,
https://doi.org/10.1007/978-3-031-65300-1_8

8.1 Diabetes Mellitus and Onychomycoses

The predisposing factors for tinea pedis and tinea unguium (onychomycosis) include primarily circulatory disorders in the lower extremities, as well as metabolic diseases such as diabetes mellitus. Diabetes mellitus is a risk factor for tinea pedis or onychomycosis. In a podiatric center at a university hospital in Japan, of 2476 patients, 337 (13.6%) had tinea pedis and 346 (14%) had onychomycosis [1]. Approximately 75% in each of these groups suffered from both dermatophytoses simultaneously. Regression analysis showed that older age, male gender, diabetes, and circulatory problems in the lower extremities were independent risk factors for tinea pedis. In contrast, diabetic peripheral neuropathy (DPN) was a risk factor for onychomycosis. Previous studies have shown that people with diabetes have a significantly higher risk of bacterial and fungal infections compared to patients with gastroesophageal reflux [2].

A national database analysis in the USA focused on the association between onychomycosis and age, gender, and underlying diseases [3]. Patients with onychomycosis were more likely to suffer from obesity, tinea pedis, peripheral vascular disease, venous insufficiency, varicosis, diabetes mellitus, and human immunodeficiency virus (HIV) infection compared to control subjects.

However, on the other hand, there is hardly any medical knowledge about foot and nail fungus among the population. This was the result of an online questionnaire study in Saudi Arabia that focused on the association of diabetes mellitus with tinea pedis and tinea unguium [4].

Among 300 patients with diabetes in India, 34% had mycologically and/or histopathologically confirmed onychomycosis [5]. Most of them suffered from distolateral subungual onychomycosis (78%). A pathogen could be detected by culture in almost 56%. Of these, almost 50% had non-dermatophyte mold (NDM). This was followed by *Candida* species (approx. 30%) and dermatophytes (approx. 22%).

In a prospective study [6], the prevalence of onychomycosis in diabetics (type 2) was 22%, most infections were caused by dermatophytes, and yeast fungi were found in only four cases. Of the 1245 Taiwanese patients with diabetes mellitus, 383 had onychomycosis, corresponding to a prevalence of 30.76% [7]. Older age, male gender, metabolic syndrome, obesity, elevated triglyceride levels, and poor glycemic control (increased HbA1c) were associated with onychomycosis. Another important risk factor is diabetes mellitus: depending on the study, onychomycosis prevalences for type 2 diabetics are up to 22% [6, 7] or even 51% [8].

Of 95 type 1 diabetics (average duration of illness 35.8 years) in Germany, 82.1% had changes on their feet that were suspicious of mycosis, and in 84.6% this suspicion could also be confirmed with native preparation and mycological culture [9]. Twenty-eight patients had nail mycosis, and another 28 had combined skin and nail mycosis. In a cross-sectional study from Japan, 51.3% of diabetics suffered from toenail onychomycosis [8]. The thickness of the nails correlated significantly with a higher HbA1c value. Onychomycosis was significantly more common when feet were not washed daily.

8.2 Onychomycosis in Diabetes and Chronic Hemodialysis

Thirty-nine percent of 100 patients on chronic hemodialysis had onychomycosis [10]. The most common pathogens were dermatophytes (approx. 70%), *Candida* spp. (15%), and nondermatophyte molds (NDM, 15%). *Trichophyton interdigitale* was the most common pathogen, followed by *Candida* species and *Trichophyton rubrum*. The risk of onychomycosis increased by 1.9% with each year of life. Diabetics on hemodialysis are 88% more likely to develop onychomycosis than nondiabetics.

In a recent study on onychomycosis in hemodialysis patients from Brazil, male gender, older age, and obesity were shown to be the main risk factors associated with onychomycosis [11]. And the patients with diabetes mellitus had a higher propensity for onychomycosis outbreaks compared to hemodialysis patients without diabetes.

8.3 Onychomycosis Risk and Duration of Diabetes Mellitus

In addition, the risk of onychomycosis in diabetics increases with increasing duration of the underlying disease and age [9]. A study showed a significant positive correlation between the level of HbA1c and the thickness of mycotic nails. Daily foot washing has been identified as a surprisingly simple preventative measure to reduce the risk of athlete's foot and onychomycosis [8].

8.4 Higher Risk of Diabetic Foot Ulcer Due to Onychomycosis?

The connection between tinea pedis, athlete's foot, and onychomycosis with a higher likelihood of diabetic foot ulcers has long been known. Conversely, onychomycosis is also viewed as a predictor of diabetic foot syndrome [7]. Previous studies had found that people with diabetes and onychomycosis have a 1.6 times higher risk of diabetic foot ulcers [12]. However, no such significant connection could be demonstrated in a recent study [13]. In contrast, impaired sensitivity and the presence of callus were significantly associated with diabetic foot ulcers, but dry skin and onychomycosis were not.

Another systemic review on the occurrence of diabetic ulcerations of the foot and the associated factors was also unable to establish a connection to onychomycosis [14]. Among 5664 patients with diabetes, 29.18% had onychomycosis, mostly due to *Trichophyton rubrum*. A significant connection was found between onychomycosis and diabetic neuropathy as well as an increased HbA1c value. However, there was no significant association between onychomycosis and diabetic foot ulcers.

8.5 Clinical Picture

8.5.1 Tinea Pedis

The most common fungal skin infections in patients with diabetes affect the feet and toenails. Tinea pedis is a dermatophytosis that primarily affects the spaces between the toes and can then spread to the plantar area and ultimately the entire foot (Fig. 8.1). You can see blistering of the stratum corneum, scaling, reddening of the skin, and even maceration and erosion. Itching occurs relatively late in the course. Spread to other parts of the body is possible, e.g., to the trunk as tinea corporis (Fig. 8.2).

8.5.2 Onychomycosis (Tinea Unguium)

Onychomycosis is almost always associated with tinea pedis. An initially distolateral subungual onychomycosis develops over months and years into the maximum variant, total dystrophic onychomycosis, in which the nail matrix is also affected (Fig. 8.3). Clinically, onychomycosis is characterized by opacity of the nail plate and yellow-brown, sometimes dark brown discoloration of the nail substance. Subungual hyperkeratoses push the nail plate upward. The crumbly consistency and decay, or onycholysis, of the nail are also typical. Yellow stripes in the longitudinal direction are an indication of matrix involvement in onychomycosis. These subungual conglomerates of fungal mycelium, arthrospores, and keratin are also referred to as dermatophytomas or "glacial nails." Dermatophytomas are particularly problematic regarding the treatment of onychomycosis.

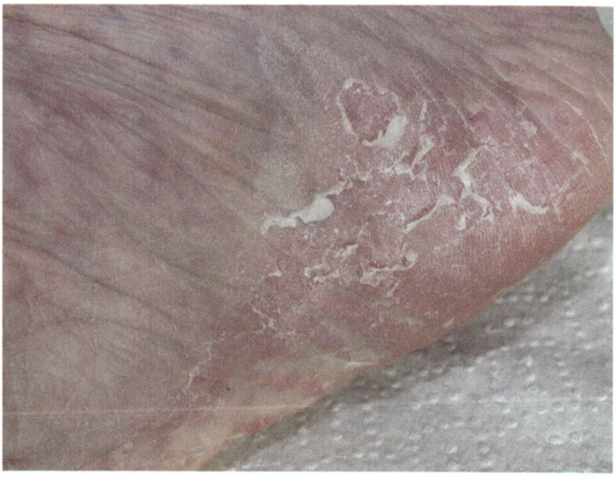

Fig. 8.1 Tinea pedis due to *Trichophyton rubrum*. Dry, hyperkeratotic, blistering, scaling lesions on erythematous skin of the foot. Sixty-five-year-old patient with diabetes mellitus type 2

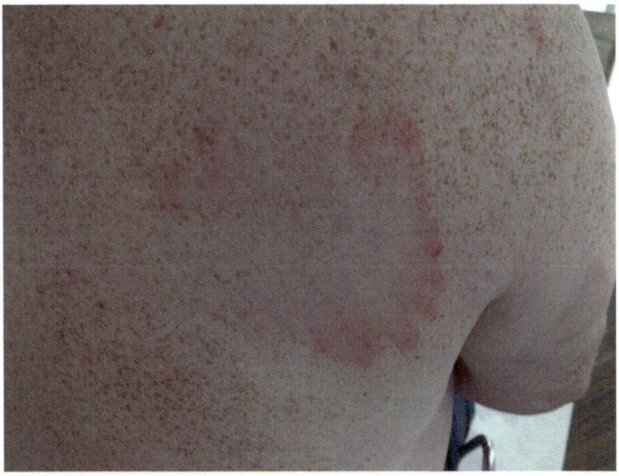

Fig. 8.2 Tinea corporis due to *Trichophyton rubrum*. Centrifugal, marginal plaque, peripherally erythematous posed, centrally flat, and pale. Sixty-five-year-old patient with diabetes mellitus type 2

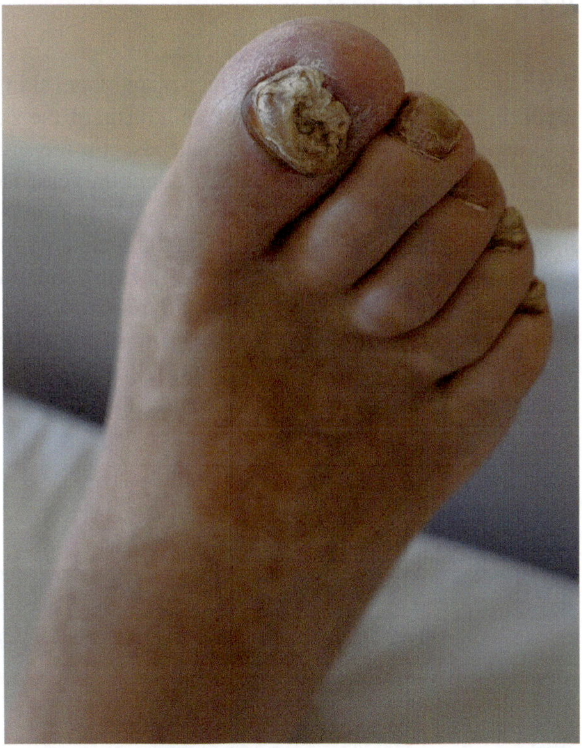

Fig. 8.3 Tinea unguium (onychomycosis) of the nail of the big toe due to *Trichophyton rubrum*. Dry, hyperkeratotic, blistering, scaling lesions on erythematous skin of the foot. Eighty-year-old patient with diabetes mellitus type 2

8.6 Pathogens of Dermatomycoses

8.6.1 Dermatophytes

Dermatophytes, or foot and nail fungi, are the main pathogens of dermatomycosis and onychomycosis. By far the most common isolated dermatophyte is *Trichophyton rubrum*, an anthropophilic fungus that is transmitted directly, but more indirectly (via surfaces when walking barefoot), from person to person (Fig. 8.4a, b). In second place is *Trichophyton interdigitale*, another anthropophilic dermatophyte (Fig. 8.5a, b). Both pathogens are capable of causing both tinea pedis and onychomycosis. Other dermatophytes, such as *Trichophyton tonsurans* or *Trichophyton violaceum*, are very rarely found around the feet and toenails.

8.6.2 Yeast Fungi

In addition, yeast fungi can often be isolated from skin areas suspected of dermatomycosis in people with diabetes. Candidiasis of the skin is then present. The skin fold areas in the interdigital area, but also on the groins or in the submammary region, are often affected. The most common yeast isolated is *Candida albicans*. There are also other *Candida* species, such as *Candida parapsilosis* or *Candida tropicalis*. However, yeast fungi are often detectable from smears of inflammatory, especially intertriginous regions, without skin candidiasis being present. This may be a temporary colonization of the inflammatory areas. Onychomycoses are also caused by yeast fungi. Here too, the distinction must be made between an infection and a colonization. An essential criterion for infection is the microscopic or histopathological evidence of fungal elements in the nail tissue.

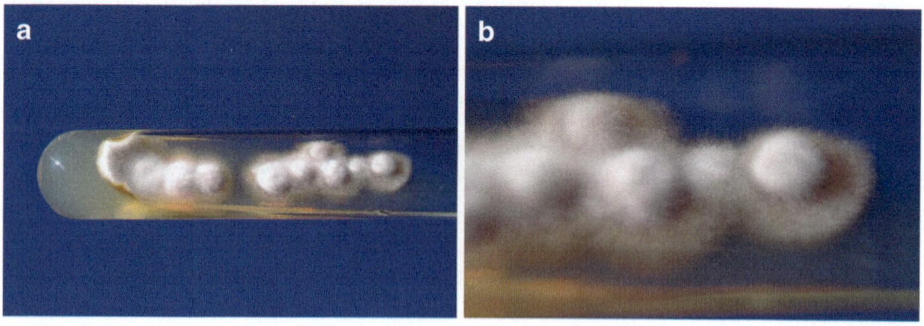

Fig. 8.4 (**a**) *Trichophyton rubrum*. White, floccose colonies in tubes with tilted agar. Sabouraud's dextrose agar containing cycloheximide. (**b**) Close picture of the culture

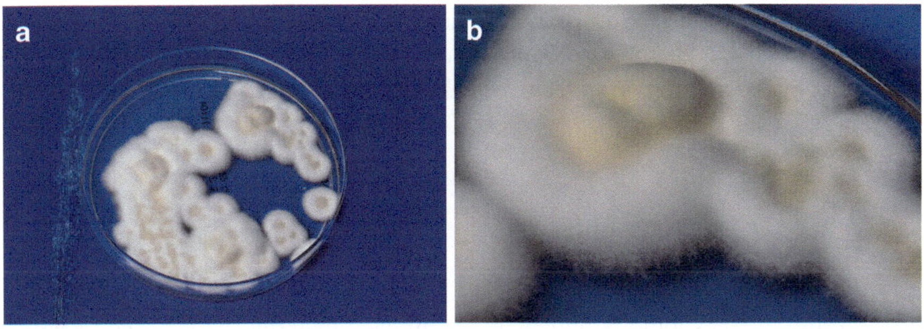

Fig. 8.5 (**a**) *Trichophyton interdigitale*. White, flat colonies, central bright yellow stained in petri dish agar plate. Sabouraud's dextrose agar without cycloheximide. (**b**) Close picture of the culture

8.7 Microbiological Detection of Fungi

8.7.1 Material Sampling

The mycological examination is essential for the diagnosis of dermatomycosis. In addition to skin scales, nail shavings are taken if onychomycosis is suspected. Skin scales can be scraped from the edges of the scaly lesions using a scalpel or a curette. For the diagnosis of onychomycosis, nail shavings should be removed from the depths, at the border to the healthy area, using a scalpel, curette, or, better still, a milling cutter. At least 20 skin flakes or nail shavings are required for an effective mycological diagnosis in the laboratory. Swabs should be used if the skin lesion is erosive and weeping. It is also possible to cultivate dermatophytes from smears.

8.7.2 Laboratory Diagnostics

Dermatomycological diagnostics are based on microscopic and cultural detection of pathogens. One rule states that local antimycotic treatment should only be carried out after a positive microscopic specimen has been obtained; if the pathogen is cultured, systemic antimycotic therapy can then be initiated [15].

8.7.3 Microscopic Specimen

The simplest method of microscopic detection of fungi in skin flakes, nail material, and hair roots is the preparation with 20% potassium hydroxide (potassium hydroxide/KOH). However, the fluorescence-optical preparation with optical brighteners from the diamino stilbene group (Blankophor® or Calcofluor®) is even more sensitive. These bind to chitin, the main component of the fungal cell wall. If fungal mycelium and spores or arthrospores are detected, onychomycosis can be assumed. However, the genus or species cannot be determined from this [16]. This requires cultural fungal detection or molecular identification of the dermatophytes underlying nail mycosis.

8.7.4 Cultural Fungal Detection

Two culture media should be inoculated from each material sample, one of which contains cycloheximide (Actidion®) to suppress mold growth. Sabouraud's dextrose agar and Kimmig agar are suitable as nutrient media. The mixture is incubated at 26–32 °C, preferably at 28 °C, for 4 weeks [17].

8.7.5 Molecular Biological Direct Detection

Molecular methods increase the sensitivity of mycological diagnostics. The polymerase chain reaction (PCR) is now used to directly detect dermatophytes from nail material and skin flakes as well as hair roots. New methods, such as PCR-ELISA (enzyme-linked immunosorbent assay), real-time PCR (RT-PCR), multiplex PCR, and PCR microarray, allow the specific detection of the underlying dermatophyte DNA but also that of yeast and mold. The decisive advantage of molecular DNA detection methods for dermatophytes lies in their speed [18]. Diagnosis down to the species level is possible within 1–2 days. The disadvantage is the significantly higher costs compared to fungal culture [19].

8.8 Treatment of Cutaneous Fungal Infections in Diabetic Patients

8.8.1 Treatment of Dermatomycoses

8.8.1.1 Tinea Pedis

Tinea pedis is in principle the domain of topical antifungal therapy. Internal treatment should only be initiated for extensive forms, especially the "moccasin" form of tinea pedis. Most antifungal substances are broad-spectrum antimycotics with effectiveness not only against dermatophytes but also against yeasts and molds.

It is important that polyenes, such as nystatin, are not active against dermatophytes, but only against yeast fungi. A variety of locally applicable antimycotics in cream, ointment, solution, spray, powder, and nail polish form are available to treat fungal skin infections. Depending on the type of tinea pedis, it is important to decide which base should be used. For interdigital tinea pedis, which is often macerated and erosive as well as secondary to bacterial infection, solutions are preferred, including powder if necessary. For rather dry and scaly forms of ringworm on the soles and backs of the feet, a cream or ointment is recommended.

Important active ingredients for the treatment of tinea pedis and tinea corporis are azoles (bifonazole, clotrimazole, miconazole, sertaconazole, etc.). There is also very good experience with the morpholine amorolfine, ciclopirox olamine, terbinafine, and naftifine.

The usual use of most topical antifungals for tinea pedis is twice daily, i.e., morning and evening. Clotrimazole should even be used two to three times a day, bifonazole, for example, once a day, and miconazole one to two times a day. Terbinafine is also only administered once a day. The treatment period covers a 4-week period, corresponding to the regeneration time of the epidermis, i.e., the "turnover" of the keratinocytes from the basal cells to the stratum corneum.

8.8.2 *Treatment of Onychomycosis*

Nail fungal infection is treated with topical and systemic (orally applied) antimycotics [20]. However, the usual nontraumatic removal of the fungal nail area using keratinolytic 40% urea ointments as the first step in the treatment of onychomycosis, which is also recommended in the guidelines, is not indicated for people with diabetes and is even contraindicated in the presence of diabetic neuropathy. An alternative is atraumatic nail removal using a milling machine in a podiatry facility. After reducing the changed nail tissue, treatment can be carried out with antifungal nail polish. Surgical extraction of nails in cases of onychomycosis is now obsolete.

8.8.3 *Topical Treatment of Onychomycosis with Antifungal Nail Polish*

Mild or moderate infections of the nails can be successfully treated with topical antifungals in the form of nail polish. This applies to nail fungal infections with involvement of up to 40% of the nail surface (according to the international consensus conference, degree of infection <50%) or infection of a maximum of three out of ten toenails. The active ingredients ciclopirox olamine and amorolfine are available in alcohol-based paint formulations. Both are broad-spectrum antimycotics with activity against dermatophytes, yeast, and molds. Acrylic varnish containing ciclopirox olamine is applied every 2 days and from the second month onward twice a week. Nail polish containing amorolfine is used once a week. Beforehand, the nail must be cleaned of nail polish residues and degreased, and the diseased parts of the nail should be reduced by filing; at least roughening the surface is recommended.

Ciclopirox olamine-containing nail polish is now also used with the water-soluble biopolymer hydroxypropyl chitosan, which, through its binding to nail keratin, enables better transport and release of the active ingredient ciclopirox olamine [21]. The application takes place daily. A similar water-soluble nail polish with the active ingredient terbinafine has recently become available in Germany. This contains terbinafine (78.22 mg terbinafine/mL nail polish) and—like the nail polish containing ciclopirox olamine mentioned above—the biopolymer hydroxypropyl chitosan. It is used daily for 4 weeks and then once a week.

8.8.4 Systemic Treatment of Onychomycosis with Oral Antifungals

According to the current German Guideline Onychomycosis from 2023 [22], it is recommended either 12 weeks of terbinafine (1 × 1 tablet of 250 mg/day) or fluconazole (150 mg once per week) for 6–12 months (toenails) or 3–6 months (fingernails) or until healing. The third option is itraconazole, either continuously or as pulse therapy. The application of the pulse therapy is 2 × 200 mg itraconazole (2 × 2 capsules/day) for 1 week, followed by a 3-week break. A total of three to a maximum of four pulses are specified. Alternatively, itraconazole can also be given continuously for onychomycosis. For onychomycosis of the toenails, 200 mg itraconazole as hard capsule is used daily for 3 months. The more absorbable super bioavailability itraconazole (SUBA-itraconazole) is available in Germany. Half the dose of conventional itraconazole can be used here, which is two capsules of 50 mg (= 100 mg) each day for 12 weeks for tinea unguium (onychomycosis). The best therapeutic results can be achieved when combined topical and systemic antifungal treatment is used [23].

References

1. Ogawa T, Matsuda A, Ogawa Y, et al. Risk factors for the development of tinea pedis and onychomycosis: real-world evidence from a single-podiatry center, large-scale database in Japan. J Dermatol. 2024;51:30–9.
2. Wang YR, Margolis D. The prevalence of diagnosed cutaneous manifestations during ambulatory diabetes visits in the United States, 1998–2002. Dermatology (Basel). 2006;212:229–34.
3. Albucker SJ, Falotico JM, Choo Z-N, et al. Risk factors and treatment trends for onychomycosis: a case-control study of onychomycosis patients in the all of us research program. J Fungi (Basel). 2023;9:9.
4. Khalifa A, Alreshidi IG, Alaradi LA, et al. Tinea unguium and tinea pedis and their correlation with diabetes mellitus in the general population in the hail region, Saudi Arabia: a cross-sectional study. Cureus. 2023;15:e40116.
5. Agrawal S, Singal A, Grover C, et al. Clinico-mycological study of onychomycosis in Indian diabetic patients. Indian Dermatol Online J. 2023;14:807–13.

6. Saunte DML, Holgersen JB, Haedersdal M, et al. Prevalence of toe nail onychomycosis in diabetic patients. Acta Derm Venereol. 2006;86:425–8.
7. Chang S-J, Hsu S-C, Tien K-J, et al. Metabolic syndrome associated with toenail onychomycosis in Taiwanese with diabetes mellitus. Int J Dermatol. 2008;47:467–72.
8. Takehara K, Oe M, Tsunemi Y, et al. Factors associated with presence and severity of toenail onychomycosis in patients with diabetes: a cross-sectional study. Int J Nurs Stud. 2011;48:1101–8.
9. Eckhard M, Lengler A, Liersch J, et al. Fungal foot infections in patients with diabetes mellitus—results of two independent investigations. Mycoses. 2007;50(Suppl 2):14–9.
10. Lamb FM, Ottonelli Stopiglia CD, Vetoratto G, et al. Frequency of onychomycoses in chronic renal failure patients undergoing hemodialysis in Porto Alegre, Brazil. Acta Dermatovenerol Croat. 2013;21:19–23.
11. Bersano JMQB, Cordeiro MG, Marson FAL. Prevalence and risk predictors of onychomycosis in patients on hemodialysis: an observation, prospective, and unicenter study in Brazil. Front Med (Lausanne). 2023;10:1268324.
12. Boyko EJ, Ahroni JH, Cohen V, et al. Prediction of diabetic foot ulcer occurrence using commonly available clinical information: the Seattle diabetic foot study. Diabetes Care. 2006;29:1202–7.
13. Naemi R, Balasubramanian G, Darvel T, et al. Predicting diabetic foot ulceration using routinely collected data in a foot clinic. What level of prognostic accuracy can be achieved? Diabetes Metab Res Rev. 2023;39:e3674.
14. Navarro-Pérez D, Tardáguila-García A, García-Oreja S, et al. Onychomycosis associated with diabetic foot syndrome: a systematic review. Mycoses. 2023;66:459–66.
15. Nenoff P, Krüger C, Schaller J, et al. Mycology—an update. Part 2: dermatomycoses: clinical picture and diagnostics. J Dtsch Dermatol Ges. 2014;12:749–77.
16. Nenoff P, Klonowski E, Uhrlaß S, et al. Dermatomykosen—Klinik, Erreger und Diagnostik [Clinical picture, causative agents and diagnostics of dermatomycoses]. Dermatologie (Heidelberg). 2023;74:974–93.
17. Mehlhorn C, Uhrlaß S, Klonowski E, et al. Konventionelle und molekulare Diagnostik bei Onychomykose—Teil 1: Konventionelle Differenzierung von Dermatophyten—*Trichophyton rubrum, Trichophyton interdigitale* [Conventional and molecular diagnostics in onychomycosis-part 1: Conventional differentiation of dermatophytes-*Trichophyton rubrum, Trichophyton interdigitale*]. Dermatologie (Heidelb). 2023;75:134.
18. Vazheva GZ, Zisova LG, Becheva EA, et al. In search of dermatophytes—frequency and etiology of fungal infections in patients with and without diabetes mellitus. Folia Med (Plovdiv). 2022;64:922–31.
19. Mehlhorn C, Uhrlaß S, Klonowski E, et al. Konventionelle und molekulare Diagnostik bei Onychomykose—Teil 2 : Molekulare Identifizierung der ursächlichen Dermatophyten mit Polymerasekettenreaktion und Sequenzanalyse der ITS(„internal transcribed spacer")-Region der ribosomalen Desoxyribonukleinsäure [Conventional and molecular diagnostics in onychomycosis-part 2: Molecular identification of causative dermatophytes by polymerase chain reaction and sequence analysis of the internal transcribed spacer region of ribosomal DNA]. Dermatologie (Heidelb). 2023.
20. Piraccini BM, Starace M, Rubin AI, et al. Onychomycosis: recommendations for diagnosis, assessment of treatment efficacy, and specialist referral. The CONSONANCE consensus project. Dermatol Ther (Heidelb). 2022;12:885–98.
21. Piraccini BM, Iorizzo M, Lencastre A, et al. Ciclopirox hydroxypropyl chitosan (HPCH) nail lacquer: a review of its use in onychomycosis. Dermatol Ther (Heidelb). 2020;10:917–29.
22. Nenoff P, Reinel D, Mayser P, et al. S1-guideline onychomycosis. J Dtsch Dermatol Ges. 2023;21:678–94.
23. Effendy I, Mayer J, Nenoff P, et al. Combination therapy of severe onychomycoses—recommendations of an expert panel. Akt Dermatol. 2020;46:311–8.

Chapter 9
Cutaneous Bacterial Infections in Diabetes and Treatment

Evgenia Makrantonaki and Christos C. Zouboulis

Abstract Diabetes mellitus (DM) is a debilitating, life-limiting disease. According to recent estimates, 415 million adults currently suffer from the disease. This number is expected to rise to 642 million by 2040. Skin disorders can often predict the onset of this metabolic disorder. Uncontrolled hyperglycaemia impairs the overall immunity of the diabetic patient, involving various mechanistic pathways, resulting in the diabetic skin being immunocompromised and prone to bacterial infections. Among others, diabetic foot infections are very common. There are specific microbes that are associated with each type of infection, and the presence of these microbes is an indication of the specific type of infection. In this chapter we have focused on the association of DM with different types of bacterial skin infections and resistance patterns to antimicrobial agents commonly used in the treatment of diabetes-associated infections.

9.1 Introduction

Diabetes mellitus is a challenging public health problem. An estimated 415 million adults worldwide have the disease, and this number is expected to rise to 642 million by 2040, according to the International Diabetes Federation. In Europe, there are currently 59.8 million people with diabetes, 10.3% of whom are men and 9.6%

E. Makrantonaki (✉)
Departments of Dermatology, Venereology, Allergology and Immunology, Dessau Medical Center, Brandenburg Medical School Theodor Fontane, Dessau, Germany

Derma Center Wildeshausen, Wildeshausen, Germany

Department of Dermatology and Allergology, Ulm University, Ulm, Germany

C. C. Zouboulis
Departments of Dermatology, Venereology, Allergology and Immunology, Dessau Medical Center, Brandenburg Medical School Theodor Fontane, Dessau, Germany

European Hidradenitis Suppurativa Foundation e.V., Dessau, Germany
e-mail: christos.zouboulis@klinikum-dessau.de

K. Fritz, G.-S. Tiplica (eds.), *Cutaneous Manifestations in Diabetes*,
https://doi.org/10.1007/978-3-031-65300-1_9

women aged 20–79, and diabetes accounts for about 11% of deaths per year in this age group. The disease's economic impact on national health systems is enormous. Treatment of diabetes and its complications accounts for between 5 and 20% of total national health expenditure. Although the risk factors and prevention measures are well known, the prevalence of diabetes has been steadily on the rise in all age groups. This is mainly due to increasing overweight and sedentary lifestyles [1].

Interestingly, a large number of diabetic patients remain undiagnosed, and in some cases, if DM is not managed properly, patients are likely to become progressively ill, as high glucose blood levels can damage the blood vessels, the heart, the eyes, the kidney and the nerves. Skin, the most visible organ of our body, often presents the first warning signals for this metabolic disorder and can be used as a good predictor marker for evaluating not only the risk of developing diabetes but also treatment success. In this chapter, we address the effects of DM on skin and the most common diabetes-associated bacterial skin infections which may predict or accompany this disease.

9.2 Pathophysiology of Bacterial Infections in DM

DM is characterized by an inability to transport the protein insulin, leading to an increase in serum glucose levels in the blood and a consequent decrease in cellular glucose levels. In both type 1 and type 2 diabetes, this is due to an immune complex-mediated attack on the insulin-producing beta cells of the pancreas or to defects in the secretion of insulin [2, 3].

In 30–70% of people with DM, pathological skin lesions are reported in the literature [4], among them bacterial infections. Hyperglycaemia impairs both innate and adaptive immunity through a variety of mechanisms. Disturbed humoral and cellular mechanisms often observed in diabetics may explain their high susceptibility to infection. Reduced levels of complement C4, increased levels of tumour necrosis factor-α (TNF-α), interleukin-6 (IL-6) and interleukin-8 (IL-8) with reduced response to stimulation may be some of the mechanisms (Fig. 9.1). Cellular mechanisms such as impaired chemotaxis and phagocytosis of polymorphonuclear cells and neutrophils, impaired killing by polymorphonuclear cells and reduced proliferative response of lymphocytes to pathogens such as *Staphylococcus aureus* may also be involved [5, 6]. The situation is further complicated by peripheral vascular disease and diabetic neuropathy. Dysregulation of immune cell chemotaxis and proliferation also result from decreased production of substance P and nerve growth factor in patients with diabetic neuropathy [7]. The migration of leukocytes is impaired in denervated tissue [8].

Additionally, a number of biochemical processes contribute to the disease process. There may be changes in the extracellular matrix as a result of functional deficits in proteins. This is mainly due to non-enzymatic glycation of proteins, lipids and nucleic acids by increased glucose levels. This leads to the formation of advanced glycation end products (AGEs) [9]. AGEs may directly affect the biological activity of skin cells, and it has been illustrated that AGEs can decrease keratinocyte cell viability and migration [10], reduce the proliferation ability of dermal fibroblasts and induce their apoptosis [11] and premature cellular senescence [12–14]. Furthermore, AGEs accumulation disturbs the elastic network and microvasculature [15, 16].

Recent evidence suggests that in diabetes, the inflammatory response is inappropriately amplified and prolonged early in wound healing. Proinflammatory genes and transcription factors are upregulated in DM in addition to increased oxidative stress [17]. This results in the persistent presence in the wound of vastly increased numbers of dysfunctional, hyperpolarized macrophages that fail to transition to a pro-healing phenotype [18, 19]. As macrophages release important mediators within the wound, their recruitment is essential for diabetic wound [20]. Contributing to this process are systemic chronic inflammation, poor angiogenesis and lymphangiogenesis in DM skin. Consequently, chronic, superinfected, non-healing wounds occur, and they are a major problem in DM patients.

Furthermore, reduced epidermal lipid synthesis, lamellar body production, stratum corneum hydration and antimicrobial peptide expression have also been associated with high HbA1c levels [21], leading to a deterioration in skin barrier function and predisposing the skin to xerosis and cutaneous infection [22]. Sweat gland function is often impaired. Initially, thermoregulatory sweating is reduced, particularly on the arms and legs. As the neuropathic condition progresses, sweating is reduced over the whole body (global anhidrosis). Typically, the skin is dry and appears overheated due to the lack of cooling function of sweat making skin more prone to bacterial infections [23] (Fig. 9.1).

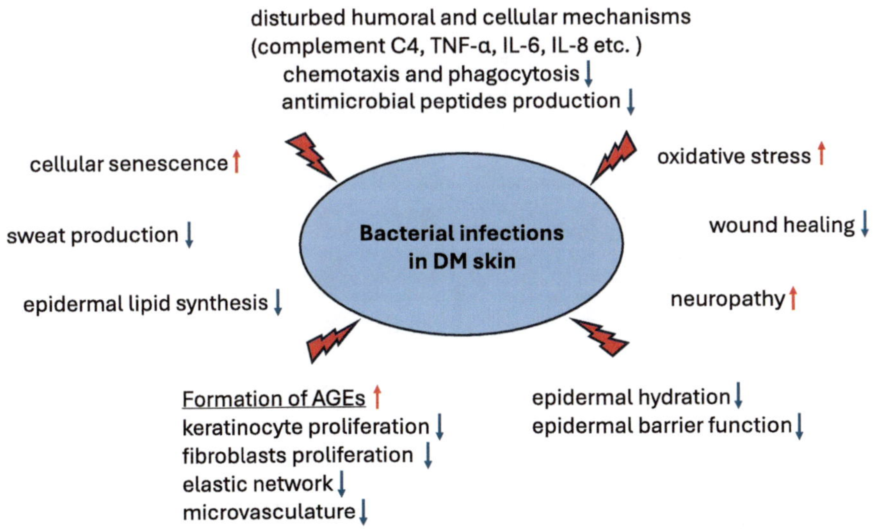

Fig. 9.1 Illustration of common pathomechanisms affecting skin in DM patients. Consequently, skin becomes prone to bacterial infections, among them *S. aureus* (culture in the middle of the figure), *Streptococcus pyogenes* and several Gram-negative bacteria

9.3 DM-Associated Bacterial Skin Infections

Bacterial skin infections are very common in DM patients, and among these infections, folliculitis, furuncles, carbuncles, abscesses, erysipelas and cellulitis (phlegmon) are the most frequent (Fig. 9.2a–h). Early signs of uncontrolled DM include therapy-resistant folliculitis and relapsing furuncles and abscesses. Erysipelas is defined as a non-purulent infection. It is thought to be caused primarily by *beta-haemolytic* streptococci. Clinical signs include a bright red rash and early fever or chills. A limited soft tissue infection (cellulitis) is usually caused by *Staphylococcus aureus*, is often due to chronic wounds and presents with a more violaceous red colour and only rarely with an initial fever or chills. Severe cellulitis is a purulent, partially necrotic infection that extends through tissue borders to fascia. These infections can occur in any anatomical site and are a major cause of morbidities and occasionally mortality in people with DM [18]. The most common site is the foot. In the United States and the United Kingdom, the reported prevalence of diabetic foot ulcers is as high as 10% [24]. This common complication occurs in 15% of all DM patients and accounts for more than 80% of all lower leg amputations [25] (Fig. 9.2). Foot infections in DM patients account for approximately 111,000 hospitalizations per year in America [26]. According to the Infectious Disease Society of America (IDSA) guidelines, infection is present if there is obvious purulent

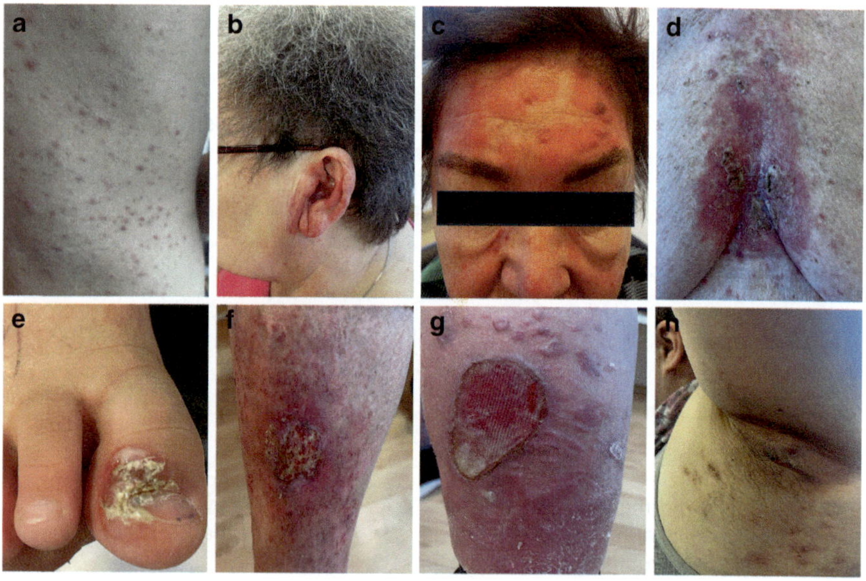

Fig. 9.2 Common bacterial infections in DM patients. (**a**) Therapy-resistant folliculitis (back region), (**b**) erysipelas (*S. aureus* (+)/ear), (**c**) erysipelas (*S. aureus* (+)/face), (**d**) impetiginized eczema (*S. aureus* (+)/breast region), (**e**) paronychia (*S. aureus* (+)/digitus I, foot), (**f**) ulcus accompanied by wound healing disorder after trauma (*S. aureus* (+)/lower leg), (**g**) bullous erysipelas (*S. pyogenes* (+)/lower leg), (**h**) fistules and erythrasma (brownish colour) (axillary region)

drainage and/or the presence of two or more signs of inflammation (erythema, pain, tenderness, warmth or induration) [27]. Systemic signs of infection include anorexia, nausea, vomiting, fever, chills, night sweats, change in mental status and a recent worsening of glycaemic control. Hypothermia (<36 °C) or fever (38 °C), hypotension, tachycardia and tachypnoea are considered signs of severe infection and sepsis [28]. However, patients with DM may have an impaired neuroinflammatory response and not manifest typical signs of infection [27]. 82% of patients admitted for osteomyelitis (OM) were afebrile on admission often failing to mount a physiological response to infection [29]. Therefore, secondary signs of infection must be assessed such as exudate production, delayed wound healing and wound breakdown. Detailed wound descriptions such as length, width and depth of the wound, colour and consistency of drainage and character of wound base (granular, fibrous or necrotic) should be documented. The lower extremity can also be elevated for 5 min to assess for dependent rubor since erythema associated with infection typically does not resolve with elevation. Osteomyelitis should be considered if bone is visible or palpable in the base of an ulcer [28]. For the management of these infections and the prevention of their suspected complications, knowledge of the microorganisms associated with diabetic foot ulcer infections is of great importance. In a study of 84 randomly selected hospital patients with severe diabetic foot infections, a polymicrobial flora was found in 83% of cultures, with an average of 2.8 species per sample and a 3:1 ratio of aerobic to anaerobic bacteria [30]. *Staphylococcus epidermidis*, *Staphylococcus aureus* and *Streptococcus* species were most common. Anaerobic bacteria included *Peptostreptococcus magnus* and *Bacteroides fragilis* [30]. In further studies, the most common organisms isolated from diabetic wound, particularly in mild to moderate diabetic foot infections, showed to be aerobic Gram-positive cocci [31]. *Staphylococcus aureus*, *group B* streptococci, *enterococci* and facultative Gram-negative bacilli were identified in cultures of limb-threatening infections. *Pseudomonas aeruginosa* was particularly identified in macerated wounds, and obligate anaerobes were present in necrotic or gangrenous infections [32]. Among hospitalized patients, methicillin-resistant *Staphylococcus aureus (MRSA)* prevalence in diabetic foot infections was 15–30% depending on geography [33].

In a retrospective cohort study matching over 500,000 DM patients to non-diabetic controls, the risk of nearly every type of infection studied was higher among DM patients with the highest risk ratios seen for osteomyelitis (RR = 4.39; 95% CI 3.80–5.06), followed by sepsis (RR = 2.45; 95% CI 2.23–2.68), postoperative infections (RR = 2.02, 95% CI 1.80–2.27) and cellulitis (RR = 1.81; 95% CI 1.76–1.86) [34]. In a cross-sectional study, DM patients were inclined to have chronic ulcers, brown spots on the legs and pruritus at a 7.46-fold higher risk (AOR 7.46; 95% CI, 3.86–14.43; $P < 0.001$) than non-diabetic patients. Furthermore, they exhibited marginally higher risks of bacterial infection, scabies or skin tags [35].

In a large, unselected population consisting of 457 patients with insulin-dependent (IDDM) or non-insulin-dependent diabetes mellitus (NIDDM), the prevalence and the main clinical characteristics of skin disorders were documented. The most frequent skin lesions observed in IDDM patients among others were vitiligo and psoriasis, followed by xerosis, warts, eczema and *Candida* infections, without differences among patients with good, fair or poor metabolic control. On the other hand, in NIDDM patients the most frequent skin lesions were infections and diabetic dermopathy, observed in 20.6 and in 12.5% of all patients, respectively. Psoriasis, pruritus, xerosis, lichen and cutaneous complications of diabetes treatment were also observed, while other skin lesions were rare. Moreover, the frequency of skin infections was significantly higher in poorly controlled patients than in those with a good metabolic control [36].

In a recent study evaluating skin infections caused by coryneform bacteria such as erythrasma, it was shown that infections affected both male and female patients equally and were more commonly detected in patients with a BMI >23 kg/m^2 (62.5%) and in people with DM (50%) [37]. Wood's lamp examination forms an indispensible tool to diagnose erythrasma in DM patients. Typical localizations for erythrasma are the axillary and genital region (Fig. 9.2h).

9.4 Treatment of Bacterial Skin Infections in Diabetic Patients

The treatment of bacterial infections in DM is very challenging and depends entirely on the correct diagnosis of the infection and the bacteria involved. Firstly, it is important to consider the severity of the infection and distinguish between superficial and deep-seated infections [27, 38, 39]. In addition, as mixed infections are common in DM, treatment should be based on the pathogens involved, and the spectrum of antibiotics should be adjusted accordingly. The S2k guidelines for skin and soft tissue infections [39] suggest a therapeutic plan for the treatment of mild to severe bacterial infections based on evidence-based clinical trials. In general, for severe infections with systemic signs or signs of sepsis, especially in critical sites such as the face and hands, immunosuppression and comorbidities, parenteral treatment with higher doses of antibiotics should be considered.

Furuncles and carbuncles, often caused by methicillin-susceptible *(MSSA)* or methicillin-resistant *Staphylococcus aureus (MRSA)*, should be incised when they form, and additional antibiotic treatment is indicated if the surrounding soft tissue is erythematous and indurated and systemic signs are present. First-line agents include cefazolin 1 g IV t.i.d. or flucloxacillin 1 g IV t.i.d., and second-line agents include cefuroxime (1.5 g IV t.i.d.) or clindamycin IV (0.6–1.2 g t.i.d.) [40, 41]. For abscesses, which are usually caused by MSSA and MRSA after incision, drainage and surgical management, antibiotics that could be considered, depending on severity, are cefazolin, flucloxacillin and clindamycin. For mixed infections caused by anaerobes or Gram-negative pathogens, first-line treatment should include ampicillin/sulbactam [42] or amoxicillin/clavulanic acid [43], and second-line treatment should include piperacillin/tazobactam followed by oral amoxicillin/clavulanic acid. In cases of penicillin allergy, ciprofloxacin plus metronidazole or moxifloxacin could be used [39].

For erysipelas, usually caused by *β-haemolytic* streptococci or, in some cases, *Staphylococcus aureus*, the first-line treatment for uncomplicated cases is penicillin G (1.2–1.5 million IU t.i.d.) and, for more complicated cases, high-dose penicillin G (ten million IU IV t.i.d.) followed by oral penicillin V (1.2–1.5 million IU t.i.d.). Higher doses of penicillin G have also been recommended [44]. Depending on the severity of the disease, the minimum duration of treatment is 7–10 days to avoid the risk of reinfection. Second-line therapy includes flucloxacillin (1 g q.i.d.) and cefuroxime (0.75–1.5 g t.i.d.). In cases of penicillin allergy, clindamycin (0.6–1.2 g t.i.d.), clarithromycin (0.5 g b.i.d.) or moxifloxacin 0.4 g once daily can be alternatively used [39].

For limited soft tissue infections, e.g. due to chronic non-healing wounds, mostly caused by *Staphylococcus aureus*, cefazolin (0.5 g q.i.d to 1-2 b.i.d.) or flucloxacillin 1 g t.i.d to q.i.d. should be considered as first-line therapy [39]. Clindamycin (0.6–1.2 g t.i.d.) may also be used for deep-seated infections with anaerobic organisms, while cefuroxime (0.75–1.5 g t.i.d.) may be recommended for Gram-negative organisms and trimethoprim/sulfamethoxazole (160/800 mg PO b.i.d.) for MRSA/MSSA contamination [39].

Severe necrotizing, deep-seated soft tissue infections are acutely life-threatening and require rapid and broad antibiotic therapy against *Staphylococcus aureus* and anaerobic and/or Gram-negative bacteria followed by immediate surgical debridement. According to disease severity, cefuroxime (1.5–3 g t.i.d.) or cefazolin (1–2 g t.i.d.) or flucloxacillin (1 g t.i.d. up to q.i.d.) could be considered. In case of no response, clindamycin (0.6–1.2 g t.i.d.) in combination with rifampicin (0.2–0.2 g t.i.d.) or fosfomycin (4–5 g b.i.d. up to t.i.d.) or fusidic acid (0.5 g t.i.d. up to q.i.d.) is recommended [39]. In cases of suspected mixed infections with no response to prior treatment and relevant comorbidities, piperacillin/tazobactam (4.5 g t.i.d. up to q.i.d.) followed if necessary by amoxicillin/clavulanic acid (1.5–3 g t.i.d.) or ampicillin/sulbactam (1.2 g t.i.d. up to q.i.d.) PO could be used. Imipenem/cilastatin (1 g t.i.d. up to q.i.d.) or meropenem (1 g t.i.d.) or ertapenem (1 g once daily) is a further option [39].

For the common foot infections seen in severe, uncontrolled DM patients, the following antibiotics are suggested: for superficial infections, high-dose cefuroxime, especially if Gram-negative bacteria are involved (0.75–1.5 g t.i.d. and 3 g t.i.d. in severe cases), or cefazolin (1–2 g t.i.d.). Second-line treatment includes amoxicillin/clavulanic acid (1.2 g t.i.d. to q.i.d.) or ampicillin/sulbactam (1.5 g to 3 g t.i.d.). In cases of penicillin allergy, moxifloxacin 0.4 g once daily may be a good alternative [27, 38]. Deep-seated foot infections, which are often contaminated with Enterobacteriaceae and anaerobes in addition to *Staphylococcus aureus* or streptococci, should be treated with aminopenicillin plus beta-lactamase inhibitor or moxifloxacin or piperacillin/tazobactam (4.5 g t.i.d. or q.i.d.) [45, 46] or ciprofloxacin (0.4 g b.i.d.) or levofloxacin (0.5 g once daily) plus metronidazole (0.5 g t.i.d.) (to cover anaerobes) or carbapenems. Particular attention should be paid to methicillin-resistant *Staphylococcus aureus* contamination [39].

In general, a 2–4-week course of antibiotic therapy is started for both mild and severe diabetic foot infections. It is administered intravenously. Antibiotic therapy is continued for a further 4–6 weeks. Surgical management of moderate to severe diabetic foot infections includes drainage, debridement of non-viable soft tissue and bone and aggressive incision. Adjunctive therapies that include the use of negative pressure wound therapy, hyperbaric oxygen and the use of antibiotic-impregnated beads are also very promising [47]. Revascularization is also a high priority in the management of the infected diabetic foot in the context of multidisciplinary care [48]. Regular foot examination and appropriate footwear [49] are recommended as important measures that people with diabetes should take to control diabetic foot infections.

References

1. Makrantonaki E, Jiang D, Hossini AM, Nikolakis G, Wlaschek M, Scharffetter-Kochanek K, et al. Diabetes mellitus and the skin. Rev Endocr Metab Disord. 2016;17(3):269–82. https://doi.org/10.1007/s11154-016-9373-0.
2. Halban PA, Polonsky KS, Bowden DW, Hawkins MA, Ling C, Mather KJ, et al. Beta-cell failure in type 2 diabetes: postulated mechanisms and prospects for prevention and treatment. Diabetes Care. 2014;37(6):1751–8. https://doi.org/10.2337/dc14-0396.
3. Canivell S, Gomis R. Diagnosis and classification of autoimmune diabetes mellitus. Autoimmun Rev. 2014;13(4–5):403–7. https://doi.org/10.1016/j.autrev.2014.01.020.
4. Meurer M, Stumvoll M, Szeimies RM. Skin changes in diabetes mellitus. Der Hautarzt; Zeitschrift fur Dermatologie, Venerologie, und verwandte Gebiete. 2004;55(5):428–35. https://doi.org/10.1007/s00105-004-0726-3.
5. Gallacher SJ, Thomson G, Fraser WD, Fisher BM, Gemmell CG, MacCuish AC. Neutrophil bactericidal function in diabetes mellitus: evidence for association with blood glucose control. Diabet Med. 1995;12(10):916–20.
6. Rajagopalan S. Serious infections in elderly patients with diabetes mellitus. Clin Infect Dis. 2005;40(7):990–6. https://doi.org/10.1086/427690.
7. Alavi A, Sibbald RG, Mayer D, Goodman L, Botros M, Armstrong DG, et al. Diabetic foot ulcers: part I. Pathophysiology and prevention. J Am Acad Dermatol. 2014;70(1):1.e1–18.; quiz 9–20. https://doi.org/10.1016/j.jaad.2013.06.055.
8. Quattrini C, Jeziorska M, Malik RA. Small fiber neuropathy in diabetes: clinical consequence and assessment. Int J Low Extrem Wounds. 2004;3(1):16–21. https://doi.org/10.1177/1534734603262483.
9. Singh VP, Bali A, Singh N, Jaggi AS. Advanced glycation end products and diabetic complications. Korean J Physiol Pharmacol. 2014;18(1):1–14. https://doi.org/10.4196/kjpp.2014.18.1.1.
10. Zhu P, Yang C, Chen LH, Ren M, Lao GJ, Yan L. Impairment of human keratinocyte mobility and proliferation by advanced glycation end products-modified BSA. Arch Dermatol Res. 2011;303(5):339–50. https://doi.org/10.1007/s00403-010-1102-z.
11. Alikhani Z, Alikhani M, Boyd CM, Nagao K, Trackman PC, Graves DT. Advanced glycation end products enhance expression of pro-apoptotic genes and stimulate fibroblast apoptosis through cytoplasmic and mitochondrial pathways. J Biol Chem. 2005;280(13):12087–95. https://doi.org/10.1074/jbc.M406313200.
12. Berge U, Behrens J, Rattan SI. Sugar-induced premature aging and altered differentiation in human epidermal keratinocytes. Ann N Y Acad Sci. 2007;1100:524–9. https://doi.org/10.1196/annals.1395.058.

13. Ravelojaona V, Robert AM, Robert L. Expression of senescence-associated beta-galactosidase (SA-beta-gal) by human skin fibroblasts, effect of advanced glycation end-products and fucose or rhamnose-rich polysaccharides. Arch Gerontol Geriatr. 2009;48(2):151–4. https://doi.org/10.1016/j.archger.2007.12.004.
14. Sejersen H, Rattan SI. Dicarbonyl-induced accelerated aging in vitro in human skin fibroblasts. Biogerontology. 2009;10(2):203–11. https://doi.org/10.1007/s10522-008-9172-4.
15. Petrofsky J, Lee H, Trivedi M, Hudlikar AN, Yang CH, Goraksh N, et al. The influence of aging and diabetes on heat transfer characteristics of the skin to a rapidly applied heat source. Diabetes Technol Ther. 2010;12(12):1003–10. https://doi.org/10.1089/dia.2010.0152.
16. Petrofsky JS, McLellan K, Bains GS, Prowse M, Ethiraju G, Lee S, et al. Skin heat dissipation: the influence of diabetes, skin thickness, and subcutaneous fat thickness. Diabetes Technol Ther. 2008;10(6):487–93. https://doi.org/10.1089/dia.2008.0009.
17. Giacco F, Brownlee M. Oxidative stress and diabetic complications. Circ Res. 2010;107(9):1058–70. https://doi.org/10.1161/CIRCRESAHA.110.223545.
18. Wicks K, Torbica T, Mace KA. Myeloid cell dysfunction and the pathogenesis of the diabetic chronic wound. Semin Immunol. 2014;26(4):341–53. https://doi.org/10.1016/j.smim.2014.04.006.
19. Maruyama K, Asai J, Ii M, Thorne T, Losordo DW, D'Amore PA. Decreased macrophage number and activation lead to reduced lymphatic vessel formation and contribute to impaired diabetic wound healing. Am J Pathol. 2007;170(4):1178–91. https://doi.org/10.2353/ajpath.2007.060018.
20. Brancato SK, Albina JE. Wound macrophages as key regulators of repair: origin, phenotype, and function. Am J Pathol. 2011;178(1):19–25. https://doi.org/10.1016/j.ajpath.2010.08.003.
21. Park HY, Kim JH, Jung M, Chung CH, Hasham R, Park CS, et al. A long-standing hyperglycaemic condition impairs skin barrier by accelerating skin ageing process. Exp Dermatol. 2011;20(12):969–74. https://doi.org/10.1111/j.1600-0625.2011.01364.x.
22. Sakai S, Kikuchi K, Satoh J, Tagami H, Inoue S. Functional properties of the stratum corneum in patients with diabetes mellitus: similarities to senile xerosis. Br J Dermatol. 2005;153(2):319–23. https://doi.org/10.1111/j.1365-2133.2005.06756.x.
23. Vinik AI, Freeman R, Erbas T. Diabetic autonomic neuropathy. Semin Neurol. 2003;23(4):365–72. https://doi.org/10.1055/s-2004-817720.
24. Reiber GE, Vileikyte L, Boyko EJ, del Aguila M, Smith DG, Lavery LA, et al. Causal pathways for incident lower-extremity ulcers in patients with diabetes from two settings. Diabetes Care. 1999;22(1):157–62. https://doi.org/10.2337/diacare.22.1.157.
25. Arsanjani Shirazi A, Nasiri M, Yazdanpanah L. Dermatological and musculoskeletal assessment of diabetic foot: a narrative review. Diabetes Metab Syndr. 2016;10:S158. https://doi.org/10.1016/j.dsx.2016.03.004.
26. Jeffcoate WJ, Lipsky BA. Controversies in diagnosing and managing osteomyelitis of the foot in diabetes. Clin Infect Dis. 2004;39(Suppl 2):S115–22. https://doi.org/10.1086/383272.
27. Lipsky BA, Berendt AR, Cornia PB, Pile JC, Peters EJ, Armstrong DG, et al. Infectious Diseases Society of America clinical practice guideline for the diagnosis and treatment of diabetic foot infections. Clin Infect Dis. 2012;54:e132.
28. Hobizal KB, Wukich DK. Diabetic foot infections: current concept review. Diabet Foot Ankle. 2012;3:18409. https://doi.org/10.3402/dfa.v3i0.18409.
29. Armstrong DG, Lavery LA, Sariaya M, Ashry H. Leukocytosis is a poor indicator of acute osteomyelitis of the foot in diabetes mellitus. J Foot Ankle Surg. 1996;35(4):280–3. https://doi.org/10.1016/s1067-2516(96)80075-5.
30. Diamantopoulos EJ, Haritos D, Yfandi G, Grigoriadou M, Margariti G, Paniara O, et al. Management and outcome of severe diabetic foot infections. Exp Clin Endocrinol Diabetes. 1998;106(4):346–52. https://doi.org/10.1055/s-0029-1211996.
31. Calhoun JH, Overgaard KA, Stevens CM, Dowling JP, Mader JT. Diabetic foot ulcers and infections: current concepts. Adv Skin Wound Care. 2002;15(1):31–42.; quiz 4–5. https://doi.org/10.1097/00129334-200201000-00011.

32. Lipsky BA, Berendt AR, Deery HG, Embil JM, Joseph WS, Karchmer AW, et al. Diagnosis and treatment of diabetic foot infections. Plast Reconstr Surg. 2006;117:212S.
33. Eleftheriadou I, Tentolouris N, Argiana V, Jude E, Boulton AJ. Methicillin-resistant *Staphylococcus aureus* in diabetic foot infections. Drugs. 2010;70(14):1785–97. https://doi.org/10.2165/11538070-000000000-00000.
34. Shah BR, Hux JE. Quantifying the risk of infectious diseases for people with diabetes. Diabetes Care. 2003;26(2):510–3.
35. Tseng HW, Ger LP, Liang CK, Liou HH, Lam HC. High prevalence of cutaneous manifestations in the elderly with diabetes mellitus: an institution-based cross-sectional study in Taiwan. J Eur Acad Dermatol Venereol JEADV. 2015;29(8):1631–5. https://doi.org/10.1111/jdv.12664.
36. Romano G, Moretti G, Di Benedetto A, Giofre C, Di Cesare E, Russo G, et al. Skin lesions in diabetes mellitus: prevalence and clinical correlations. Diabetes Res Clin Pract. 1998;39(2):101–6.
37. Pinto M, Hundi GK, Bhat RM, Bala NK, Dandekeri S, Martis J, et al. Clinical and epidemiological features of coryneform skin infections at a tertiary hospital. Indian Dermatol Online J. 2016;7(3):168–73. https://doi.org/10.4103/2229-5178.182351.
38. Singer AJ, Dagum AB. Current management of acute cutaneous wounds. N Engl J Med. 2008;359(10):1037–46. https://doi.org/10.1056/NEJMra0707253.
39. Sunderkotter C, Becker K, Eckmann C, Graninger W, Kujath P, Schofer H. S2k guidelines for skin and soft tissue infections excerpts from the S2k guidelines for "calculated initial parenteral treatment of bacterial infections in adults—update 2018". J Dtsch Dermatol Ges. 2019;17(3):345–69. https://doi.org/10.1111/ddg.13790.
40. Chen AE, Carroll KC, Diener-West M, Ross T, Ordun J, Goldstein MA, et al. Randomized controlled trial of cephalexin versus clindamycin for uncomplicated pediatric skin infections. Pediatrics. 2011;127(3):e573–80. https://doi.org/10.1542/peds.2010-2053.
41. Schofer H, Bruns R, Effendy I, Hartmann M, Jappe U, Plettenberg A, et al. Diagnosis and treatment of *Staphylococcus aureus* infections of the skin and mucous membranes. J Dtsch Dermatol Ges. 2011;9(11):953–67. https://doi.org/10.1111/j.1610-0387.2011.07786.x.
42. Chan JC. Ampicillin/sulbactam versus cefazolin or cefoxitin in the treatment of skin and skin-structure infections of bacterial etiology. Adv Ther. 1995;12(2):139–46.
43. Matthews P, Alpert M, Rahav G, Rill D, Zito E, Gardiner D, et al. A randomized trial of tigecycline versus ampicillin-sulbactam or amoxicillin-clavulanate for the treatment of complicated skin and skin structure infections. BMC Infect Dis. 2012;12:297. https://doi.org/10.1186/1471-2334-12-297.
44. Kilburn SA, Featherstone P, Higgins B, Brindle R. Interventions for cellulitis and erysipelas. Cochrane Database Syst Rev. 2010;2010(6):CD004299. https://doi.org/10.1002/14651858.CD004299.pub2.
45. Gyssens IC, Dryden M, Kujath P, Nathwani D, Schaper N, Hampel B, et al. A randomized trial of the efficacy and safety of sequential intravenous/oral moxifloxacin monotherapy versus intravenous piperacillin/tazobactam followed by oral amoxicillin/clavulanate for complicated skin and skin structure infections. J Antimicrob Chemother. 2011;66(11):2632–42. https://doi.org/10.1093/jac/dkr344.
46. Schaper NC, Dryden M, Kujath P, Nathwani D, Arvis P, Reimnitz P, et al. Efficacy and safety of IV/PO moxifloxacin and IV piperacillin/tazobactam followed by PO amoxicillin/clavulanic acid in the treatment of diabetic foot infections: results of the RELIEF study. Infection. 2013;41(1):175–86. https://doi.org/10.1007/s15010-012-0367-x.
47. Singh N, Armstrong DG, Lipsky BA. Preventing foot ulcers in patients with diabetes. JAMA. 2005;293(2):217–28. https://doi.org/10.1001/jama.293.2.217.
48. Reiber GE, Raugi GJ. Preventing foot ulcers and amputations in diabetes. Lancet. 2005;366(9498):1676–7. https://doi.org/10.1016/S0140-6736(05)67674-X.
49. Bus SA, van Netten JJ, Kottink AI, Manning EA, Spraul M, Woittiez AJ, et al. The efficacy of removable devices to offload and heal neuropathic plantar forefoot ulcers in people with diabetes: a single-blinded multicentre randomised controlled trial. Int Wound J. 2018;15(1):65–74. https://doi.org/10.1111/iwj.12835.

Chapter 10
Skin Infestations in the Diabetic Patients: Scabies

Sandra Widaty, Carmen Salavastru, and Caroline Oktarina

Abstract Scabies is a neglected tropical disease caused by an infestation of *Sarcoptes scabiei* var. *hominis*. Various studies highlight the close association between crusted scabies and diabetes mellitus. In immunocompromised patients, such as diabetic patients, there are immunosuppression and reduced skin sensation which facilitate crusted scabies development. Classic scabies presents as itchy skin lesions in typical distribution areas, while crusted scabies manifests as generalized hyperkeratotic skin lesions with thick crusts and numerous fissures. While classic scabies presents with intense pruritus, the pediatric population and crusted scabies patients are reported to have less intense pruritus. Classic scabies can be diagnosed based on the criteria developed by the International Alliance for the Control of Scabies, and the severity classification can be determined based on the criteria developed by Davis et al. Treatment failure can occur while treating scabies. Hence, comprehensive treatment is necessary, not only providing pharmacological management but also nonpharmacological management.

Scabies is a dermatological disorder, considered as a neglected tropical disease by the World Health Organization (WHO), caused by infestation of *Sarcoptes scabiei* var. *hominis* [1, 2]. In immunocompromised patients, such as diabetic patients, a more severe variant of scabies, crusted scabies (also known as Norwegian scabies), can manifest [1].

S. Widaty (✉) · C. Oktarina
Department of Dermatology and Venereology, Faculty of Medicine, Universitas Indonesia, Cipto Mangunkusumo Hospital, Jakarta, Indonesia

C. Salavastru
Department of Pediatric Dermatology, Carol Davila University of Medicine and Pharmacy, Colentina Clinical Hospital, Bucharest, Romania

K. Fritz, G.-S. Tiplica (eds.), *Cutaneous Manifestations in Diabetes*,
https://doi.org/10.1007/978-3-031-65300-1_10

10.1 Epidemiology

A systematic review in 2022 reported that the prevalence of scabies varied between 0.18 and 76.9% worldwide. Indonesia, a tropical country located in the Southeast Asia, reports the highest prevalence, which was 76.9% in school children population. In terms of scabies prevalence in general population, Ghana and Fiji showed the highest prevalence (71% and 41.7%, respectively) [3]. The worldwide epidemiology for crusted scabies has not been reported yet [1]. A 5-year study in several long-term care hospices in South Korea reported that crusted scabies occurred in 22.8% of the patients. There were 66 patients with average age of 77.6 ± 12.4 years old [4]. Another study in Australia reported that 80 patients suffered from 92 crusted scabies occurrences. Of all patients, 50% of them had diabetes mellitus [5]. A retrospective study in France reported 95 crusted scabies patients within 6 years, 13.6% of them had history of diabetes mellitus [6]. These findings highlight the close association between crusted scabies and diabetes mellitus.

10.2 Pathogenesis

Scabies belongs to the Arthropoda phylum, Chelicerata subphylum, Arachnida class, Acari order, and Astigmata suborder [7]. *S. scabiei* has life cycle of 9–15 days, starting from an egg to a larva to a nymph to an adult mite. This obligate parasite digs burrows until the lower part of stratum corneum. Female mites have longer life span compared to male mites, which is approximately 2 months. When detached from the hosts, the mites can endure 24–36 h in the environment with relative humidity of 40–80% and temperature of 21 °C [1].

In the case of crusted scabies, the number of mites increases profusely, causing a severe and highly transmissible scabies. *S. scabiei* is known to produce numerous allergens, namely, apolipoprotein, cysteine protease, glutathione S-transferase, paramyosin, and serine protease. These allergens are also produced by house dust mites which belong in the same suborder. This is linked to the itch presentation, which is always complained by the patients [7].

The cysteine proteases are thought to facilitate in digging burrow and keratin digestion. In crusted scabies cases, the increase of cysteine proteases leads to a decrease of T-helper (Th)1 response and an increase of Th2 and Th17 responses along with interleukin (IL)-4, IL-5, IL-13, and IL-17 secretion. The immunoglobulin (IgE) increases exceedingly as well. In the skin, CD8 T cells become the major effector cells. This differs from classic scabies, in which Th1 response and CD4 T cells hold the major roles [7, 8].

The interactions between cytokines result in itch as the most common complaint of scabies patients. In classic scabies, the prurireceptors are activated by Th1 immune response, in the forms of IL-2 and interferon (IFN)-γ. On the other hand, in crusted scabies, the prurireceptors are activated by IL-31 [9]. Nocturnal pruritus is one of the characteristic findings in scabies due to intensified mites' activity nocturnally. Hyperkinesis and allokinesis occur when the mites move vigorously while delivering eggs and scybala (feces). This induces the noradrenergic system and leads to hypersensitivity of the nerves and pruritus exacerbation [10]. The mite constituents might also induce itch through direct actions, which include [9]:

(a) Triggering Toll-like receptor (TLR)3, TLR4, and TLR7
(b) Triggering protease-activated receptor (PAR)-2
(c) Induction of mast cell activation mediated by IgE, which produces tumor necrosis factor (TNF)-α, histamine, and tryptase
(d) Production of prostaglandins and leukotrienes

Recent studies also denote the role of microbiota in scabies infestation. Metagenomic studies on *S. scabiei* eggs revealed that *Klebsiella* and *Streptomyces* were the predominant bacteria in the mite gut. *Streptomyces* is thought to help complex carbohydrate degradation which facilitates keratin digestion and yields antimicrobial properties which eliminate harmful bacteria for the mite gut environment. *Klebsiella*'s roles have not been established yet, but it is known to increase fertility of another arthropod (*Ceratitis capitata*). On the hosts' skin, *S. scabiei* infestation is linked to an increase of *Staphylococcus aureus* colonization, which corresponds with high incidence with *S. aureus* secondary infections [11].

In immunocompromised patients, such as diabetic patients, there are immunosuppression and reduced skin sensation which facilitate crusted scabies development. High number of mites induced keratin overproduction which manifests as thick crusts and hyperkeratotic lesions. These hyperkeratotic lesions are also linked to the increased IL-4 production [1].

10.3 Clinical Presentation

Classic scabies presents as itchy skin lesions in typical distribution area. The lesions varied from papules, nodules, excoriation, eczematization, impetiginization, and lichenification (Fig. 10.1). The predilection sites for classic scabies include finger webs, wrists, armpits, breasts, abdomen, genitalia, and buttocks. The itch is more severe at night (nocturnal pruritus). On the other hand, crusted scabies manifests as generalized hyperkeratotic skin lesions with thick crusts and numerous fissures. While classic scabies presents with intense pruritus, the pediatric population and crusted scabies patients are reported to have less intense pruritus. However, this might be disregarded since most patients have neurological disorders and difficulty to scratch or communicate their symptoms [2, 10].

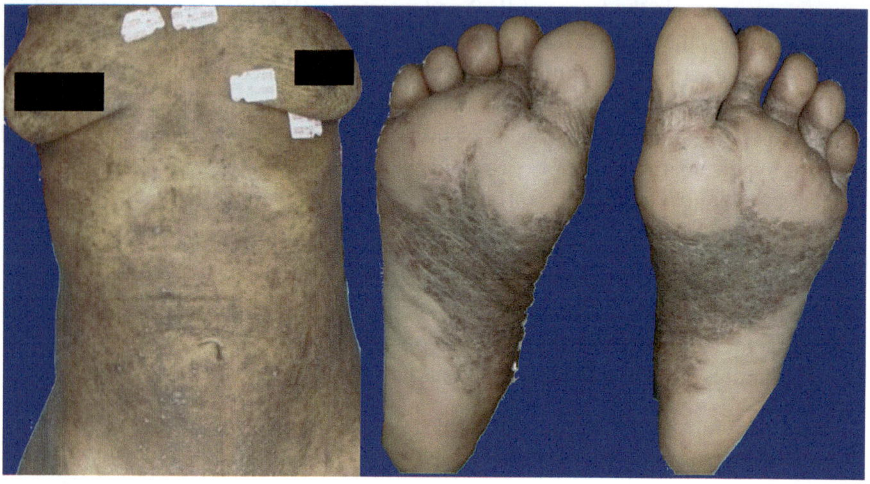

Fig. 10.1 A case of scabies in a 58-year-old diabetic patient with lesions found on the arms, neck, trunk, hands, and feet

Itch is a dominant feature, even in crusted scabies cases [12, 13]. Previous study in diabetic patients showed that itch is one of the most predominant symptoms. Diabetic patients have 16.5 times more risk of experiencing itch compared to non-diabetic patients. Neuropathic pruritus commonly causes generalized pruritus in the trunk and groin which coincidentally matches the predilection of scabies infestation [10, 14]. The scabies itch is usually described as burning, stinging, or crawling. This intense itch leads to unintentional scratch which results in excoriations as one of the most common findings in scabies patients [10].

10.4 Diagnosis

The classic scabies can be diagnosed based on the criteria developed by the International Alliance for the Control of Scabies (2020) in 2020. The criteria are shown in Table 10.1 [15].

In addition to the diagnosis, particularly for crusted scabies, there is a severity classification by Davis et al. as shown in Table 10.2 [16].

Table 10.1 Scabies diagnostic criteria by the International Alliance for the Control of Scabies

A. Confirmed scabies Presence of one or more criteria A1. Mites, eggs, or feces identified on light microscope of the skin specimens (Fig. 10.2) A2. Mites, eggs, or feces identified in vivo through high-powered imaging device A3. Mites identified in vivo through dermoscopy
B. Clinical scabies Presence of one or more criteria B1. Scabies burrows B2. Typical lesions including male genitalia B3. Typical lesions in a typical distribution and presence of two history features (pruritus and history of positive contact)
C. Suspected scabies Presence of one or more criteria C1. Typical lesions in a typical distribution and presence of one history feature (pruritus or history of positive contact) C2. Atypical lesions in an atypical distribution and presence of two history features (pruritus and history of positive contact)

Cited with modification from the study by Engelman et al. [15]

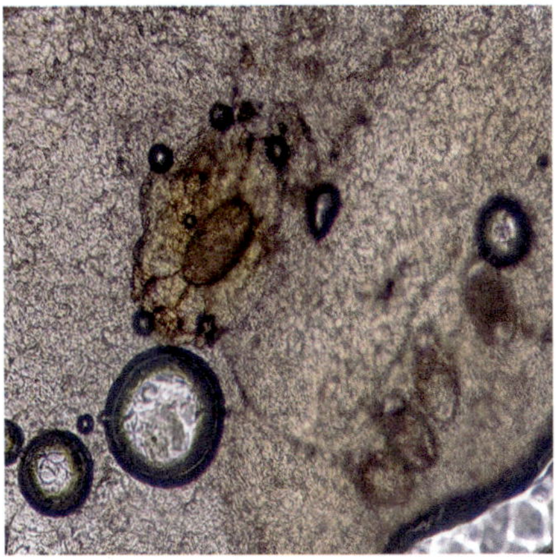

Fig. 10.2 *Sarcoptes scabiei* var. *hominis* in direct microscopic examination from skin scrapping

Table 10.2 Severity classification of crusted scabies

A. Distribution and extent of crusting
1. Wrists, web spaces, feet only (<10% total body surface area)
2. Above plus forearms, lower legs, buttocks, trunk, or 10–30% TBSA
3. Above plus scalp or >30% TBSA
B. Crusting/shedding
1. Mild crusting (<5 mm depth of crust), minimal skin shedding
2. Moderate (5–10 mm) crusting, moderate skin shedding
3. Severe (>10 mm), profuse skin shedding
C. Past episodes
1. Never had it before
2. 1–3 prior hospitalizations for crusted scabies or depigmentation of elbows, knees
3. ≥4 prior hospitalizations for crusted scabies or depigmentation as above plus legs/back or residual skin thickening/ichthyosis
D. Skin condition
1. No cracking or pyoderma
2. Multiple pustules and/or weeping sore and/or superficial skin cracking
3. Deep skin cracking with bleeding, widespread purulent exudates
Grade 1: Total score 4–6
Grade 2: Total score 7–9
Grade 3: Total score 10–12

Cited from Davis et al. [16]

10.5 Treatment

Scabies treatment should be comprehensive, not only providing pharmacological management but also nonpharmacological management. The nonpharmacological management emphasizes on education for close contact treatment and fomites management. All close contacts should be treated concomitantly with the patients to prevent reinfection. The fomites, including clothes, towels, bedsheets, etc., should be washed with hot water (>50 °C), dry-cleaned, or stored inside a plastic case for 1 week. The principles for scabies pharmacological treatment are summarized in Table 10.3 [2].

Table 10.3 Scabies pharmacological treatment

Classic scabies		Crusted scabies	
First-line treatment			
Permethrin 5% cream	Whole body application, repeat in 7–14 days	Permethrin 5% cream or benzyl benzoate 25% lotion and oral ivermectin	Whole body application for 7 days, then twice weekly until cured
Oral ivermectin	0.2 mg/kg, repeat in 7 days, taken with food		0.2 mg/kg on day 1, 2, and 8. Severe cases might need more doses on day 9, 15, 22, and 29
Benzyl benzoate 10–25% lotion	Whole body application for 2 consecutive days, repeat in 7 days		
Second-line treatment			
Malathion 0.5% aqueous lotion	Whole body application, cleanse after 24 h, repeat in 7 days		
Ivermectin 1% lotion	Whole body application		
Sulfur 6–33% cream, lotion, or ointment	Whole body application for 3 consecutive days		
Synergized pyrethrin foam	Whole body application for 3 consecutive days		

Cited with modification from Widaty et al. [2]

10.6 Prognosis

Treatment failure can occur while treating scabies. A meta-analysis reported that the prevalence of treatment failure was 15.2% worldwide with higher number in children compared to adults (18.6% vs 14.1%). The higher treatment failure rates were shown by the administration of crotamiton (27.7%), benzyl benzoate (25.3%), and lindane (18.1%). Various factors are thought to play a role in the treatment failure, including patient's characteristics, disease characteristics (severe diseases), drug characteristics, and treatment implementation challenges. Patient's characteristics include female, cognitive disorders, immobility, and behavioral disorders. Drug characteristics include single-dose administration, inadequate dose, single treatment, drug resistance, inadequate potency, and prolonged interval between treatments. The challenges in implementing treatment are corticosteroid use during treatment, lack of hygiene, no fomites management, contact history, delayed treatment, and no close contact treatment [17].

References

1. Niode NJ, Adji A, Gazpers S, et al. Crusted scabies, a neglected tropical disease: case series and literature review. Infect Dis Rep. 2022;14(3):479–91.
2. Widaty S, Miranda E, Cornain EF, Rizky LA. Scabies: update on treatment and efforts for prevention and control in highly endemic settings. J Infect Dev Ctries. 2022;16(2):244–51.
3. Schneider S, Wu J, Tizek L, Ziehfreund S, Zink A. Prevalence of scabies worldwide—an updated systematic literature review in 2022. J Eur Acad Dermatol Venereol. 2023;37(9):1749–57.
4. Kim DH, Yun SY, Park YC, Kang SA, Yu HS. Prevalence of scabies in long-term care hospitals in South Korea. PLoS Negl Trop Dis. 2020;14(8):e0008554.
5. Mackenzie CD, Hasan T, Krause VL, James C, Currie BJ. Crusted scabies; a 2-year prospective study from the Northern Territory of Australia. PLoS Negl Trop Dis. 2020;14(12):e0008994.
6. Skayem C, Majda A, Gary C, et al. Severe scabies: a French multi-centre study involving 95 patients with crusted and profuse disease and review of the literature. Acta Derm Venereol. 2023;103:adv00878.
7. Sanchez-Borges M, Gonzalez-Aveledo L, Capriles-Hulett A, Caballero-Fonseca F. Scabies, crusted (Norwegian) scabies and the diagnosis of mite sensitisation. Allergol Immunopathol (Madr). 2018;46(3):276–80.
8. Bhat SA, Walton SF, Ventura T, et al. Early immune suppression leads to uncontrolled mite proliferation and potent host inflammatory responses in a porcine model of crusted versus ordinary scabies. PLoS Negl Trop Dis. 2020;14(9):e0008601.
9. Stander S, Stander S. Itch in scabies-what do we know? Front Med (Lausanne). 2021;8:628392.
10. Kim HS, Hashimoto T, Fischer K, Bernigaud C, Chosidow O, Yosipovitch G. Scabies itch: an update on neuroimmune interactions and novel targets. J Eur Acad Dermatol Venereol. 2021;35(9):1765–76.
11. Taylor S, Fischer K. Understanding the role of the scabies mite microbiota in the development of novel control strategies. J Cell Immunol. 2021;3(2):122–7.
12. Lause M, Libson K, Korman AM, et al. Crusted scabies at a tertiary care center: case series and cautionary tale. JAAD Case Rep. 2023;41:17–21.
13. Wang Y, Liu Y, Long FQ. Crusted scabies mimicking psoriasis in a patient with type 1 diabetes mellitus. An Bras Dermatol. 2021;96(3):385–6.
14. Tseng HW, Ger LP, Liang CK, Liou HH, Lam HC. High prevalence of cutaneous manifestations in the elderly with diabetes mellitus: an institution-based cross-sectional study in Taiwan. J Eur Acad Dermatol Venereol. 2015;29(8):1631–5.
15. Engelman D, Yoshizumi J, Hay RJ, et al. The 2020 international alliance for the control of scabies consensus criteria for the diagnosis of scabies. Br J Dermatol. 2020;183(5):808–20.
16. Davis JS, McGloughlin S, Tong SY, Walton SF, Currie BJ. A novel clinical grading scale to guide the management of crusted scabies. PLoS Negl Trop Dis. 2013;7(9):e2387.
17. Mbuagbaw L, Sadeghirad B, Morgan RL, et al. Failure of scabies treatment: a systematic review and meta-analysis. Br J Dermatol. 2024;190(2):163–73.

Chapter 11
Common Skin Manifestations Related to Obesity

Seher Eren, Klaus Fritz, and Carmen Salavastru

Abstract Obesity, with a body mass index (BMI) over 30 kg/m^2, is a growing health concern worldwide, manifesting from early childhood to midlife and stemming from diverse causes including genetics, endocrine disorders, and psychosocial factors. This complex condition not only leads to metabolic issues like insulin resistance and type 2 diabetes mellitus but also precipitates a range of dermatological changes. These skin manifestations include cellulite, acanthosis nigricans, and skin tags linked to insulin resistance, hyperandrogenism, striae from skin overextension, and complications arising from peripheral vascular disease, such as stasis pigmentation and lymphedema. Additionally, the relationship between obesity and skin issues extends to changes in skin barrier function, sebaceous and sweat gland activity, and an increase in the thickness of the stratum corneum, the outermost layer of the epidermis, leading to conditions such as keratosis pilaris and plantar hyperkeratosis. These comprehensive findings underscore the intricate connection between obesity and skin health, highlighting the need for holistic approaches in treatment and management.

S. Eren (✉)
Hautärzte am Marktplatz, Dr. Bettinger und Kollegen, Karlsruhe, Germany
e-mail: contact@drsehereren.com

K. Fritz
Dermatology and Laser Consulting, Landau, Germany

Carol Davila University of Medicine and Pharmacy, Bucharest, Romania
e-mail: drklausfritz@drklausfritz.com

C. Salavastru
Carol Davila University of Medicine and Pharmacy, Bucharest, Romania

Colentina Clinical Hospital, Bucharest, Romania

Pediatric Dermatology Discipline, Dermato-oncology Research Facility, Bucharest, Romania

K. Fritz, G.-S. Tiplica (eds.), *Cutaneous Manifestations in Diabetes*,
https://doi.org/10.1007/978-3-031-65300-1_11

11.1 Introduction

Obesity, defined by a body mass index (BMI) exceeding 30 kg/m^2, is becoming an increasingly common health issue. It can manifest at any stage, from early childhood to adulthood, though it is most frequently observed in middle age [1].

Obesity arises from a complex interplay of various factors. While rare, primary endocrine disorders like Cushing's syndrome are seldom the root cause; more commonly, obesity leads to conditions such as hyperinsulinemia and diabetes. A genetic component often plays a role, typically involving a combination of multiple genes, which, in certain environments, can increase the propensity for excessive fat accumulation. Additionally, specific rare genetic mutations, such as leptin deficiency or melanocortin receptor abnormalities, can cause severe obesity from a young age. Behavioral and psychosocial elements also significantly contribute to the development of obesity [2].

One frequently observed outcome of obesity is the development of insulin resistance, which often leads to type 2 diabetes mellitus [1]. Skin complications are also prevalent in individuals with type 1 diabetes. Observations indicate that patients with type 2 diabetes are more prone to developing skin lesions, often infection-related, in contrast to those with type 1 diabetes who tend to have lesions that are more autoimmune in nature. For those with type 2 diabetes, these infection-driven skin issues often correlate with inadequate metabolic control, as evidenced by elevated HbA1c levels [3].

Initial indications of disease may manifest as skin symptoms, potentially emerging well before diabetes mellitus is diagnosed. In diabetic patients, effective control of blood sugar levels is key to the management of dermatological conditions [4].

Obesity often co-occurs with several comorbidities, including hypertension, cardiovascular diseases, polycystic ovary syndrome, and obstructive sleep apnea syndrome. Additionally, it is linked to an increased risk of breast and colorectal cancers and is frequently associated with psychological and orthopedic issues, as well as various skin disorders. It has a multifaceted impact on skin physiology, influencing aspects such as skin barrier functionality, activity of sebaceous glands and sebum production, sweat gland function, lymphatic system, collagen's structure and its functionality, wound healing processes, as well as microcirculation, macrocirculation, and the characteristics of subcutaneous fat. Dermatological manifestations frequently observed in obesity can be categorized based on their pathophysiological origins. These include conditions related to insulin resistance (IR), hyperandrogenism, issues arising from skin folds, mechanical factors, and complications stemming from hospitalization [5, 6].

Obesity markedly impacts skin physiology by altering the skin barrier, evidenced by changes in the hydration of the stratum corneum and varying patterns of transepidermal water loss (TEWL), driven by adipokines and leptin. These hormones, chiefly secreted by adipose cells, modulate the activity of keratinocytes and the structure of collagen. This leads to compromised wound healing and aggravated skin conditions due to collagen's inability to adapt to expanding skin areas. Elevated

Table 11.1 Classification of skin changes in obesity, categorized according to their underlying causes

Insulin resistance	Mechanical	Inflammatory	Metabolic	Infectious	Hospitalization
Acrochordons	Adiposis dolorosa	Hidradenitis suppurativa	Tophaceous gout	Candida	Pressure ulcers
Acanthosis nigricans	Plantar hyperkeratosis	Psoriasis	Hyperandrogenism and acne	Intertrigo	Wound healing
Keratosis pilaris	Cellulite	Rosacea		Necrotizing cellulitis/ fasciitis	
Hirsutism	Lymphedema	Atopic dermatitis			
Insulin resistance syndrome	Striae distensae				
	Chronic venous insufficiency				

Adapted and modified from Yosipovitch [6], Hirt [7], and Hidalgo [8]

levels of androgens, insulin, and growth factors in obese individuals intensify sebum production, thereby exacerbating acne. Beyond the skin barrier, obesity significantly influences sweat and blood circulation systems, resulting in increased sweating from larger skin folds and thicker subcutaneous fat, which predisposes to skin conditions like intertrigo. Microvascular issues associated with obesity, such as microangiopathy, hypertension, and chronic venous disease, can lead to dermatological problems including varicose eczema and ulceration. Moreover, obesity may heighten the risk of conditions like hidradenitis suppurativa, rosacea, psoriasis, and atopic dermatitis, where inflammation is notably involved [7]. Considering all these explanations, classifications of skin changes seen in obesity, categorized according to their underlying causes, can be summarized in an overview (Table 11.1).

This section will discuss common skin manifestations related to obesity, including acanthosis nigricans, acrochordons, keratosis pilaris, striae distensae, cellulite, and plantar hyperkeratosis.

11.2 Acrochordon (Skin Tag)

Acrochordons, also known as skin tags, are small, soft, often flesh-colored, or dark brown benign growths, typically appearing on the neck, axilla, and groin. These common dermal connective tissue neoplasms are more prevalent in middle-aged and elderly individuals and are characterized by their pedunculated shape [9, 10].

Histologically, skin tags are distinguished by a reduction in collagen fibers and the presence of dilated blood capillaries [11].

Typically, skin tags are asymptomatic; however, they can become irritable and painful due to fibrosis, necrosis, or secondary infections, especially when subjected to mechanical trauma. In uncommon instances, rubbing or scratching of these tags may lead to abrasion, bleeding, and the formation of crusts [12].

Skin tags are often observed in conjunction with conditions such as obesity, type 2 diabetes mellitus, pregnancy, dyslipidemia, hypertension, and insulin resistance [13, 14].

Multiple skin tags are commonly seen in individuals who are obese or have non-insulin-dependent diabetes; a shared underlying factor in these conditions is insulin resistance. The growth of fibroblasts in skin tags appears to be a result of hyperinsulinemia, which activates insulin-like growth factor (IGF-1) receptors located on their surfaces. There is also a close association between the presence of skin tags and elevated fasting insulin levels [11]. In recent years, there has been an observed association between skin tags and abnormalities in glucose metabolism, particularly type 2 diabetes, as well as an increase in adipose tissue deposition [15].

Typically, the treatment for skin tags involves methods like radio cautery, snip excision, or cryosurgery for their excision and removal. For smaller skin tags, laser treatments, such as nanosecond Q-switched Nd:YAG or CO_2 laser, are also employed [16].

11.3 Acanthosis Nigricans

Acanthosis nigricans (AN) is typically identified by thick, velvety, hyperpigmented plaques, predominantly found in intertriginous, flexural, and less commonly extensor areas of the skin. This condition is more prevalent in high-risk groups, like African-Americans, Hispanics, and Native Americans, but can occur in all races. AN is frequently a dermatologic indicator of systemic diseases, often linked to insulin resistance, diabetes mellitus, obesity, internal malignancies, endocrine disorders, and reactions to certain drugs [17].

The severity of acanthosis nigricans (AN) is positively correlated with fasting insulin levels [18]. The pathogenesis of AN is thought to involve elevated insulin levels binding to insulin-like growth factor 1 receptors (IGF-1Rs) on keratinocytes and fibroblasts, leading to the proliferation of these cells and the formation of visible plaques and papillomatosis. Furthermore, high insulin levels increase circulating free IGF-1, promoting keratinocyte growth and differentiation [19].

The treatment approach for AN is increasingly holistic, targeting both the cutaneous symptoms and the underlying disease or contributing medication. Non-pharmacological interventions, such as weight loss and exercise, are emphasized to enhance insulin sensitivity in cases of insulin-resistant AN. Management of AN is complex due to its association with underlying systemic diseases. Initial evaluation in AN patients involves screening for insulin resistance syndrome, which is characterized by obesity, dyslipidemia, hypertension, and type 2 diabetes mellitus. Diagnostic tests should include a fasting lipid panel, glucose and insulin levels, a complete blood count, and liver function tests [20].

11.4 Keratosis Pilaris

Keratosis pilaris (KP) is a widely recognized, benign condition of the hair follicles, marked by small, keratinous papules in a pattern centered around hair follicles, often accompanied by varying levels of erythema [21]. These keratotic papules typically cluster on the extensor surfaces of the upper arms, upper legs, and buttocks, although they can also manifest on the face and trunk [22].

The papules in keratosis pilaris can appear either in clusters or be dispersed and often present with slight erythema around the hair follicles. They have the potential to lead to post-inflammatory changes, including hyperpigmentation and pitted scarring [21].

Keratosis pilaris is notably widespread among the general population, yet its incidence and severity are higher in individuals with conditions such as atopic dermatitis and diabetes mellitus [23].

An elevated body mass index (BMI) and related health issues, such as diabetes, pregnancy, and hormonal imbalances, are frequently linked with the occurrence of KP [24]. The development of keratosis pilaris is believed to be influenced by insulin resistance and the excessive activation of the insulin-like growth factor 1 receptor on keratinocytes [25].

KP has a genetic basis, typically inherited in an autosomal dominant manner with varying degrees of penetrance. Beyond the classic presentation of KP, there are rare subtypes, including keratosis pilaris rubra (KPR), erythromelanosis follicularis faciei et colli (EFF), and the keratosis pilaris atrophicans (KPA) spectrum. Treatment approaches for KP are diverse, spanning from topical emollients and keratolytic agents like lactic acid, salicylic acid, and urea cream, which have shown differing levels of effectiveness, to the increasingly popular use of laser treatments. A combination of 2% salicylic acid in 20% urea cream has proven effective for local therapy. Additionally, topical tretinoin therapy can be employed, particularly when other treatment modalities fall short [22, 26].

Laser therapy, particularly with Q-switched neodymium-doped yttrium aluminum garnet (Nd:YAG) or pulsed dye laser, has shown effectiveness in treating keratosis pilaris cases resistant to conventional treatments, especially subtypes like keratosis pilaris rubra and keratosis pilaris atrophicans. These laser types are adept at addressing erythema, while fractional CO_2 laser therapy is more suitable for treating atrophy and scarring. However, laser treatment may lead to temporary side effects such as erythema and edema posttreatment, and there is a potential risk of post-inflammatory pigmentary changes [27].

11.5 Striae Distensae

Striae, commonly known as stretch marks, are often seen in individuals with obesity, during pregnancy, and in association with rapid weight fluctuations, including both increases and decreases. They are also linked with conditions such as Cushing's syndrome, infections, and Marfan's syndrome and prolonged treatment with adrenocorticotropic hormone (ACTH) and adrenocortical steroids. Topical steroid application, particularly under occlusion, intense slimming diets, and even normal physiological states, as seen in athletes, can lead to the development of striae. Elevated levels of steroid hormones exert a catabolic effect on fibroblasts, reducing collagen deposition in the dermal matrix [28, 29].

Striae distensae (SD) typically evolve from red or purple, raised, wavy lesions known as striae rubra, which gradually fade into white, atrophic lesions with a wrinkled surface, referred to as striae alba. Commonly appearing on the arms, thighs, abdomen, and lumbosacral area, striae can also affect other regions, including the face and flexures, especially in cases related to Cushing's syndrome or steroid therapy. During pregnancy, they are most frequently seen on the abdomen and breasts. In obese patients, striae tend to be lighter in color, less atrophic, and narrower compared to those associated with Cushing's syndrome. Rare, severe, and extensive striae may lead to ulceration or tearing. In children, striae distensae-like lesions can sometimes present as scarring alopecia [30].

Histologically, striae distensae in their earlier, immature stages often display a pink or red hue, known as striae rubra. As they undergo atrophic changes over time, they typically acquire a white coloration, termed striae alba. The histological profile of stretch marks resembles that of scar tissue, and the development of SD is akin to the processes observed in wound healing or scar formation [31].

Initial histopathological changes in the dermis during the early stages of striae distensae can be observed through electron microscopy, including the degranulation of mast cells and activation of macrophages, which leads to elastolysis in the mid-dermis. The release of enzymes by mast cells, particularly elastases, is believed to be a critical initiating factor in the pathogenesis of SD. In addition to these inflammatory processes, changes in the content of collagen, elastin, and fibrillin have been identified. The reorganization of fibrillin and elastin is thought to play a significant role in the development of SD, and those predisposed to SD may have an inherent deficiency in fibrillin [32].

Various treatment methods for striae distensae, ranging from multiple topical applications to lasers and energy-based devices, have been reported with differing degrees of success. However, the majority of available literature comprises small-scale studies, case reports, and a limited number of controlled, double-blind trials. Several studies have found tretinoin and retinoic acid to be beneficial in treating striae distensae. In the early stages of SD, these agents are thought to work by stimulating fibroblasts, thereby increasing collagen levels in the tissue. They have also been found effective in treating striae rubra, although common side effects include transient erythema and scaling. Additionally, hyaluronic acid has been shown to be effective in SD treatment due to its role in boosting collagen production. The effectiveness of these topical treatments for SD is reported to be moderate, and prolonged use of these drugs is often necessary. Consequently, the efficacy of topical agents in both the prevention and treatment of SD remains a subject of debate [33].

Lasers and light-based therapies are emerging as noninvasive options showing some success in the treatment of SD. They are effective in targeting vascular chromophores in striae rubra and stimulating the production of collagen and elastin in striae alba. A thorough literature review was conducted to compile data on laser and light treatments for SD, revealing that these methods can significantly enhance the appearance of both striae rubra and striae alba. Typically, striae rubra respond better to treatment and can be effectively managed with various lasers without significant adverse effects. Fractional lasers show the most promising results for repigmentation and collagen induction in striae alba, while other lasers offer temporary repigmentation. Combining lasers with other treatments, such as topical agents and additional energy devices, has also shown encouraging initial results [34].

11.6 Cellulite

Cellulite, also known as gynoid lipodystrophy, is characterized by an orange peel-like skin dimpling. It commonly affects individuals after adolescence and predominantly occurs in areas more prone to female-pattern fat deposition, such as the upper outer thighs, posterior thighs, buttocks, breasts, lower abdomen, upper arms, and the nape. Based on the best available evidence, this condition is understood to be a disorder involving both the subcutaneous fat layer and the overlying superficial skin [35–37].

Cellulite differs distinctly from obesity. Obesity is defined by the hypertrophy and hyperplasia of adipose tissue, which can occur in various body parts, not exclusively confined to the pelvis, thighs, or abdomen. In contrast, cellulite, predominantly but not exclusively found in the pelvis, thighs, and abdomen, arises from a combination of ultrastructural, inflammatory, histochemical, morphological, and biochemical alterations that culminate in the skin's padded and orange peel-like appearance [38].

Cellulite formation is characterized by several key structural components: adipocytes and fat cell groupings arranged in clusters, surrounded by connective tissue bands; connective tissue septae that link the underlying muscle to the subdermal layer; and cells located within these confines that cause the connective tissue to swell and stretch. As the process advances, the connective tissue experiences contraction and sclerosis, leading to skin being held at a non-flexible length, even as surrounding tissue may further expand from weight or water gain [39].

The underlying causes of cellulite are diverse and not fully understood. Present evidence suggests that endothelial dysfunction and microcirculation disturbances are significant contributors to its development. Compounding factors such as vascular and endocrine system disorders, alongside a genetic predisposition, may exacerbate the condition [40].

Maintaining a healthy diet and regular exercise regime does not consistently prevent cellulite, a condition many find cosmetically displeasing. This has spurred numerous treatment efforts, from topical applications and massage therapies to surgical interventions like liposuction and subcision, all aimed at enhancing microcirculation and diminishing cellulite, yet often yielding less than ideal results. In recent developments, nonablative lasers and radiofrequency systems have emerged as promising options, enhancing skin texture through selective heating of the dermis, which promotes the formation of new collagen [41].

11.7 Plantar Hyperkeratosis

Hyperkeratosis is characterized by an increased thickness of the stratum corneum, the outermost layer of the epidermis, resulting from either hypertrophy or hyperplasia of its cells. This thickening primarily involves keratinocytes or corneocytes, which constitute the majority of the cells in this epidermal layer. The enhanced thickness of the skin due to hyperkeratosis allows for a broader distribution of mechanical stresses, serving as a natural, symptom-free mechanism (physiological hyperkeratosis) to shield both the skin and underlying soft tissues from mechanical damage.

Pathological hyperkeratosis occurs when there's an accumulation of keratinized material to the extent that it induces tissue damage and pain, potentially through the release of inflammatory mediators or the pressure exerted by the central keratin plug on the nerves beneath. Plantar hyperkeratotic lesions are frequently observed beneath the metatarsophalangeal joints (MPJs), and numerous studies have pinpointed their development in regions subjected to increased plantar pressure [42, 43].

Plantar hyperkeratosis predominantly occurs in individuals with a high BMI, specifically between 35 and 40 kg/m^2 [44].

Reducing the heightened pressure through weight loss is advised as the primary treatment strategy. Meanwhile, protective insoles can help alleviate symptoms during the process of weight reduction [45].

References

1. Shipman AR, Millington GWM. Obesity and the skin. Br J Dermatol. 2011;165(4):743–50.
2. Scheinfeld NS. Obesity and dermatology. Clin Dermatol. 2004;22(4):303–9.
3. Paron NG, Lambert PW. Cutaneous manifestations of diabetes mellitus. Prim Care. 2000;27(2):371.
4. Karadag AS, Ozlu E, Lavery MJ. Cutaneous manifestations of diabetes mellitus and the metabolic syndrome. Clin Dermatol. 2018;36(1):89.

5. Gomez AP, Memije MV, Tamayo MT, Carreon AR. Skin disorders in overweight and obese patients and their relationship with insulin. Actas Dermosifiliogr (Engl Ed). 2014;105(2):178–85.
6. Yosipovitch G, DeVore A, Dawn A. Obesity and the skin: skin physiology and skin manifestations of obesity. J Am Acad Dermatol. 2007;56(6):901–16.
7. Hirt PA, Castillo DE, Yosipovitch G, Keri JE. Skin changes in the obese patient. J Am Acad Dermatol. 2019;81(5):1038–40.
8. Hidalgo LG. Dermatological complications of obesity. Am J Clin Dermatol. 2002;3:503–4.
9. Erdoğan BŞ, Aktan Ş, Rota S, Ergin Ş, Evliyaoğlu D. Skin tags and atherosclerotic risk factors. J Dermatol. 2005;32(5):371.
10. Farag AGA, Abdu Allah AMK, El-Rebey HS, Mohamed Ibraheem KI, Mohamed ASED, Labeeb AZ, Haggag MM. Role of insulin-like growth factor-1 in skin tags: a clinical, genetic and immunohistochemical study in a sample of Egyptian patients. Clin Cosmet Investig Dermatol. 2019;12:255.
11. Barbato MT, Criado PR, Silva AKD, Averbeck E, Guerine MB, Sá NBD. Association of acanthosis nigricans and skin tags with insulin resistance. An Bras Dermatol. 2012;87:101–2.
12. Malarmangai E, Vardhan KH, Manoharan K. Clinical evaluation of acrochordons and its association in systemic diseases. Ann Roman Soc Cell Biol. 2021;25:1429–41.
13. Vincent KD, Abramovits W. Acrochordons (skin tags). In: Dermatological cryosurgery and cryotherapy. Springer; 2016. p. 595–7.
14. Köseoğlu HG, Bozca BC, Başsorgun Cİ, Sarı R, Akbaş SH, Karakaş AA. The role of insulin-like growth factor in acrochordon etiopathology. BMC Dermatol. 2020;20(1):1.
15. Kurniawati Y, Devi M, Yakub K, Affandi K, Marlina A. Correlation of serum lipid profile with leptin levels of skin tags patients. J Phys Conf Ser. 2019;1246(1):012022.
16. Pandey A, Sonthalia S. Skin tags. Treasure Island (FL): StatPearls Publishing; 2019.
17. Higgins SP, Freemark M, Prose NS. Acanthosis nigricans: a practical approach to evaluation and management. Dermatol Online J. 2008;14(9):2.
18. Phiske MM. An approach to acanthosis nigricans. Indian Dermatol Online J. 2014;5(3):239.
19. Puri N. A study of pathogenesis of acanthosis nigricans and its clinical implications. Indian J Dermatol. 2011;56(6):678.
20. Patel NU, Roach C, Alinia H, Huang WW, Feldman SR. Current treatment options for acanthosis nigricans. Clin Cosmet Investig Dermatol. 2018;11:407–13.
21. Wang MA, Wilson A, Murrell DF. A review of the scoring and assessment of keratosis pilaris. Skin Appendage Disord. 2023;1:241.
22. Hwang S, Schwartz RA. Keratosis pilaris: a common follicular hyperkeratosis. Cutis. 2008;82(3):177.
23. Svoboda SA, Shields BE. Cutaneous manifestations of nutritional excess: pathophysiologic effects of hyperglycemia and hyperinsulinemia on the skin. Cutis. 2021;107(2):74–8.
24. Wang JF, Orlow SJ. Keratosis pilaris and its subtypes: associations, new molecular and pharmacologic etiologies, and therapeutic options. Am J Clin Dermatol. 2018;19(5):739.
25. Barnes CJ, Davis L, Bergman R, Boehncke WH, Buerger C, Boehncke S, Mashiach J. Hautveränderungen bei Adipositas. Adipositas-Ursachen, Folgeerkrankungen, Therapie. 2010;4(04):176–81.
26. Maghfour J, Ly S, Haidari W, Taylor SL, Feldman SR. Treatment of keratosis pilaris and its variants: a systematic review. J Dermatol Treat. 2022;33(3):1231–42.
27. Drivenes JL, Vasilescu IC, Bygum A. Keratosis pilaris. Tidsskrift for Den norske legeforening. 2023;143:513.
28. Nigam PK. Striae cutis distensae. Int J Dermatol. 1989;28(7):426–8.
29. Khater MH, Khattab FM, Abdelhaleem MR. Treatment of striae distensae with needling therapy versus CO_2 fractional laser. J Cosmet Laser Ther. 2016;18(2):75–9.
30. Singh G, Kumar LP. Striae distensae. Indian J Dermatol Venereol Leprol. 2005;71:370.
31. Elsaie ML, Baumann LS, Elsaaiee LT. Striae distensae (stretch marks) and different modalities of therapy: an update. Dermatol Surg. 2009;35(4):563–73.

32. Al-Himdani S, Ud-Din S, Gilmore S, Bayat A. Striae distensae: a comprehensive review and evidence-based evaluation of prophylaxis and treatment. Br J Dermatol. 2014;170(3):535.
33. Lokhande AJ, Mysore V. Striae distensae treatment review and update. Indian Dermatol Online J. 2019;10(4):380.
34. Aldahan AS, Shah VV, Mlacker S, Samarkandy S, Alsaidan M, Nouri K. Laser and light treatments for striae distensae: a comprehensive review of the literature. Am J Clin Dermatol. 2016;17:239.
35. Sadick N. Treatment for cellulite. Int J Womens Dermatol. 2019;5(1):68.
36. Avram MM. Cellulite: a review of its physiology and treatment. J Cosmet Laser Ther. 2004;6(4):181–5.
37. Emanuele E, Minoretti P, Altabas K, Gaeta E, Altabas V. Adiponectin expression in subcutaneous adipose tissue is reduced in women with cellulite. Int J Dermatol. 2011;50(4):412.
38. Khan MH, Victor F, Rao B, Sadick NS. Treatment of cellulite: part I. Pathophysiology. J Am Acad Dermatol. 2010;62(3):362.
39. Rossi AM, Katz BE. A modern approach to the treatment of cellulite. Dermatol Clin. 2014;32(1):52.
40. Tokarska K, Tokarski S, Woźniacka A, Sysa-Jędrzejowska A, Bogaczewicz J. Cellulite: a cosmetic or systemic issue? Contemporary views on the etiopathogenesis of cellulite. Adv Dermatol Allergol Postępy Dermatologii i Alergologii. 2018;35(5):448.
41. Alster TS, Tanzi EL. Cellulite treatment using a novel combination radiofrequency, infrared light, and mechanical tissue manipulation device. J Cosmet Laser Ther. 2005;7(2):82.
42. Spink MJ, Menz HB, Lord SR. Distribution and correlates of plantar hyperkeratotic lesions in older people. J Foot Ankle Res. 2009;2(1):2.
43. García CA, Soler FC. Plantar hyperkeratotic patterns in older patients. Int J Gerontol. 2017;11(4):239–43.
44. Barnes CJ, Davis L, Bergman R, Boehncke WH, Buerger C, Boehncke S, Mashiach J. Hautveränderungen bei Adipositas. Adipositas-Ursachen, Folgeerkrankungen, Therapie. 2010;4(04):180.
45. Yosipovitch G, DeVore A, Dawn A. Obesity and the skin: skin physiology and skin manifestations of obesity. J Am Acad Dermatol. 2007;56(6):908.

Chapter 12
Eruptive Xanthoma

Seher Eren, Klaus Fritz, and Carmen Salavastru

Abstract Eruptive xanthomas, a distinct dermatological manifestation in patients with diabetes, underscore the relationship between systemic diseases and skin health. Manifesting as benign lesions made up of foam cell clusters in the skin, tendons, and subcutaneous tissues, they serve as markers for hyperlipidemias, often in the context of poorly controlled diabetes mellitus. Eruptive xanthomas typically emerge as orange-yellow papules with a firm texture and an erythematous border, primarily appearing on the buttocks, posterior thighs, elbows, and the lumbar region—areas especially prone to increased pressure. The development of these lesions points to a dysfunction in lipid transport mechanisms, leading to an abnormal accumulation of lipids in skin tissues due to factors like endothelial dysfunction, disturbances in microcirculation, and a genetic predisposition to lipid metabolism disorders. Controlling hyperlipidemia and diabetes through dietary changes, weight control, exercise, and pharmacotherapy is crucial for the regression of xanthomas.

S. Eren (✉)
Hautärzte am Marktplatz, Dr. Bettinger und Kollegen, Karlsruhe, Germany
e-mail: contact@drsehereren.com

K. Fritz
Dermatology and Laser Consulting, Landau, Germany

Carol Davila University of Medicine and Pharmacy, Bucharest, Romania
e-mail: drklausfritz@drklausfritz.com

C. Salavastru
Carol Davila University of Medicine and Pharmacy, Bucharest, Romania

Colentina Clinical Hospital, Bucharest, Romania

Pediatric Dermatology Discipline, Dermato-oncology Research Facility, Bucharest, Romania

K. Fritz, G.-S. Tiplica (eds.), *Cutaneous Manifestations in Diabetes*,
https://doi.org/10.1007/978-3-031-65300-1_12

12.1 Eruptive Xanthomas

Some skin disorders and some benign skin lesions can appear more frequently in diabetic patients, among them are xanthomas, especially eruptive xanthomas.

Xanthomas are foam cell clumps formed in the connective tissue of the skin, tendons, and subcutaneous tissues that manifest as cutaneous findings in hyperlipidemias [1]. These individuals typically have higher plasma lipid levels than nondiabetics, particularly when their diabetes control is inadequate [2].

Eruptive xanthomas present as sudden outbreaks of orange-yellow papules, typically 1–4 mm in diameter, with indurated texture and an erythematous border due to capillary dilation, commonly appearing on the buttocks, posterior thighs, elbows, and lumbar region, where over time, the erythema fades, leaving either normal skin or mild post-inflammatory pigmentation (Figs. 12.1 and 12.2) [3, 4]. Eruptive xanthomas can cause itchiness, and in certain cases, the Koebner phenomenon might be observed as positive [5]. Xanthoma diagnosis typically relies on clinical assessment. If clinical findings are inconclusive, a skin biopsy is recommended for histopathological verification [6].

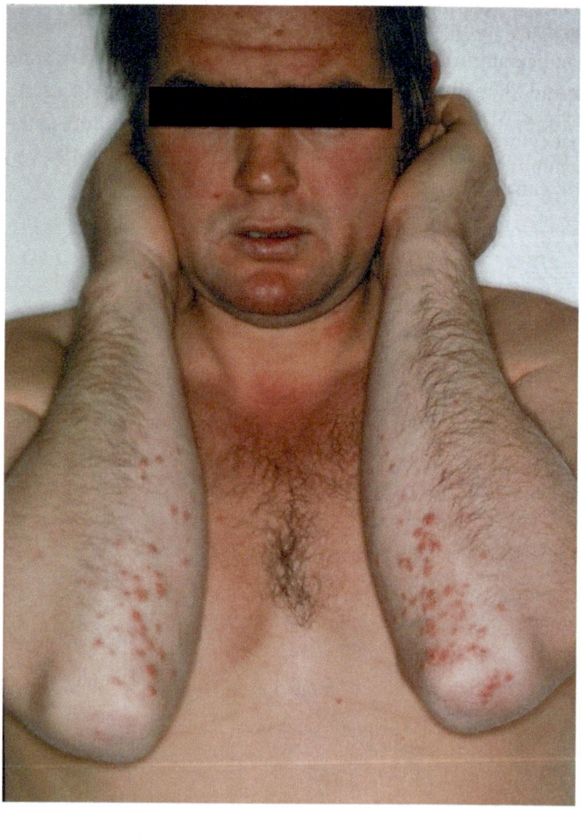

Fig. 12.1 The widespread involvement of eruptive xanthomas on the extensor part of the arm

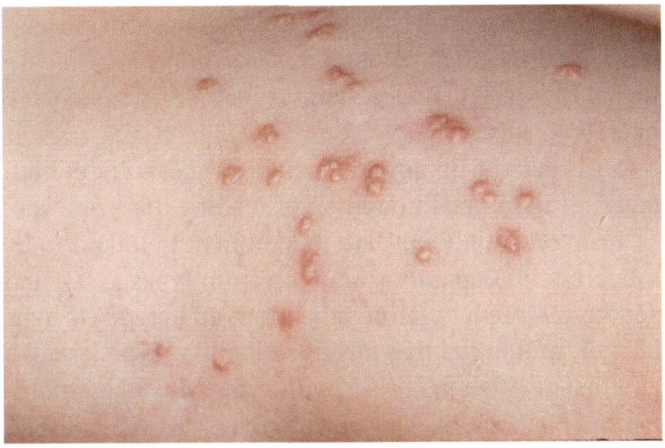

Fig. 12.2 The typical appearance of eruptive xanthomas characterized by orange-yellow papules, with an indurated texture and an erythematous border

Xanthomas originate from a dysfunction in lipid transport, involving cholesterol, triglycerides, or phospholipids, leading to their excessive accumulation in skin tissues. This process begins with increased lipid leakage into connective tissue from blood vessels. Monocytes and macrophages in these areas ingest these lipids via receptors or phagocytosis, forming foam cells. Key factors in xanthoma development include increased lipid concentrations in connective tissue, varying lipoprotein types at normal blood levels, greater lipid extravasation due to factors like vascular permeability and chronic inflammation, local lipid synthesis and storage in histiocytes, and disruption in reverse cholesterol transport [4, 7].

Lipoproteins, comprising lipids and proteins, are macromolecular aggregates that enable lipid compatibility with the aqueous body's fluids. These are made up of nonpolar lipids (like triglycerides and cholesteryl esters), polar lipids (such as phospholipids and free cholesterol), and apolipoproteins, which are amphiphilic proteins binding to lipids and plasma. They play a crucial role in solubilizing lipids in plasma, facilitating the transport of triglycerides—a key energy source—for synthesis, utilization, and storage, as well as cholesterol transportation for absorption, synthesis, metabolism, and elimination. The plasma contains five lipoprotein classes: chylomicrons (CM), very low-density lipoproteins (VLDL), low-density lipoproteins (LDL), intermediate-density lipoproteins (IDL), and high-density lipoproteins (HDL), each differing in composition, size, and density [8].

Lipid abnormalities in type 1 diabetes mellitus are primarily associated with inadequate control of blood glucose, and the most common issue is the presence of high levels of triglycerides in the blood. The management of blood glucose and the levels of plasma triglycerides are closely linked in type 1 diabetes mellitus. This connection results from the body's inability to effectively clear chylomicrons and VLDL-C due to a reduction in the activity of the lipoprotein lipase enzyme. Fortunately, this situation can be reversed with improvements in the management of diabetes. Lipid abnormalities in individuals with type 2 diabetes mellitus occur at twice the rate compared to those without diabetes, and they are more intricate when compared to individuals with type 1 diabetes mellitus. This complexity arises due to the interactions involving obesity, insulin resistance, and hyperinsulinemia—common factors associated with this condition. The most prevalent lipid abnormalities linked to type 2 diabetes mellitus include elevated triglyceride levels and a decrease in HDL-C levels [9].

Disorders of lipoprotein metabolism can affect both the function and the plasma levels of individual lipoproteins, leading to a wide spectrum of dyslipidemias [10].

Eruptive xanthomas are predominantly linked to hypertriglyceridemia and chylomicronemia, mainly stemming from types I, III, and V hyperlipidemia. Eruptive xanthomas are less frequently observed in type IV hyperlipidemia, but they can also be seen in familial hypertriglyceridemia. Type I, caused by a deficiency in lipoprotein lipase, often manifests with symptoms like eruptive xanthomas, lipemia retinalis, and pancreatitis, and triglyceride levels typically exceed 1000 mg/dL. Type V, or familial hyperlipoproteinemia, results from increased production of VLDL and chylomicrons, presenting in adults potentially alongside conditions such as diabetes mellitus, hypertension, hyperuricemia, pancreatitis, and polyneuropathy, with triglyceride levels above 500 mg/dL. Both types I and V are not typically linked to early onset of atherosclerosis. Type III hyperlipidemia, or familial dysbetalipoproteinemia, involves reduced clearance of VLDL and chylomicrons, leading to eruptive xanthomas, particularly on elbows and palmar creases. Patients generally show elevated levels of both cholesterol and triglycerides, over 250 mg/dL, heightening the risk of premature atherosclerosis [11]. Table 12.1 and Fig. 12.3 briefly summarize hyperlipidemias and their associated genetic or secondary diseases, as well as the mostly observed cutaneous manifestations [12–14].

Secondary forms of hyperlipoproteinemia occur as a result of other diseases or medication. Eruptive xanthomas, often linked with severe hypertriglyceridemia, may indicate chylomicronemia syndrome. Diabetes often leads to secondary hypertriglyceridemia [15]. Causes of hypertriglyceridemia include diseases such as inadequately controlled diabetes mellitus, obesity, alcoholism, and renal insufficiency under hemodialysis therapy, as well as drug therapies with systemic corticosteroids, retinoids, or thiazide diuretics. Secondary hypercholesterolemia often occurs in association with nephrotic syndrome, hypothyroidism, or cholestasis. These dermatological signs such as eruptive xanthomas are valuable for clinicians in identifying hypertriglyceridemia and insulin resistance caused by obesity or diabetes mellitus and in detecting genetic conditions affecting lipoprotein metabolism [4, 16, 17]. The information box below lists other diseases and medications that cause hyperlipidemias associated with eruptive xanthomas.

Eruptive xanthomas are important markers for systemic issues like uncontrolled diabetes and hypertriglyceridemia, aiding in the prevention of pancreatitis and heart diseases. Further analysis of apolipoproteins aids in risk assessment and tailoring specific management strategies for cardiovascular conditions [18].

Adequate treatment necessitates rigorous control of the underlying hyperlipidemia. This includes following a diet low in fats and rapidly absorbed carbohydrates, weight reduction, and maintaining regular exercise, especially in patients with insulin resistance, apart from drug therapy. With adequate reduction of serum lipid levels, regression of xanthomas can be anticipated within 3–6 months [15, 17].

Table 12.1 Types of hyperlipoproteinemia, related lipid abnormalities, associated primary and secondary diseases, and cutaneous manifestations

Hyperlipoproteinemia phenotype	Laboratory definition	Defects	Associated with genetic disorders	Mostly observed cutaneous manifestations	Clinical manifestations
Type I	Hyperchylomicronemia Triglycerides ↑↑	Lipoprotein lipase deficiency ApoCII deficiency	Familial apoprotein CII deficiency Familial hyperchylomicronemia	Eruptive xanthomas	Lipemia retinalis, recurrent bouts of abdominal pain and pancreatitis, hepatosplenomegaly
Type IIa	Total cholesterol ↑ Triglycerides ↔ LDL ↑	LDL receptor deficiency	Familial hypercholesterolemia	Xanthelasma Tendon xanthomas Interdigital planar xanthomas	Corneal arcus, premature coronary artery, and peripheral arterial atherosclerotic disease
Type IIB	Total cholesterol ↑ Triglycerides ↑ VLDL ↑ LDL ↑	Decreased LDL receptor and increased ApoB	Familial combined hyperlipidemia		Increased risk for premature coronary atherosclerosis
Type III	Total cholesterol ↑ Triglycerides ↑ HDL ↓	Defect in Apo E 2 synthesis	Dysbetalipoproteinemia	Tuberous xanthomas, palmar xanthomas	Premature coronary peripheral vascular disease
Type IV	VLDL ↑ Triglycerides ↑ Total cholesterol ↑ /↔	Increased VLDL production and decreased elimination	Familial hypertriglyceridemia Familial combined hyperlipidemia	Eruptive xanthomas	Acute pancreatitis
Type V	Chylomicronemia VLDL ↑ TG ↑	Increased VLDL production and decreased lipoprotein lipase	Familial hypertriglyceridemia Familial multiple lipoprotein-type hyperlipidemia	Eruptive xanthomas	Abdominal pain, with or without acute pancreatitis Atherosclerosis Premature coronary artery and peripheral vascular disease

Adapted and modified from Flynn [12], Beaumont [13], and Gotto [14]

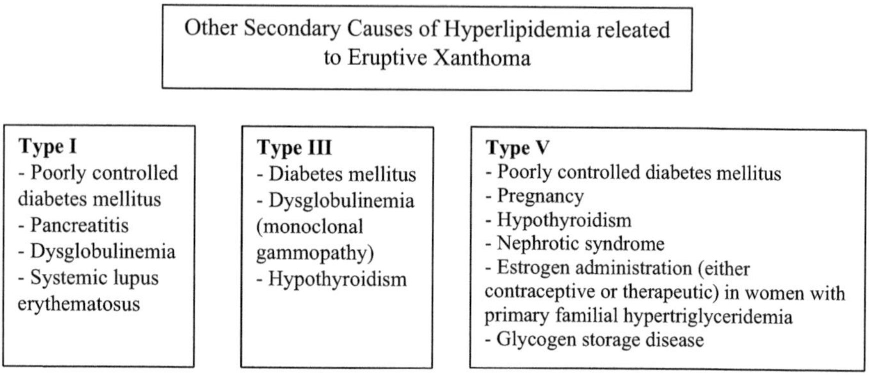

Fig. 12.3 Some secondary causes of hyperlipidemia. Adapted and modified from Gotto [14]

References

1. Zhao C, Kong M, Cao L, Zhang Q, Fang Y, Ruan W, Bi Q. Multiple large xanthomas: a case report. Oncol Lett. 2016;12(6):4327.
2. Dunn FL. Hyperlipidemia and diabetes. Med Clin N Am. 1982;66(6):1347.
3. Cornelius CE. Disappearance of eruptive xanthoma following carbohydrate restriction. Arch Dermatol. 1967;96(1):45–50.
4. Zak A, Zeman M, Slaby A, Vecka M. Xanthomas: clinical and pathophysiological relations. Biomed Pap Med Fac Univ Palacky Olomouc Czech Repub. 2014;158(2):184.
5. Solak B, Kara RO, Acikgoz SB, Kosem M. First and only symptom of undiagnosed diabetes mellitus: eruptive xanthoma. Case Rep. 2015;2015:bcr2015212160.
6. Lee SY, Sheth CA. Eruptive xanthoma associated with severe hypertriglyceridemia and poorly controlled type 1 diabetes mellitus. J Community Hosp Intern Med Perspect. 2019;9(4):344–6.
7. Renner R, Teuwen I, Harth W, Treudler R, Simon JC. Eruptive Xanthome bei Hypertriglyzeridämie: eruptive xanthomas with hypertriglyceridemia. Hautarzt. 2008;59:995–9.
8. Shattat GF. A review article on hyperlipidemia: types, treatments and new drug targets. Biomed Pharmacol J. 2015;7(1):400.
9. O'Brien T, Nguyen TT, Zimmerman BR. Hyperlipidemia and diabetes mellitus. Mayo Clin Proc. 1998;73(10):969–76.
10. Steinhagen-Thiessen E, Kassner U. 421 Störungen des Lipoproteinmetabolismus. In: Suttorp N, Möckel M, Siegmund B, et al., editors. Harrisons Innere Medizin. 19th ed. Berlin: ABW Wissenschaftsverlag; 2016.
11. Summa, C., Igor Chaplik, D. O., Gropper, C., Hoffman, C., & Hwang, R. (2003). Eruptive xanthoma occurring with type III hyperlipidemia: a case report and review of the literature. Am Osteopathic Coll Dermatol. 70.
12. Flynn PD. Xanthomas and abnormalities of lipid metabolism and storage. 9th ed. Rook's textbook of dermatology; 2016. p. 1–13.
13. Beaumont JL, Carlson LA, Cooper GR, Fejfar Z, Fredrickson DS, Strasser T. Classification of hyperlipidaemias and hyperlipoproteinaemias. Bull World Health Organ. 1970;43(6):891–915.
14. Gotto AM Jr, Jones PH, Scott LW. The diagnosis and management of hyperlipidemia. Dis Mon. 1986;32(5):245–311.
15. Villalón G, Martín JM, Monteagudo C, Alonso V, Montesinos E, Jordá E. Eruptive xanthomas after onset of diabetes mellitus. Actas Dermo-Sifiliograficas. 2008;99(5):426–7.

16. Ohtaki S, Ashida K, Matsuo Y, Moritaka K, Iwata S, Nagayama A, Nomura M. Eruptive xanthomas as a marker for metabolic disorders: a specific form of xanthoma that reflects hypertriglyceridemia. Clin Case Rep. 2022;10(4):e05671.
17. Roller E, Schulte KW, Hengge U, Ruzicka T, Kuhn A, Megahed M. Eruptive xanthomas. Hautarzt. 2004;55:978–80.
18. Munoz NR, Agwuegbo CC, Gauhar F. Eruptive xanthomas precipitated by severe hypertriglyceridemia from diabetes and alcohol use. Cureus. 2023;15(8):e43288.

Chapter 13
Granuloma Annulare

María Gamo Guerrero and Elena Conde Montero

Abstract Granuloma annulare is a cutaneous granulomatous inflammatory disease, whose pathogenesis is poorly understood. It has been associated to several triggers, mostly to diabetes mellitus. In this chapter it is discussed the evidence on the association with those different pathologies and presents the different clinical subtypes with their histological clues. At the end, the different treatments that have shown efficacy are described, underlining that this is a therapeutic challenge.

13.1 Introduction

Granuloma annulare (GA) is a cutaneous granulomatous inflammatory dermatosis with a benign and self-limited course.

The prevalence of GA in the general population is estimated to be 0.1–0.4%, with women predominance and with a higher proportion of patients affected in the first three decades of life [1, 2].

Its pathogenesis is poorly understood and its duration may be variable, which is unpredictable. Most of the reported cases of GA are sporadic. Several morphological forms and clinical subtypes have been described in the literature, including generalized, localized, subcutaneous, and perforating GA. Moreover, it can affect any part of the skin.

Etiology of granuloma annulare (GA) is not clear. Even if it has been associated with several triggers, the exact mechanism by which these factors influence the development of the disease is unknown. GA has been associated with a variety of comorbidities, including diabetes mellitus, thyroid disorders, dyslipidemia, underlying malignancies, and tuberculosis. There are also reports associating the appearance of GA with bacillus Calmette–Guérin vaccination. However, little data from controlled studies are available to validate these associations. Even if the

M. Gamo Guerrero · E. Conde Montero (✉)
Department of Dermatology, Hospital Universitario Infanta Leonor y Virgen de la Torre, Madrid, Spain

K. Fritz, G.-S. Tiplica (eds.), *Cutaneous Manifestations in Diabetes*,
https://doi.org/10.1007/978-3-031-65300-1_13

relationship between GA and diabetes mellitus is the most reported, as physiopathology is unclear, it is still controversial [1–3].

Even if some reports have concluded that no association exists [4], various studies support the association. In a study conducted by Studer et al. [5], 12% of 84 patients with GA (localized or generalized) were diabetic, while the prevalence of diabetes mellitus among the regional population was estimated to be 5%. The same team also demonstrated that diabetic patients were more frequently involved by the chronic relapsing form of GA than nondiabetic patients [6]. Kidd et al. [7] demonstrated that glucose tolerance may be reduced and insulin levels increased in patients with GA. Moreover, simultaneous appearance of necrobiosis lipoidica, GA, and diabetes mellitus in a same patient has been reported [8].

Finally, a case–control study was recently conducted on 28 consecutive GA patients. Six out of 28 patients with GA (21.4%) and 5 out of 41 individuals in the control group (12.1%) proved to have diabetes mellitus [2].

13.2 Clinical Manifestations

GA can present with a variety of clinical findings. The most common one is localized GA and is characterized by erythematous or skin-colored non-scaly papules and plaques often in an annular configuration, rope-like border, and central clearing [9–11]. It is often located on the extremities, especially on the lateral and dorsal hands and feet. There is usually no pruritus or other symptoms associated with the lesions [11] (Fig. 13.1).

About 15% of patients with GA have generalized cutaneous lesions [10]. Generalized GA presents with numerous flesh-colored papules in an annular configuration, often pruritic, on the trunk and extremities [11, 12]. A relationship between generalized GA and diabetes mellitus has been suggested as we mentioned

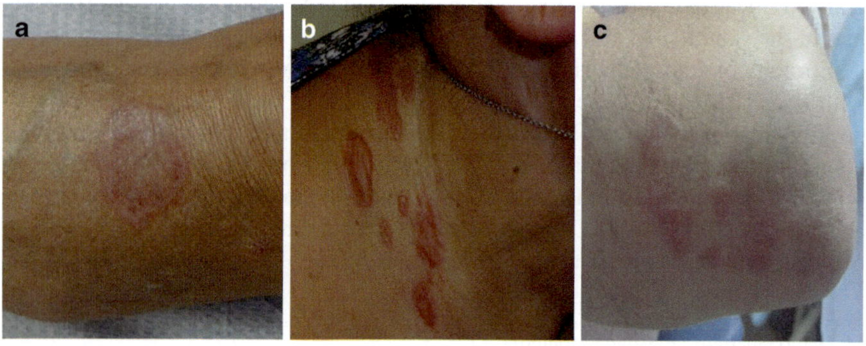

Fig. 13.1 Localized granuloma annulare is characterized by erythematous annular plaques that may be singular (**a**) or multiple (**b**, **c**). It is essential to make the differential diagnosis with other common annular skin conditions, as tinea corporis, pityriasis rosea, annular lichen planus, nummular eczema, or psoriasis

before [13, 14]. The lesions may precede the signs and symptoms of diabetes [15]. This subtype is often resistant to topical regular treatment and for it, systemic therapy may be required [11, 12, 15] (Fig. 13.2).

Another subtype of GA, seen nearly exclusively in children from 1 to 14 years, is the subcutaneous variant. Painless, firm subcutaneous nodules on the scalp or extremities characterize this entity, also known as pseudorheumatoid nodule [11, 16, 17] (Fig. 13.3).

Atypical variants of GA have also been reported. The patch variant of GA presents with smooth erythematous to brownish macules that may involve large areas of skin on the extremities and trunk, with no evidence of papules or induration [11, 12]. Perforating GA is a rare presentation of disease and is characterized by papules with a central crust or scale and an umbilicated center. These lesions, often localized on the trunk and upper and lower limbs, may be pruritic or painful [3, 12, 18].

13.3 Histopathology

Histologically, two main patterns are described. The classic one is the palisading pattern, characterized by a central zone of necrobiotic collagen with mucin deposition surrounded by palisading histiocytes and varying numbers of lymphocytes and eosinophils [3, 12, 19–21] (Fig. 13.4). Mucin deposition can be highlighted with Alcian Blue or colloidal iron stains [21]. The most frequent variant is the interstitial or "incomplete" pattern (seen in the 70% of cases) [22]. In this form, scattered histiocytes are seen between a surrounding collagen bundle in the upper and the mid-dermis, giving the appearance of a "busy dermis" [3, 9, 21, 23].

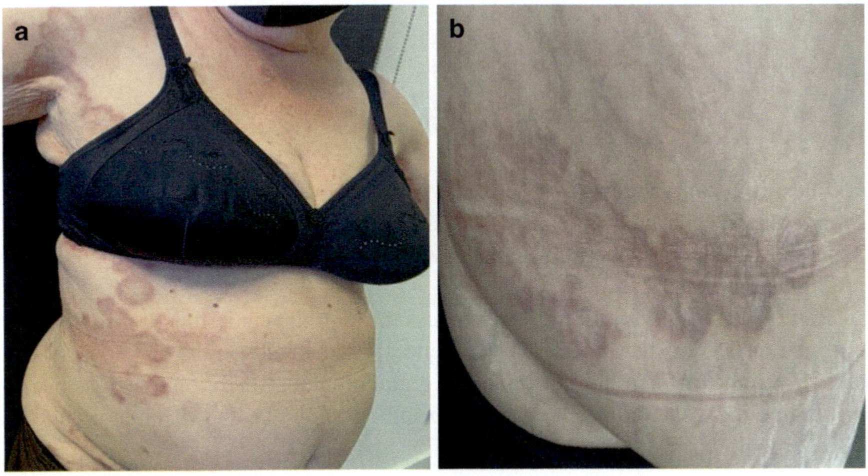

Fig. 13.2 Generalized granuloma annulare presents with widespread annular polycyclic erythematous plaques on the trunk (**a**, **b**)

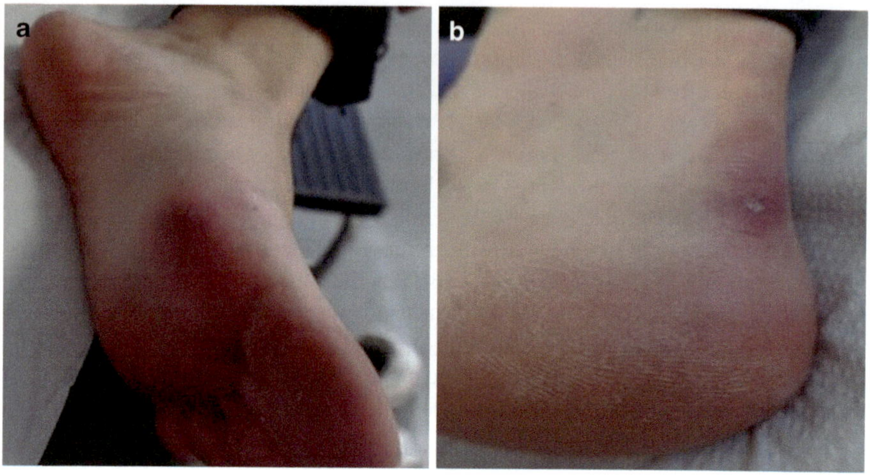

Fig. 13.3 Subcutaneous granuloma annulare is more common in children and presents as a firm, painless nodule on the extremities (**a**, **b**)

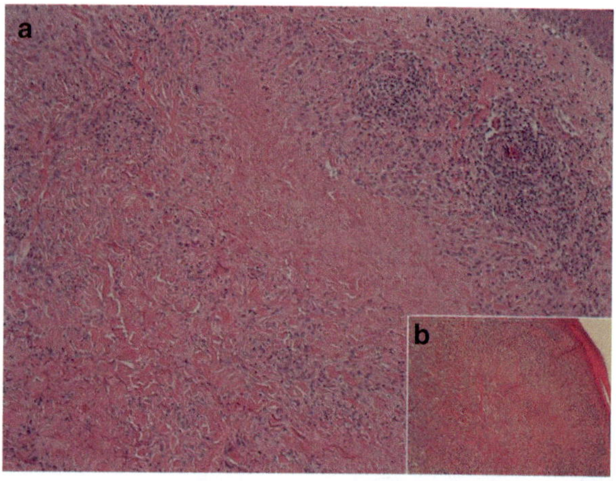

Fig. 13.4 HE × 10. (**a**) Central zone of necrobiotic collagen surrounded by palisading histiocytes in the papillary dermis. (**b**) Deposition of mucin between the collagen bundles

Interstitial pattern may be associated with patch (rather than papular/plaque) presentation [17]. The subcutaneous tissue can also be involved, consisting of a central zone of necrotic collagen surrounded by palisading histiocytes and mononuclear inflammatory cells [21, 24].

Rarely, in GA, perforation of the process through the epidermis (transepidermal elimination) occurs [1, 21, 22]. The presence of mucin aids in the diagnosis of GA and also in the differentiation from other granulomatous conditions, such as necrobiosis lipoidica, sarcoidosis, necrobiotic xanthogranuloma, and rheumatoid nodule ("red granulomas") [3, 25].

13.4 Differential Diagnosis

The differential diagnosis of GA is broad; therefore, a skin biopsy is recommended for clinicopathological correlation when GA is suspected [1]. GA can be mistaken for other common annular skin conditions, as tinea corporis, pityriasis rosea, annular lichen planus, nummular eczema, annular elastolytic giant cell granuloma (actinic granuloma), psoriasis, or erythema migrans of Lyme disease. One of the keys to distinguish GA from these annular lesions is the absence of desquamation as well as associated pustules or vesicles, and the shiny erythematous-violaceous or brownish surface [11, 18, 26].

In the differential diagnosis of generalized lesions, secondary syphilis, arthropod bites, and eruptive xanthomas and histiocytomas should be included.

Subcutaneous lesions must be distinguished from rheumatoid nodules, sarcoidosis, panniculitis, and infection in the proper clinical context [1].

13.5 Treatment

Various treatment strategies have been suggested in the literature [27]. However, as GA is normally self-resolving, an unbiased assessment of therapeutic response is not easy.

Although treatment with high potency topical corticosteroids (with or without occlusion) is widespread, this treatment strategy is frequently ineffective.

Several treatments have been used to treat generalized GA. Potassium iodide is a traditional treatment that has been shown to have positive results [28]. Regarding phototherapy, good results have been reported with UVA, using both oral and topical psoralens, and narrowband UVB [29, 30]. Moreover, cyclosporin [31] and infliximab have been effective in recalcitrant cases [32].

References

1. Thornsberry LA, English JC. Etiology, diagnosis, and therapeutic management of granuloma annulare: an update. Am J Clin Dermatol. 2013;14(4):279–90. https://doi.org/10.1007/s40257-013-0029-5.
2. Alirezaei P, Farshchian M. Granuloma annulare: relationship to diabetes mellitus, thyroid disorders and tuberculin skin test. Clin Cosmet Investig Dermatol. 2017;10:141–5.
3. Keimig EL. Granuloma annulare. Dermatol Clin. 2015;33(3):315–29.
4. Nebesio CL, Lewis C, Chuang T-Y. Lack of an association between granuloma annulare and type 2 diabetes mellitus. Br J Dermatol. 2002;146(1):122–4. https://doi.org/10.1046/j.0007-0963.2001.04527.x.
5. Studer EM, Calza AM, Saurat JH. Precipitating factors and associated diseases in 84 patients with granuloma annulare: a retrospective study. Dermatology. 1996;193(4):364–8.

6. Kidd GS, Graff GE, Davies BF, McDermott MT, Aeling JL, Hofeldt FD. Glucose tolerance in granuloma annulare. Diabetes Care. 1985;8(4):380–4. https://doi.org/10.2337/diacare.8.4.380.
7. Binazzi M, Simonetti S, Simonetti V. Granuloma annulare, necrobiosis lipoidica, and diabetic disease. Int J Dermatol. 1988;27(8):576–9.
8. Davison JE, Davies A, Moss C, Kirk JMW, Taibjee SM, Agwu JC. Links between granuloma annulare, necrobiosis lipoidica diabeticorum and childhood diabetes: a matter of time? Pediatr Dermatol. 2010;27(2):178–81. https://doi.org/10.1111/j.1525-1470.2010.01099.x.
9. Dabski K, Winkelmann RK. Generalized granuloma annulare. Histopathol Immunopathol. 1989;20(1):28–39. https://doi.org/10.1016/S0190-9622(89)70004-9.
10. Muhlbauer JE. Granuloma annulare. J Am Acad Dermatol. 1980;3(3):217–30. https://doi.org/10.1016/S0190-9622(80)80181-2.
11. Schmieder SJ, Harper CD, Schmieder GJ. Granuloma annulare. In: StatPearls [Internet]. Treasure Island (FL): StatPearls Publishing; 2023.
12. Piette EW, Rosenbach M. Granuloma annulare: clinical and histologic variants, epidemiology, and genetics. J Am Acad Dermatol. 2016;75(3):457–65. https://doi.org/10.1016/j.jaad.2015.03.054.
13. Andersen BL, Verdich J. Granuloma annulare and diabetes mellitus. Clin Exp Dermatol. 1979;4(1):31–7. https://doi.org/10.1111/j.1365-2230.1979.tb01588.x.
14. Yun JH, Lee JY, Kim MK, Seo YJ, Kim MH, Cho KH, Kim MB, Lee WS, Lee KH, Kim YC, Lee SJ, Choi GS, Won YH, Ihm CW, Yoon TYSO. Clinical and pathological features of generalized granuloma annulare with their correlation: a retrospective multicenter study in Korea. Ann Dermatol. 2009;21(2):113. Epub 2009 May 31. https://doi.org/10.5021/ad.2009.21.2.113.
15. Agrawal P, Pursnani N, Jose R, Farooqui M. Granuloma annulare: a rare dermatological manifestation of diabetes mellitus. J Family Med Prim Care. 2019;8(10):3419–21. https://doi.org/10.4103/jfmpc.jfmpc_616_19. PMID: 31742181; PMCID: PMC6857419.
16. Felner EI, Steinberg JB, Weinberg AG. Subcutaneous granuloma annulare: a review of 47 cases. Pediatrics. 1997;100(6):965–7. https://doi.org/10.1542/peds.100.6.965. PMID: 9374565.
17. Grogg KL, Nascimento AG. Subcutaneous granuloma annulare in childhood: clinicopathologic features in 34 cases. Pediatrics. 2001;107(3):E42. https://doi.org/10.1542/peds.107.3.e42.
18. Cyr PR. Diagnosis and management of granuloma annulare. Am Fam Physician. 2006;74(10):1729–34.
19. Chaitra V, Inchara YK, Rajalakshmi T, Antony M. Granuloma annulare—histology reconsidered. Indian J Dermatol Venereol Leprol. 2010;76(5):568–9. https://doi.org/10.4103/0378-6323.69050.
20. Stefanaki K, Tsivitanidou-Kakourou T, Stefanaki C, Valari M, Argyrakos T, Konstantinidou CV, Karentzou O, Katsambas A. Histological and immunohistochemical study of granuloma annulare and subcutaneous granuloma annulare in children. J Cutan Pathol. 2007;34(5):392–6. https://doi.org/10.1111/j.1600-0560.2006.00626.x.
21. Elston DM, Ferringer T, Ko CK, Peckham S, High WA, DiCaudo DJ. Dermatopathology. 2nd ed. London: Elsevier; 2013. ISBN 978-0-7020-5527-0.
22. Johnston RB. Weedon's skin pathology essentials. 2nd ed. London: Elsevier; 2017. ISBN 978-0-7020-6830-0.
23. Chatterjee D, Kaur M, Punia RPS, Bhalla M, Handa U. Evaluating the unusual histological aspects of granuloma annulare: a study of 30 cases. Indian Dermatol Online J. 2018;9(6):409–13. https://doi.org/10.4103/idoj.IDOJ_75_18. PMID: 30505780; PMCID: PMC6233004.
24. Aichelburg MC, Pinkowicz A, Schuster C, Volc-Platzer B, Tanew A. Patch granuloma annulare: clinicopathological characteristics and response to phototherapy. Br J Dermatol. 2019;181(1):198–9. https://doi.org/10.1111/bjd.17606. Epub 2019 Mar 13. PMID: 30609014; PMCID: PMC6850090.
25. Lynch JM, Barrett TL. Collagenolytic (necrobiotic) granulomas: part II—the 'red' granulomas. J Cutan Pathol. 2004;31(6):409–18. https://doi.org/10.1111/j.0303-6987.2004.00208.x.
26. Trayes KP, Savage K, Studdiford JS. Annular lesions: diagnosis and treatment. Am Fam Physician. 2018;98(5):283–91.

27. Piette EW, Rosenbach M. Granuloma annulare: pathogenesis, disease associations and triggers, and therapeutic options. J Am Acad Dermatol. 2016;75(3):467–79. https://doi.org/10.1016/j.jaad.2015.03.055.
28. Caserio RJ, Eaglstein WH, Allen CM. Treatment of granuloma annulare with potassium iodide. J Am Acad Dermatol. 1984;10:294–5.
29. Batchelor R, Clark S. Clearance of generalized papular umbilicated granuloma annulare in a child with bath PUVA therapy. Pediatr Dermatol. 2006;23:72–4. https://doi.org/10.1111/j.1525-1470.2006.00175.x.
30. Setterfield J, Huilgol SC, Black MM. Generalised granuloma annulare successfully treated with PUVA. Clin Exp Dermatol. 1999;24:458–60. https://doi.org/10.1046/j.1365-2230.1999.00532.x.
31. Spadino S, Altomare A, Cainelli C, et al. Disseminated granuloma annulare: efficacy of cyclosporine therapy. Int J Immunopathol Pharmacol. 2006;19:433–8. https://doi.org/10.1177/039463200601900219.
32. Hertl MS, Haendle I, Schuler G, Hertl M. Rapid improvement of recalcitrant disseminated granuloma annulare upon treatment with the tumour necrosis factor-alpha inhibitor, infliximab. Br J Dermatol. 2005;152:552–5. https://doi.org/10.1111/j.1365-2133.2005.06371.x.

Chapter 14
Metabolic Effects on the Skin Produced by Obesity: Necrobiosis Lipoidica

Kirsi Isoherranen and Nicolas Kluger

Abstract Necrobiosis lipoidica is an uncommon granulomatous inflammatory disorder involving collagen degeneration. It is linked with diabetes, but not all patients have it. Typical clinical picture is symmetrical well-demarcated yellow-brown plaques with violaceous borders. Diagnosis is usually clinical, but biopsy may be needed for differential diagnosis. There are no guidelines about the treatment. Corticosteroids are widely used, and phototherapy is also a valid option. The future will show the role of JAK inhibitors in the treatment.

Abbreviations

NL	Necrobiosis lipoidica
MAL-PDT	Methyl aminolevulinate-photodynamic therapy
ALA-PDT	Aminolevulinic acid-photodynamic therapy

14.1 Introduction

Necrobiosis lipoidica (NL) is an uncommon granulomatous inflammatory skin disease involving collagen degeneration. It mainly affects middle-aged women and can be idiopathic or related to diabetes. Patients with diabetes tend to develop NL younger than patients without [1]. The landmark studies of the disease have been performed in the 1960s–1980s, and these studies are the cornerstone for understanding and diagnosing this disease process [2]. Recent studies have helped build the knowledge base about this disease and treatment options. However, there is a huge

K. Isoherranen (✉) · N. Kluger
Department of Dermatology, Helsinki University Hospital, Helsinki, Germany
e-mail: kirsi.isoherranen@hus.fi; nicolas.kluger@hus.fi

K. Fritz, G.-S. Tiplica (eds.), *Cutaneous Manifestations in Diabetes*,
https://doi.org/10.1007/978-3-031-65300-1_14

need for robust clinical trials in the field. The clinical course of this disease is variable and difficult to predict; some patients will experience a chronic disease process and others will have fast and spontaneous resolution [2].

14.2 Epidemiology

NL is rare and its exact prevalence is unknown. The prevalence of diabetes at the time of NL diagnosis has been estimated to be somewhere between 30 and 60% [3]. The incidence of NL in individuals with diabetes is only 0.3–1.2%; NL precedes diabetes in up to 14%, appears simultaneously in up to 24%, and occurs after diabetes in 62% of cases [2]. There is a female predominance in individuals affected by the disease, but ulcerated lesions appear more frequently in men [4, 5]. Pediatric cases with type 1 diabetes (T1DM) have been also reported [6].

14.3 Pathophysiology

The primary cause of NL is an immune-mediated vascular disease, but the precise pathophysiology underlying NL has not been discovered [4]. The role of genetics remains to be elucidated [7]. The pathogenesis likely involves impaired neutrophil migration, collagen abnormalities, microangiopathy, and granuloma formation. Vascular abnormalities seen in NL lesions are thickening of the vessel walls, fibrosis, and endothelial proliferation, and these changes were found to be more prominent in diabetic patients than nondiabetics [8]. Collagen abnormalities include absent cross striations and loss of collagen and elastin [9]. Thickening of the basement membrane is thought to appear due to increased cross-linking of collagen caused by the higher levels of lysyl oxidase [10]. Immunoglobulin deposition, such as of fibrin, immunoglobulin M (IgM), and C3, at the dermoepidermal junction of blood vessels has been shown in immunofluorescence studies [11]. Granuloma formation has been thought to occur as result of defective neutrophil migration resulting in macrophage accumulation and granuloma formation [12]. Diabetic microangiopathy has been suspected as a cause for ulcerated NL [5].

14.4 Clinical Picture

NL lesions are usually bilateral and symmetrical, affecting the extensor sides of the lower leg [4]. Rarely, NL may locate on the face, scalp, trunk, groin, or upper extremities [13]. Lesions are typically characterized by well-demarcated yellow-brown plaques with violaceous borders with central waxy atrophic appearance and telangiectasias (Figs. 14.1 and 14.2). Telangiectasias are more frequent in patients with diabetes, especially with T1DM [1]. Firstly, lesions appear as small, firm, red-brown papules that evolve into atrophic plaques over time. Some lesions have minimal symptoms, but 25–33% of cases develop painful ulcerations [5] (Figs. 14.3 and 14.4). Ulcerated NL is frequently associated with comorbidities, such as diabetes, arterial hypertension, obesity, and hypercholesterolemia [5]. Of note, a rare form of perforative NL with transepithelial elimination of material from the dermis has been exclusively described among patients with diabetes [14].

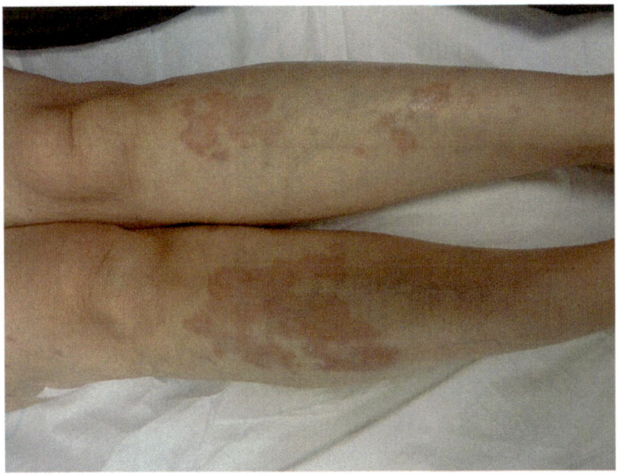

Fig. 14.1 Bilateral, non-ulcerated necrobiosis lipoidica (NL) lesions in lower legs

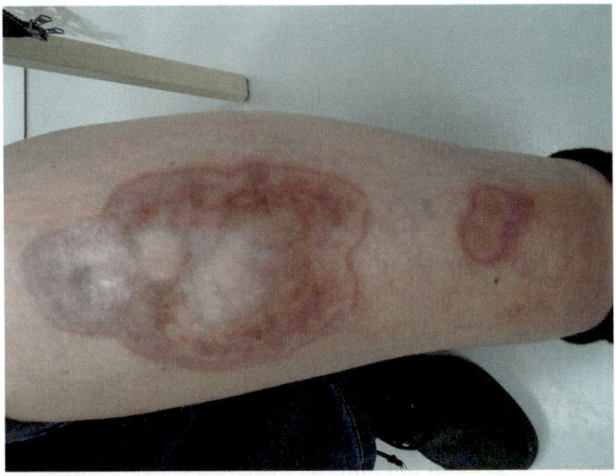

Fig. 14.2 Waxy and atrophic NL lesions

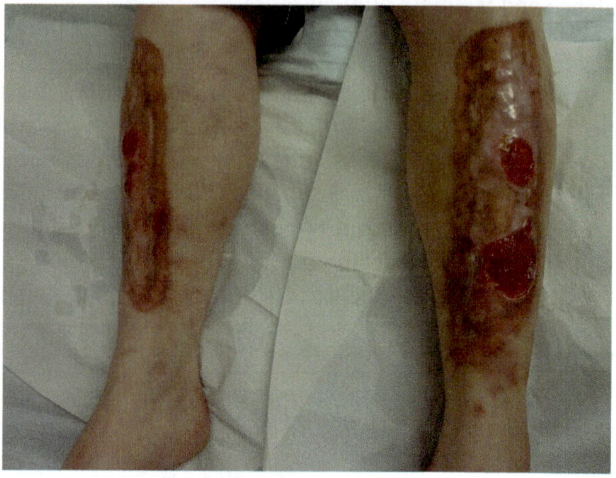

Fig. 14.3 Bilateral ulcerated NL lesions

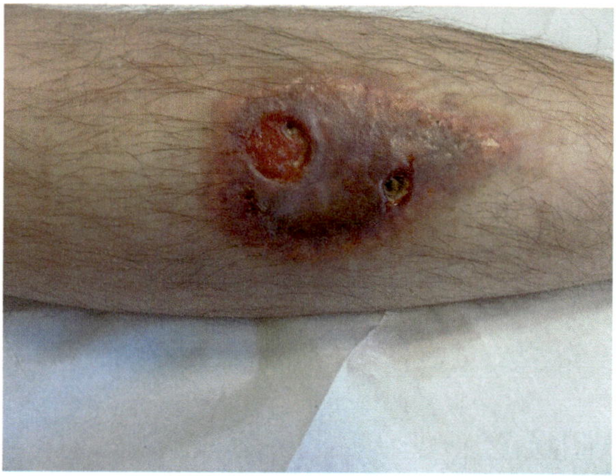

Fig. 14.4 Ulcerated, longstanding NL lesion on the right leg

14.5 Diagnosis

Prompt and accurate diagnosis of NL is a key to appropriate treatment and monitoring. The diagnosis of NL is usually clinical. Dermoscopy can provide additional clues to the diagnostic such as arborizing telangiectasias and hairpin vessels and whitish structures (degenerated collagen) [15].

Atypical presentations (small lesions of early onset, unusual localization, or ulcerations) may delay the diagnosis. A biopsy may be necessary to rule out sarcoidosis, erythema nodosum, necrobiotic xanthogranuloma (NXG), chronic venous ulcers, or granuloma annulare [2, 13]. Investigations should also include screening of comorbidities, such as diabetes, obesity, and vascular disease [4]. In addition, thyroid disorders and inflammatory diseases, such as Crohn's disease, ulcerative colitis, and rheumatoid arthritis, should be excluded.

Histopathologically, NL is characterized by granulomatous inflammation that is palisaded horizontally, with a pattern of "layers of a cake" which contain dermal fibrosis and eosinophilic necrobiotic collagen. There is also perivascular inflammation that is composed of lymphocytes, plasma cells, and histiocytes [16]. Uncommon features include asteroid bodies, cholesterol clefts, lipid droplets, and lipomembranous fat necrosis [17]. There are some differences in the histopathology of patients with and without DM. Acanthosis of the epidermis and neutrophilic infiltration are more commonly seen in patients with diabetes, whereas naked (sarcoid-like) granulomas and eosinophils are more common in nondiabetic patients [18].

14.6 Treatment

Currently, there are no guidelines on the treatment of NL. The disease course is often indolent, and treatment is based on patients' concerns. Each treatment option demonstrates both advantages and disadvantages that should be discussed with the patient. Cosmesis is an important aspect, as even when NL heals, post-inflammatory hyperpigmentation and atrophy are persistent. If there is no ulceration or symptoms, it is reasonable not to treat NL, as 17% of lesions may resolve spontaneously [2].

Optimization of glucose control is important in patients with diabetes, as well as additional lifestyle modifications, including smoking cessation and avoidance of trauma [2]. However, it is admitted that glucose regulation does not affect the progression of NL [13]. Coexistent venous insufficiency should be treated, and compression therapy is the cornerstone of treatment as well [19], as it controls edema, prevents ulceration, promotes ulcer healing, and protects from trauma.

Corticosteroids are the standard treatment of NL, even if they often show unsatisfactory results [19, 20]. They can be provided topically, intralesionally, and systemically in most resistant cases. Topical steroids decrease the inflammation of active lesions but should be avoided in inactive atrophic lesions, as they may exacerbate the atrophy and increase the risk of new ulcerations [2, 21, 22]. Although systemic steroids can cause hypertension and hyperglycemia, a short-term course is usually effective in producing resolution of active lesions. Intralesional corticosteroid is recommended in solitary lesions, and it should be targeted to the borders to avoid exacerbation of atrophy. Topical tacrolimus, a calcineurin inhibitor, has been shown to be effective in resolving ulceration associated with NL [3, 19, 23] and the best response seen in early inflammatory stages.

Traditional systemic agents include cyclosporine, methotrexate, and mycophenolate mofetil. The use of cyclosporine has been limited due to recurrence of ulcers after discontinuation of the drug and side effects such as hypertension, hyperkalemia, and nephrotoxicity. Cyclosporine has been used at a dosage of 2–4 mg/kg/day [2, 24]. One case study reported ulcer healing with methotrexate, titrated up to a dose of 15 mg weekly, but reduction in methotrexate dose led to disease flare-up. Healing was achieved with the addition of cyclosporine (4 mg/kg) to the methotrexate/pentoxifylline regime [25]. There are no published cases of monotherapy with methotrexate. The advantage of mycophenolate mofetil is its minimal nephrotoxicity, with the main adverse effect being gastrointestinal discomfort. However, recurrence has been reported after its discontinuation as well [26].

Fumaric acid esters have showed promising results [27, 28]. However, their use is limited by their side effects and their availability mainly in German-speaking countries.

Ultraviolet phototherapy, especially topical psoralen-UVA (PUVA), has been widely used in NL lesions. PUVA decreases inflammation and decreases the active inflamed borders, but has no clinical effects on atrophic areas [2]. The largest amount of published data regarding the treatment of NL using topical PUVA therapy exists. Approximately two-thirds of cases achieved a partial or complete response [3]. Also photodynamic therapy [methyl aminolevulinate-photodynamic therapy (MAL-PDT) and aminolevulinic acid-photodynamic therapy (ALA-PDT)] has shown good efficacy [19]. Other laser and light therapies include pulsed dye laser and UVA1 and lastly CO_2 laser [29]. However, due to diverse exposure times and energy settings, larger and more standardized studies on laser and light therapies are needed to establish a clear consensus on these treatment options.

The role of TNF-α inhibitors is tempting due to the role of TNF in the formation of granulomas [30]. Infliximab, etanercept, and adalimumab have been used, and around 70% of patients treated with TNF-α inhibitors achieved a complete response [3, 31]. Recently, reports about the use of JAK inhibitors have been published. Ruxolitinib and tofacitinib were found to be effective in ulcerated NL [32, 33]. Also topical application of JAK inhibitors might be the future treatment of NL.

14.7 Prognosis

Long-standing ulcerated NL is a risk factor for cutaneous malignancies, especially squamous cell carcinomas [34, 35]. Therefore, NL lesions should be monitored for transformation to malignancy.

References

1. Severson KJ, Costello CM, Brumfiel CM, Patel MH, Butterfield RJ, Nelson SA, et al. Clinical and morphological features of necrobiosis lipoidica. J Am Acad Dermatol. 2022;86(5):1133–5.
2. Sibbald C, Reid S, Alavi A. Necrobiosis lipoidica. Dermatol Clin. 2015;33(3):343–60.
3. Jockenhöfer F, Kröger K, Klode J, Renner R, Erfurt-Berge C, Dissemond J. Cofactors and comorbidities of necrobiosis lipoidica: analysis of the German DRG data from 2012. J Dtsch Dermatol Ges. 2016;14:277–84.
4. Hashemi DA, Brown-Joel ZO, Tkachenko E, Nelson CA, Noe MH, Imadojemu S, et al. Clinical features and comorbidities of patients with necrobiosis lipoidica with or without diabetes. JAMA Dermatol. 2019;155(4):455–9.

5. Erfurt-Berge C, Seitz AT, Rehse C, Wollina U, Schwede K, Renner R. Update on clinical and laboratory features in necrobiosis lipoidica: a retrospective multicentre study of 52 patients. Eur J Dermatol. 2012;22(6):770–5.
6. Berman HS, Shabihkhani M, Hogeling M. Pediatric necrobiosis lipoidica: case report and review of the literature. Dermatol Online J. 2021;27(7):d327754363.
7. Hawryluk EB, Izikson L, English JC 3rd. Non-infectious granulomatous disease: an evidence-based update to important clinical questions. Am J Clin Dermatol. 2010;11:171–81.
8. Quimby SR, Muller SA, Schroeter AL. The cutaneous immunopathology of necrobiosis lipoidica diabeticorum. Arch Dermatol. 1988;124:1364–71.
9. Oikarinen A, Mörtenhumer M, Kallioinen M, Savolainen E-R. Necrobiosis lipoidica: ultrastructural and biochemical demonstration of a collagen defect. J Invest Dermatol. 1987;88(2):227–32.
10. Markey AC, Tidman MJ, Rowe PH, Missen GA, Macdonald DM. Aggressive ulcerative necrobiosis lipoidica associated with venous insufficiency, giant-cell phlebitis and arteritis. Clin Exp Dermatol. 1988;13:252–4.
11. Ullman S, Dahl MV. Necrobiosis lipoidica. An immunofluorescence study. Arch Dermatol. 1977;113:1671–3.
12. Kota SK, Jammula S, Kota SK, Meher LK, Modi KD. Necrobiosis lipoidica diabeticorum: a case-based review of literature. Indian J Endocrinol Metab. 2012;16:614–20.
13. Reid SD, Ladizinski B, Baibergenova A, Alavi A. Update on necrobiosis lipoidica: a review of etiology, diagnosis, and treatment options. J Am Acad Dermatol. 2013;69(5):783–91.
14. Kluger N, Segretin C, Jegou MH. Nécrobiose lipoïdique perforante [Perforating necrobiosis lipoidica]. Ann Dermatol Venereol. 2017;144(2):158–60.
15. Pellicano R, Caldarola G, Filabozzi P, Zalaudek I. Dermoscopy of necrobiosis lipoidica and granuloma annulare. Dermatology. 2013;226(4):319–23.
16. Lehman JS, Sokumbi O, Peters MS, Bridges AG, Comfere NI, Gibson LE, et al. Histopathologic features of noninfectious granulomatous disorders involving the skin. Hum Pathol. 2020;103:127–45.
17. Gibson LE, Reizner GT, Winkelmann RK. Necrobiosis lipoidica diabeticorum with cholesterol clefts in the differential diagnosis of necrobiotic xanthogranuloma. J Cutan Pathol. 1988;15(1):18–21.
18. Johnson E, Patel MH, Brumfiel CM, Severson KJ, Bhullar P, Boudreaux B, et al. Histopathologic features of necrobiosis lipoidica. J Cutan Pathol. 2022;49:692–700.
19. Nihal A, Caplan AS, Rosenbach M, Damsky W, Mangold AR, Shields BE. Treatment options for necrobiosis lipoidica: a systematic review. Int J Dermatol. 2023;62(12):1529–37.
20. Peckruhn M, Tittelbach J, Elsner P. Update: treatment of necrobiosis lipoidica. J Dtsch Dermatol Ges. 2017;15(2):151–7.
21. Petzelbauer P, Wolff K, Tappeiner G. Necrobiosis lipoidica: treatment with systemic corticosteroids. Br J Dermatol. 1992;126:542–5.
22. Erfurt-Berge C, Heusinger V, Reinfoldt-Jockenhöfer F, Dissemond J, Renner R. Comorbidity and therapeutic approaches in patients with necrobiosis lipoidica. Dermatology. 2022;238(1):148–55.
23. Clayton TH, Harrison PV. Successful treatment of chronic ulcerated necrobiosis lipoidica with 0.1% topical tacrolimus ointment. Br J Dermatol. 2005;152:581–2.
24. Stinco G, Parlangeli ME, De Francesco V, Frattasio A, Germino M, Patrone P. Ulcerated necrobiosis lipoidica treated with cyclosporin A. Acta Derm Venereol. 2003;83:151–3.
25. West EA, Warren RB, King CM. A case of recalcitrant necrobiosis lipoidica responding to combined immunosuppression therapy. J Eur Acad Dermatol Venereol. 2007;21:830–1.
26. Reinhard G, Lohmann F, Uerlich M, Bauer R, Bieber T. Successful treatment of ulcerated necrobiosis lipoidica with mycophenolate mofetil. Acta Derm Venereol. 2000;80:312–3.
27. Kreuter A, Knierim C, Stücker M, Pawlak F, Rotterdam S, Altmeyer P, al. Fumaric acid esters in necrobiosis lipoidica: results of a prospective noncontrolled study. Br J Dermatol. 2005;153:802–7.

28. Mrowietz U, Christophers E, Altmeyer P. Treatment of severe psoriasis with fumaric acid esters: scientific background and guidelines for therapeutic use. The German Fumaric acid Ester consensus conference. Br J Dermatol. 1999;141:424–9.
29. Rajabi-Estarabadi A, Aickara DJ, Williams NM, et al. Laser and light therapies for the treatment of necrobiosis lipoidica. Lasers Med Sci. 2021;36:497–506.
30. Kolde G, Muche JM, Schulze P, et al. Infliximab: a promising new treatment option for ulcerated necrobiosis lipoidica. Dermatology. 2003;206:180–1.
31. Zhang KS, Quan LT, Hsu S. Treatment of necrobiosis lipoidica with etanercept and adalimumab. Dermatol Online J. 2009;15:12.
32. Lee JJ, English JC III. Improvement in ulcerative necrobiosis lipoidica after Janus kinase-inhibitor therapy for polycythemia vera. JAMA Dermatol. 2018;154:733–4.
33. Janßen S, Jansen TM. Ulcerated necrobiosis lipoidica successfully treated with tofacitinib. Int J Dermatol. 2022;61(6):739–41.
34. Uva L, Freitas J, Soares de Almeida L, Vasques H, Moura C, Miguel D, et al. Squamous cell carcinoma arising in ulcerated necrobiosis lipoidica diabeticorum. Int Wound J. 2015;12(6):741–3.
35. Harvey JA, Severson KJ, Brumfiel CM, Patel MH, Butterfiel RJ, Nelson SA, et al. Necrobiosis lipoidica-associated cutaneous malignancy. J Am Acad Dermatol. 2022;86(6):1428–9.

Chapter 15
Pruritus in the Diabetic Patient

Lea-Sophie Stahl, Felix Witte, Sonja Ständer, and Aleksandra A. Stefaniak

Abstract Diabetic pruritus is defined as a manifestation of chronic pruritus due to diabetes mellitus (DM). Chronic pruritus (CP) caused by diabetes mellitus and other metabolic diseases is a clinical challenge referring to diagnostics and therapy as it usually occurs without initial skin lesions, with a lack of validated biomarkers, and as a slow but increasing onset of pruritus without clear clinical characteristics.

This book chapter reviews the current scientific understanding of chronic pruritus in the diabetic patient, considering prevalence, epidemiology, and clinical presentation.

The challenge to treat this entity lies in the complex interplay of neuropathic, metabolic, and inflammatory mechanisms influencing the underlying mechanisms of diabetic pruritus.

Therefore, the field of pruritus requires further studies to deepen the understanding of the detailed pathomechanisms to advance development of further targeted therapies.

Abbreviations

AP	Acute pruritus
CP	Chronic pruritus
CKD-aP	Chronic kidney disease-associated pruritus
DLQI	Dermatological life quality index
HADS	Hospital Anxiety and Depression Scale

L.-S. Stahl · F. Witte · S. Ständer (✉)
Department of Dermatology, Center for Chronic Pruritus, University Hospital of Münster, Münster, Germany
e-mail: Lea-sophie.stahl@ukmuenster.de; felix.witte@ukmuenster.de; Sonja.staender@ukmuenster.de

A. A. Stefaniak
Department of Dermatology, Venereology and Allergology, Wroclaw Medical University, Wrocław, Poland
e-mail: aleksandra.stefaniak@student.umed.wroc.pl

K. Fritz, G.-S. Tiplica (eds.), *Cutaneous Manifestations in Diabetes*,
https://doi.org/10.1007/978-3-031-65300-1_15

IFSI	International Forum for the Study of Itch
NRS	Numeric rating scale
SFN	Small fiber neuropathy
SSRI	Selective serotonin reuptake inhibitor
VAS	Visual analog scale

15.1 Introduction and Clinical Overview

Pruritus, a term that is rooted in the Latin "prurire" that means "to itch," describes a complex sensory phenomenon with a multifaceted etiology and significant impact on patients' quality of life. This sensation arises from the activation of the peripheral or central nervous system including intraepithelial nerves, triggering an irresistible urge to scratch, and is often accompanied by stress and discomfort.

Pruritus that lasts longer than 6 weeks is described as chronic pruritus (CP) and is much more challenging regarding therapeutic management compared to acute itching particularly because of the wide range of causes for chronic pruritus.

Despite the growing interest in the symptom and pruritus itself and ongoing efforts to differentiate its various manifestations, the available data on pruritus in the context of metabolic disturbances, e.g., in diabetes mellitus (DM), remains limited [1].

DM is a metabolic disorder that affects multiple systems of the human body. It can lead to various complications, including manifestations of the skin. The incidence of DM within the global population has been increasing for years due to lifestyle and dietary habits. Due to the increasing prevalence and severity of the consequences of this metabolic disorder, there is a rising need for further research in this field [2, 3].

However, the pathogenesis of itch in the diabetic patient remains to date inadequately elucidated. Ongoing studies contribute further insights by classification of itch characteristics and delving into potential underlying entities like DM. These efforts provide to advance our comprehension of pruritus in DM and reevaluate more targeted interventions for affected individuals [2, 4].

15.1.1 Acute Pruritus

Acute pruritus (AP) represents a transient sensory experience that plays a crucial role as a vital warning mechanism, signaling the presence of a variety of factors like insects, parasites, skin conditions, irritating plant components, or (allergic) reactions to medication like opioids, antihypertensive drugs, or uricostatics like allopurinol. Scratching as a natural response to the occurring itch sensation can alleviate these threats. In general, acute itching serves as a healthy purpose and resonates well to itch-controlling therapy options due to its transient, intense reaction to stimuli. Its duration typically varies from only a few seconds to <6 weeks and usually resolves within the elimination of the provoking trigger. Clinical manifestations of acute itching can often show erythematous skin with papules or even vesicles [1, 4, 5].

15.1.2 Chronic Pruritus

Chronic pruritus (CP) represents a frequent sensory experience, not only associated with cutaneous or systemic diseases but also occurring within the general population. The estimated lifetime prevalence of chronic pruritus measures between 22 and 25.5% [6]. It is characterized by persistence of itching lasting over 6 weeks or more.

The management of chronic pruritus is complex and challenging due to its heterogeneous clinical presentation and the fact that pruritus may be often refractory to therapy.

According to the International Forum for the Study of Itch (IFSI), the appearance of chronic pruritus can be categorized into three groups:

IFSI I: Chronic pruritus on inflamed, lesional skin

IFSI II: Chronic pruritus on normal-appearing, non-lesional skin

IFSI III: Chronic pruritus accompanied by chronic scratch lesions (Table 15.1) [5, 7]

The etiology of (chronic) pruritus can vary between dermatological, neurological, psychiatric, metabolic, and other systemic conditions. In contrast to dermatological diseases, pruritus in systemic, neuropathic, or psychiatric disorders typically manifests on normal-appearing, non-lesional skin. However, it may also lead to secondary cutaneous manifestations and (scratch) lesions [7, 8].

Table 15.1 Categorization of chronic pruritus by appearance according to IFSI [5, 7]

IFSI category	Definition	Description
IFSI I	Chronic pruritus on lesional skin	With presence of a (pathological) skin condition (*formerly: Pruritus* cum *materia*)
IFSI II	Chronic pruritus on non-lesional skin	Without initial presence of skin pathologies (*formerly: Pruritus sine materia*)
IFSI III	Chronic pruritus with chronic scratch lesions	With the predominant presence of secondary scratch lesions (e.g., *in prurigo or lichen simplex*)

15.1.3 Diabetes Mellitus

DM is recognized as a chronic metabolic disorder, not only impacting insulin availability but also causing systemic effects on the entire body of affected patients [9–12]. According to the International Diabetes Federation in 2015, 1 in 11 adults in the age range of 20–79 years, totaling 415 million patients globally, was affected by DM of any type worldwide. The reasons for the increasing global frequency of diabetes vary and include economic development, population ageing, unhealthy diets, and urbanization.

Regarding the definition from WHO, diabetes can be divided, based on the onset and etiology, into the following groups:

1. Diabetes type 1 (autoimmune/idiopathic types)
2. Diabetes type 2
3. Other forms of diabetes (e.g., caused by drugs or chemicals, endocrinopathies, exocrine pancreatic diseases, infections, genetic defects)
4. Gestational diabetes [3, 13]

A state of persistent hyperglycemia as presented in every type of DM is linked to damage and dysfunction of various organ systems including cardiovascular system, renal system, eyes, and nerves. Additionally, cutaneous disorders are represented with nearly 80% of patients suffering from DM. The appearance of cutaneous manifestations is reported to occur both before the onset and during the course of diabetes mellitus [3]. Also pruritus is a known complaint in DM. Recent attention focuses on the underlying pathophysiology of diabetic itch [3, 13].

15.2 Demographics and Epidemiology of Chronic Pruritus in Diabetes

Epidemiological studies regarding the prevalence of diabetes in a cohort of patients with chronic pruritus as well as prevalence of pruritus in diabetes patients are still rare. Studies revealed the prevalence of chronic pruritus in DM among 18.4–27.5% of patients, with a point prevalence of 13.5% and a lifetime prevalence of up to 27.5% [3, 12, 14]. However, it is crucial to acknowledge that these studies encompassed diverse populations and the methodologies employed were not consistently aligned with current standards in itch research. It remains unclear whether the studies assessed acute or chronic pruritus, and the populations studied were diverse, including patients from various diabetic groups.

In recent research conducted on the adult population afflicted with type 2 DM, the point prevalence of itching was found to be 32%, with a prevalence rate of 35.7% during the course of the disease [2]. On the other hand, in children with type 1 DM, the prevalence of pruritus over the course of the disease was 22%, with a point prevalence of itching at 12% [15].

Referring to multivariate analysis, eczema, dry skin, asthma, liver diseases, a higher body mass index, and increased anxiety scores can be determinants of CP.

However, these attributes can occur in several diseases, and diagnostically searching for the exact origin of (diabetic) pruritus can often remain unsuccessful [1].

15.2.1 Distribution and Clinical Characteristics of Diabetic Pruritus

Chronic pruritus in DM does not show a specific clinical pattern. In up to 50% of diabetic pruritus patients, pruritus has been reported to be generalized [16]. In older references, diabetic pruritus was mainly discussed as presenting as anogenital pruritus or pruritus vulvae in women that was explained by a higher incidence of fungal infections. However, this perspective is now considered outdated [2, 17].

Today, evidence suggests the trunk as the loco typico for diabetic pruritus, as reported in a large-scale survey of 2656 diabetic outpatients and 499 nondiabetic subjects. Interestingly, in this paper, diabetic pruritus was found to be associated with diabetic polyneuropathy [11]. Besides truncal pruritus, pruritus of the scalp was found correlating with the prevalence of diabetes mellitus [15, 18].

Regarding its itch characteristics, diabetic pruritus manifests with burning and sometimes stinging quality which is in line with the association to neuropathy as described in the study of H. Yamaoka and colleagues [19]. The itch intensity reported by diabetic patients with pruritus ranges from moderate to severe (6,31 ± 2,16 NRS) [2].

15.2.2 Patient-Reported Outcome and Measurement of Chronic Itch

Standardized and validated instruments for an assessment of chronic pruritus are important due to its subjective nature. The documentation of the intensity of itch and the influence of pruritus on the quality of life serves as a basis for the measurement of the treatment efficacy. The presence and intensity of itch can be evaluated via several questionnaires (Table 15.2).

The most frequently used assessment for measurement of itch intensity is the numeric rating scale (NRS) where patients have to rate their pruritus on numbers from zero (no itch) to ten (worst itch) or the visual analog scale (VAS) with an equal range but with a continuous line without numbers. To differentiate between mild, moderate, severe, and very severe itch, NRS and VAS use cutoff values of 3, 7, and 9 [22].

Table 15.2 Patient-reported outcome instruments for assessment of chronic pruritus [20, 21]

Aim	Questionnaire	Specific information and instructions for assessors
Itch intensity	Numeric rating scale (NRS) Visual analog scale (VAS)	E.g., "on a scale from 0 (no itch) to 10 (worst itch imaginable), how was your worst itch in the past 24 h?"
Life quality	ItchyQoL DLQI	22 items regarding emotions, symptoms, self-perception – Sub-scores for "symptoms," "functioning," and "emotions" – Severity of pruritus symptoms, influence on quality of life, and emotional status 10 items assessing how the dermatological issue affected the quality of life of patients in the last week Sub-scores for "symptoms," "functioning," and "emotions"
Depression or anxiety measurement	HADS	Assessment of mood disturbance within the two categories of depression and anxiety

The DLQI (dermatological life quality index) questionnaire is a widely recognized tool regarding the measurement of the impact of symptoms on patients' quality of life. Specifically, it evaluates the severity of pruritic dermatoses on the daily life including skin symptoms, functioning, and emotions. However, in case pruritus occurs on non-lesional skin, DLQI is considered as being not appropriate. For this, an own questionnaire was developed, the so-called ItchyQoL, which has 22 items.

The ItchyQoL questionnaire assesses the health-related quality of life in patients with chronic pruritus of any type and the self-perception of affected patients [23, 24].

Another questionnaire, the Hospital Anxiety and Depression Score (HADS), serves as a tool to measure signals of anxiety and depression in patients including those with chronic itch.

15.3 Overview on Main Pathogenetic Mechanisms of Diabetic Pruritus

Diabetic pruritus is notably linked to poor disease control and caused by the interplay of multiple factors (Fig. 15.1), as highlighted by several studies. In 2021, a study on 109 patients with diabetes mellitus found a prevalence of itch in 35.8% [2]. This underscores the need to address this symptom in diabetes management. DM is known to impact the nerve fiber function and this seems also to underlie generation of chronic pruritus [11]. It induces a small fiber neuropathy (SFN), a disease that can already start in the early stage of DM. Neuropathic itch fibers in the skin seem to generate either numbness or pain or a mixture of pain and itch with itch being transmitted via pruriceptors in the spinal cord.

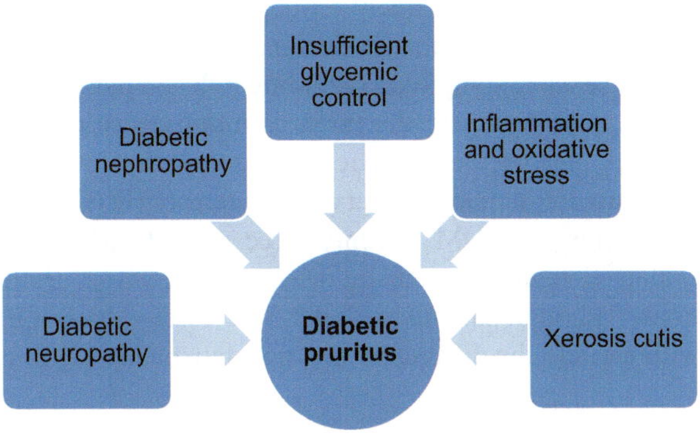

Fig. 15.1 Pathogenetic causes that can lead to diabetic pruritus

In the skin, mediator-guided activation of nerve fibers involving substance P and mast cells promotes neurogenic pathways in the transmission of itch [25].

The prevalence of diabetic polyneuropathy, and hence pruritus, correlates with glycemic control and disease duration, with evidence suggesting that intensive glycemic control can be beneficial, particularly in type 1 DM. Systemic inflammation and oxidative stress, triggered by hyperglycemia and insulin resistance, can exacerbate neuronal damage [26]. Diabetic nephropathy can also lead to pruritus, known as chronic kidney disease-associated pruritus (CKD-aP; previously called uremic pruritus), with a complex pathophysiology involving factors like skin dryness, uremic toxins, immune and neural dysregulation, and opioid mechanisms [2].

15.3.1 Neuropathic Pathways/Diabetic Neuropathy

A significant aspect of diabetic pruritus is the association between pruritus and diabetes-induced pruritus and diabetes-induced neuropathy and their shared neuropathic mechanisms.

Transmission of cutaneous itch is promoted via unmyelinated C fibers and thinly myelinated A delta fibers [27]. Free nerve endings of C fibers in the epidermis, so-called pruriceptors, are activated through specific mediators, including histamine, TSLP, leukotrienes, and interleukins (such as IL-31) [28]. The transmission of itch via C fibers results also in release of neuropeptides following neuronal activation. Key neuropeptides in this scenario are substance P and calcitonin gene-related peptide. Binding of substance P on mast cells via Mas-related G-protein-coupled receptors (Mrgpr) and blood vessels was found to induce short time vasodilatation and mast cell degranulation, leading to neurogenic inflammation and itch promotion via a histaminergic pathway [25].

Diabetic pruritus is most likely caused by direct damage to the nerve itself due to the altered tissue metabolism and associated neuroinflammation. It is assumed that skin collagen advanced glycation end products are associated with the formation of neuropathy in diabetes [29]. Associated damage of the small cutaneous C and A delta fibers with subsequent retraction of intraepidermal nerves and reduction of the total nerve fiber number is designated as small fiber neuropathy (SFN). SFN may lead to sensory symptoms including itch and pain. SFN can occur in a broad variety of diseases; however, the most common cause of SFN in developed countries is DM, as part of the diabetic polyneuropathy [30]. To date, there was one study assessing intraepidermal nerve fiber density (IENFD) as a factor contributing to itch in patients with DM. Twenty-three patients with type 2 DM were prospectively evaluated regarding itch intensity, skin dryness, IENFD, and neuropathic sensations. Although patients with itch had lower values of IENFD comparing to patients without itch, the difference was not statistically significant [31].

15.3.2 Glycemic Control

The prevalence of diabetic polyneuropathy in DM seems to correlate with glycemic control and disease duration; however, this is only evident in adult patients with a prolonged duration of DM [31, 32]. Evidence suggests that intensive glycemic control has a beneficial effect in treating diabetic polyneuropathy; interestingly, evidence is stronger for type 1 than for type 2 DM. Diabetic polyneuropathy seems to develop prior to diabetic levels of hyperglycemia (metabolic syndrome, impaired glucose tolerance), suggesting that treatment of diabetic polyneuropathy begins as early as any tendency toward development of DM is detected [33].

15.3.3 Inflammation and Oxidative Stress

Hyperglycemia and insulin resistance in DM promote systemic inflammation and oxidative stress. This activates transcriptional factors (NFkB) and downstream kinases (protein kinase C, MAPK), culminating in the release of pro-inflammatory cytokines (e.g., IL-2, IL-6, IL-8, TNFa) and chemokines, pushing the inflammatory cascade and leading to further neuronal damage and promoting neuropathic itch sensations [21, 26].

15.3.4 Diabetic Nephropathy

Diabetic nephropathy as a microvascular consequence of DM poses a further condition with pruritic potential in diabetic patients, referred to as uremic pruritus or chronic kidney disease-associated pruritus (CKD-aP). The pathophysiology of CKD-aP is not completely understood yet; however multiple pathogenetic factors are discussed, among these xerosis cutis, accumulation of uremic toxins, immune and neural dysregulation, and opioidergic mechanisms. The pathophysiological involvement of opioidergic mechanisms derives from the key role of u- and k-opioid receptors in pruritus. The current success in treating patients with CKD-aP in hemodialysis with the k-opioid receptor agonist difelikefalin supports these findings [34].

15.3.5 *Skin Dryness (Xerosis)*

There are few studies claiming that skin dryness takes part in the multimodal pathogenesis of diabetic pruritus. These data showed that dry skin was significantly more increased in patients experiencing pruritus compared to those without itch [2]. Additionally, dryness of the skin was also positive linked to elevated HbA1c in diabetic patients and neuropathic conditions as well as clinical factors like age, higher BMI, and smoking [2, 3]. This interplay between DM, pruritus, damage of nerve fibers, and general unhealthy lifestyle underscores the imperative to consider the pathogenesis of diabetic pruritus as a versatile mechanism that must be taken into account in clinical management and development of therapy models.

15.4 Clinical Management and Therapy of Diabetic Pruritus

Chronic pruritus often shows only partial symptom control or improvement through conventional therapies like antihistamines, topical therapy with emollients, and steroids due to its complex and multifactorial origin. Identification of the underlying cause of pruritus remains essential to enable targeted therapy options. However, all forms of chronic pruritus require an interdisciplinary approach for achieving a clinically measurable improvement [7].

Current consensus guidelines on pruritus therapy imply various topical and systemic therapy options (Table 15.3). These procedures shall be applied stepwise and collaboratively with the patient to ensure maximum adherence.

It is generally recommended to create a treatment plan tailored to individual considerations, including age, severity of symptoms, type of pruritus, and underlying primary condition. The plan should contain basic, topical, and when needed systemic therapy in combination [1, 28].

15.4.1 *Integrated Diabetes Management*

It is recommended to extend disease management beyond regular HbA1c control. This should include consistent monitoring of blood glucose levels with point of care testing tools to maintain them within the target range, a balanced diet, regular physical activity, and stress management. Compliance with prescribed medications and weight management are also crucial, as they positively affect blood glucose levels

Table 15.3 Overview of therapeutic options in diabetic pruritus

Therapy options	Description
Emollient utilization	Use of moisturizers (with urea/lactic acid) to restore skin barrier, retain moisture, alleviate pruritus, prevent secondary infections. Proactive care may include moisturizers with protective components
Topical treatment	First-line treatment for localized itching includes emollients (with urea), topical antipruritics (polidocanol, camphor, menthol, tannin-based products), and capsaicin patches
General treatment for pruritus	Gabapentinoids: *Caution*: *dosage is depending on general health and kidney function and must be individually determined. A common* dosage for healthy adults is, for example: 1. Gabapentin—start with 300 mg (100 mg in elderly); increase by 300 mg every 2–3 days (100 mg in elderly) to max dose of 3600 mg 2. Pregabalin—start with 75 mg (50 mg in elderly) Begin with low doses; gradually increase for antipruritic effect, typically visible after several weeks
Alternative treatment options	Non-sedating antihistamines (cetirizine, loratadine, desloratadine, fexofenadine up to 4 × standard dose) SSRIs (sertraline 25–100 mg/day, paroxetine 20–30 mg/day) can provide relief for non-dermatological itching
Additional treatment modalities	Oral lipoic acid supplementation (600 mg daily for 8 weeks) may benefit patients with diabetic itch

and insulin sensitivity and can indirectly reduce the risk of developing diabetic pruritus [28].

15.4.2 Dermatological Care in Diabetes

In DM management, skin care is imperative to prevent dry skin. Patients should avoid extreme temperatures and excessive washing that may worsen dryness. Using gentle, pH-neutral cleansers and taking shorter, lukewarm showers or baths are recommended. It is also advised to wear light, breathable clothing to minimize skin irritation [4].

15.4.3 Review of Medications

A comprehensive evaluation of the patient's medications is essential to identify any pruritogenic agents that cause itching. If pruritus is suspected to be medication-related, alternative treatments should be considered.

15.4.4 Emollient Utilization

Moisturizers, especially those with urea and lactic acid, are vital for restoring the skin barrier and retaining moisture. They can alleviate pruritus and prevent secondary infections from scratching. Proactive skin care may include moisturizers with additional protective components [35, 36].

15.4.5 Targeted Treatment for Pruritus

For localized itching, first-line treatment should include emollients like those with urea, supplemented with topical antipruritics such as polidocanol, camphor, menthol, or tannin-based products. As most patients with diabetic pruritus suffer from generalized pruritus, systemic therapies are essential. These include, in diabetic patients, for example, gabapentinoids (gabapentin, pregabalin) which could provide relief and should be considered in the treatment regimen [4].

15.4.6 Additional Treatment Modalities

Oral lipoic acid supplementation, at 600 mg daily for 8 weeks, has shown promise in treating neuropathic itch in diabetic patients [37]. While non-sedating antihistamines are in most cases without efficacy, selective serotonin reuptake inhibitors (SSRIs) can be selected as they may provide relief, although clinical studies in diabetic pruritus are missing [38, 39].

15.4.7 Treatment Application and Monitoring

Emollient therapy is an integral part of DM care. Patients with extensive pruritus may require assistance from their family or caregivers to apply topical treatments. Managing complex cases might necessitate a team approach, involving dermatologists, endocrinologists, and pain specialists. Regular follow-up appointments are crucial to assess the effectiveness of the treatment plan and to make necessary adjustments. Ongoing evaluation is essential for effective management of this complex condition.

15.5 Conclusion

In conclusion, diabetic pruritus may frequently occur in patients with any type of DM. The symptom might be often overlooked with pending early treatment management. The underlying mechanisms are most likely associated with diabetic metabolism-induced neuropathic including presence of small fiber neuropathy pathologies. This chapter underlines that the treatment of chronic pruritus necessitates a multidisciplinary diagnostic approach and the development of a personalized therapeutic strategy. This strategy should be established in collaboration with the patient, taking into account their unique medical history, symptoms, and preferences.

With the increasing incidence of metabolic disorders such as DM, it is reasonable to anticipate a rise in the prevalence of associated comorbidities and symptoms, including pruritus. Consequently, it is crucial to develop and implement standardized diagnostic and therapeutic algorithms for each comorbidity and correlated symptom [40]. These algorithms play a pivotal role in the holistic treatment of patients following a diagnosis like DM.

Standardized diagnostic and therapeutic strategies ensure comprehensive management of patients and facilitate optimized therapeutic outcomes. Despite the current limitations in our understanding and the available tools to measure diabetic pruritus, the existing data is promising, indicating that this is an area of active and future research.

Given these considerations, further studies focusing on the development of pruritus therapy are of high importance. This will not only enhance our understanding of the complex interplay of factors involved in diabetic pruritus but will also significantly contribute to the effective clinical management of this challenging symptom in the diabetic population.

References

1. Stander S, Zeidler C, Augustin M, Darsow U, Kremer AE, Legat FJ, et al. S2k guideline: diagnosis and treatment of chronic pruritus. J Dtsch Dermatol Ges. 2022;20(10):1387–402.
2. Stefaniak AA, Krajewski PK, Bednarska-Chabowska D, Bolanowski M, Mazur G, Szepietowski JC. Itch in adult population with type 2 diabetes mellitus: clinical profile, pathogenesis and disease-related burden in a cross-sectional study. Biology (Basel). 2021;10(12):1332.
3. Stefaniak AA, Chlebicka I, Szepietowski JC. Itch in diabetes: a common underestimated problem. Postepy Dermatol Alergol. 2021;38(2):177–83.
4. Weisshaar E, Szepietowski JC, Darsow U, Misery L, Wallengren J, Mettang T, et al. European guideline on chronic pruritus. Acta Derm Venereol. 2012;92(5):563–81.
5. Stander S, Weisshaar E, Mettang T, Szepietowski JC, Carstens E, Ikoma A, et al. Clinical classification of itch: a position paper of the international forum for the study of itch. Acta Derm Venereol. 2007;87(4):291–4.
6. Suilmann T, Zeidler C, Osada N, Riepe C, Stander S. Usability of validated sleep-assessment questionnaires in patients with chronic pruritus: an interview-based study. Acta Derm Venereol. 2018;98(8):722–7.

7. Pereira MP, Zeidler C, Storck M, Agelopoulos K, Philipp-Dormston WG, Zink A, et al. Challenges in clinical research and care in pruritus. Acta Derm Venereol. 2020;100(2):adv00028.
8. Kremer AE, Mettang T. Pruritus in systemic diseases: common and rare etiologies. Internist (Berl). 2019;60(8):814–20.
9. Kulzer B. Physical and psychological long-term consequences of diabetes mellitus. Bundesgesundheitsblatt Gesundheitsforschung Gesundheitsschutz. 2022;65(4):503–10.
10. Eid S, Sas KM, Abcouwer SF, Feldman EL, Gardner TW, Pennathur S, et al. New insights into the mechanisms of diabetic complications: role of lipids and lipid metabolism. Diabetologia. 2019;62(9):1539–49.
11. Yamaoka H, Sasaki H, Yamasaki H, Ogawa K, Ohta T, Furuta H, et al. Truncal pruritus of unknown origin may be a symptom of diabetic polyneuropathy. Diabetes Care. 2010;33(1):150–5.
12. Neilly JB, Martin A, Simpson N, MacCuish AC. Pruritus in diabetes mellitus: investigation of prevalence and correlation with diabetes control. Diabetes Care. 1986;9(3):273–5.
13. Aleksandra Araszkiewicz EB-S, Budzyński A, Cypryk K, Czech A, Czupryniak L, Drzewoski J, Dzida G, Dziedzic T, Franek E, Gajewska D, Górska M, Grzeszczak W, Gumprecht J, Idzior-Waluś B, Jarosz-Chobot P, Kalarus Z, Klupa T, Koblik T, Kokoszka A, Korzon-Burakowska A, Kowalska I, Krętowski A, Majkowska L, Małecki M, Mamcarz A, Mirkiewicz-Sieradzka B, Młynarski W, Moczulski D, Myśliwiec M, Narkiewicz K, Noczyńska A, Piątkiewicz P, Rymaszewska J, Sieradzki J, Solnica B, Strączkowski M, Strojek K, Szadkowska A, Szelachowska M, Wender-Ożegowska E, Wierusz-Wysocka B, Wolnik B, Wyleżoł M, Wylęgała E, Zozulińska-Ziółkiewicz D. Guidelines on the management of diabetic patients. A position of diabetes Poland. Clin Diabetol. 2019;8(1):1–95.
14. Ko MJ, Chiu HC, Jee SH, Hu FC, Tseng CH. Postprandial blood glucose is associated with generalized pruritus in patients with type 2 diabetes. Eur J Dermatol. 2013;23(5):688–93.
15. Stefaniak AA, Zubkiewicz-Kucharska A, Matusiak L, Noczynska A, Szepietowski JC. Itch in children with type 1 diabetes: a cross-sectional study. Dermatol Ther (Heidelb). 2020;10(4):745–56.
16. Bustan RS, Wasim D, Yderstraede KB, Bygum A. Specific skin signs as a cutaneous marker of diabetes mellitus and the prediabetic state—a systematic review. Dan Med J. 2017;64(1):A5316.
17. Drivsholm T, de Fine ON, Nielsen AB, Siersma V. Symptoms, signs and complications in newly diagnosed type 2 diabetic patients, and their relationship to glycaemia, blood pressure and weight. Diabetologia. 2005;48(2):210–4.
18. Bin Saif GA, Ericson ME, Yosipovitch G. The itchy scalp—scratching for an explanation. Exp Dermatol. 2011;20(12):959–68.
19. Tavee J, Zhou L. Small fiber neuropathy: a burning problem. Cleve Clin J Med. 2009;76(5):297–305.
20. Zeidler C, Raap U, Witte F, Stander S. Clinical aspects and management of chronic itch. J Allergy Clin Immunol. 2023;152(1):1–10.
21. Witte F, Zeidler C, Stander S. Management of pruritus in the elderly. Dermatologie (Heidelb). 2023;74(9):670–7.
22. Reich A, Chatzigeorkidis E, Zeidler C, Osada N, Furue M, Takamori K, et al. Tailoring the cut-off values of the visual analogue scale and numeric rating scale in itch assessment. Acta Derm Venereol. 2017;97(6):759–60.
23. Zeidler C, Steinke S, Riepe C, Bruland P, Soto-Rey I, Storck M, et al. Cross-European validation of the ItchyQoL in pruritic dermatoses. J Eur Acad Dermatol Venereol. 2019;33(2):391–7.
24. Pereïra MP, Stander S. Assessment of severity and burden of pruritus. Allergol Int. 2017;66(1):3–7.
25. Auyeung KL, Kim BS. Emerging concepts in neuropathic and neurogenic itch. Ann Allergy Asthma Immunol. 2023;131(5):561–6.
26. Pop-Busui R, Ang L, Holmes C, Gallagher K, Feldman EL. Inflammation as a therapeutic target for diabetic neuropathies. Curr Diabetes Rep. 2016;16(3):29.

27. Sutaria N, Adawi W, Goldberg R, Roh YS, Choi J, Kwatra SG. Itch: pathogenesis and treatment. J Am Acad Dermatol. 2022;86(1):17–34.
28. Misery L, Ständer S. Pruritus. Cham: Springer International Publishing; 2016.
29. Kestner RI, Stander S, Osada N, Ziegler D, Metze D. Acquired reactive perforating dermatosis is a variant of prurigo nodularis. Acta Derm Venereol. 2017;97(2):249–54.
30. Oaklander AL. Neuropathic itch. Semin Cutan Med Surg. 2011;30(2):87–92.
31. Stefaniak AA, Agelopoulos K, Bednarska-Chabowska D, Mazur G, Stander S, Szepietowski JC. Small-fibre neuropathy in patients with type 2 diabetes mellitus and its relationship with diabetic itch: preliminary results. Acta Derm Venereol. 2022;102:adv00719.
32. Baum P, Toyka KV, Bluher M, Kosacka J, Nowicki M. Inflammatory mechanisms in the pathophysiology of diabetic peripheral neuropathy (DN)-new aspects. Int J Mol Sci. 2021;22(19):10835.
33. Albers JW, Pop-Busui R. Diabetic neuropathy: mechanisms, emerging treatments, and subtypes. Curr Neurol Neurosci Rep. 2014;14(8):473.
34. Fishbane S, Jamal A, Munera C, Wen W, Menzaghi F, Investigators K-T. A phase 3 trial of Difelikefalin in hemodialysis patients with pruritus. N Engl J Med. 2020;382(3):222–32.
35. Pham HT, Exelbert L, Segal-Owens AC, Veves A. A prospective, randomized, controlled double-blind study of a moisturizer for xerosis of the feet in patients with diabetes. Ostomy Wound Manage. 2002;48(5):30–6.
36. Narbutt J, Bednarski IA, Lesiak A. The effect of an emollient with benfothiamine and Biolin prebiotic on the improvement of epidermal skin function. Postepy Dermatol Alergol. 2016;33(3):224–31.
37. Hahm JR, Kim BJ, Kim KW. Clinical experience with thioctacid (thioctic acid) in the treatment of distal symmetric polyneuropathy in Korean diabetic patients. J Diabetes Complicat. 2004;18(2):79–85.
38. O'Donoghue M, Tharp MD. Antihistamines and their role as antipruritics. Dermatol Ther. 2005;18(4):333–40.
39. Zylicz Z, Krajnik M, Sorge AA, Costantini M. Paroxetine in the treatment of severe non-dermatological pruritus: a randomized, controlled trial. J Pain Symptom Manag. 2003;26(6):1105–12.
40. Valdes-Rodriguez R, Mollanazar NK, Gonzalez-Muro J, Nattkemper L, Torres-Alvarez B, Lopez-Esqueda FJ, et al. Itch prevalence and characteristics in a Hispanic geriatric population: a comprehensive study using a standardized itch questionnaire. Acta Derm Venereol. 2015;95(4):417–21.

Chapter 16
Allergy in the Diabetic Patient

Cara Bieck and Christoph Skudlik

Abstract Allergies are physical hypersensitive reactions to normally harmless substances. For daily practice in terms of allergy in the diabetic patient, knowledge of type I allergy, the so-called immediate-type allergy, and type IV allergy, the so-called delayed-type allergy, is of importance. In diabetic patients, two main allergies are described in scientific literature: (i) allergy to insulin preparations (mainly manifesting as type I allergy) and (ii) allergy to medical devices, i.e., mainly components of glucose sensors and insulin pumps and/or their adhesives (type IV allergy). The subsequently listed exemplary allergens have been described in the case of suspected allergic contact dermatitis in diabetic patients utilizing a glucose monitoring device and/or insulin pump: 1,6-hexanediol diacrylate, 2,2′-methylenebis(6-tert-butyl-4-methylphenol) monoacrylate, 3-methyl-2-buten-1-ol, benzoylcyclohexanol, colophonium, cyanoacrylate, dimethyl adipate, dipropylene glycol diacrylate, epoxy resin, ethyl cyanoacrylate, isobornyl acrylate (IBOA), *N,N*-dimethylacrylamide, phenoxypoly(ethylenoxy) ethylacrylate, β-carboxyethyl acrylate, and γ-butyrolactone. In this, not just the plaster's glue but also the device's individual parts should be taken into consideration as potential source of exposure.

16.1 Mechanisms of Allergy

The term allergy generally describes a defensive or rather hypersensitive reaction of the body to normally harmless substances in the environment. Using the classification according to Robert Coombs and Philip Gell from 1963, different allergic

C. Bieck · C. Skudlik (✉)
Institute for Interdisciplinary Dermatological Prevention and Rehabilitation (iDerm), Osnabrück, Germany

Department of Dermatology, Environmental Medicine and Health Theory, Osnabrück University, Osnabrück, Germany
e-mail: cara.bieck@uni-osnabrueck.de; cskudlik@uni-osnabrueck.de

K. Fritz, G.-S. Tiplica (eds.), *Cutaneous Manifestations in Diabetes*,
https://doi.org/10.1007/978-3-031-65300-1_16

Table 16.1 Classification of hypersensitivity reactions. Adapted and modified from Davis [1] and Singer and Zodda [2]

Classification	Mechanism	Clinical manifestations	Timing of reaction
Type I (IgE-mediated)	Allergen IgE binds to mast cells; inflammatory mediators are released	Anaphylaxis, urticaria, angioedema	Minutes to hours post-exposure (immediate)
Type II (cytotoxic)	IgG and IgM bind to allergen on target cell, complement mediated	Neutropenia, thrombocytopenia, hemolytic anemia	Varying
Type III (immune complex)	Tissue deposition of IgG, bound to allergen, activated by complement	Serum sickness, vasculitis, glomerulonephritis	1–3 weeks post-exposure
Type IV (delayed, cell-mediated)	T lymphocytes, macrophages	Contact dermatitis	24–72 h (sometimes a few days beyond) post-exposure

IgE immunoglobulin E, *IgG* immunoglobulin G, *IgM* immunoglobulin M

reaction types can be described (Table 16.1). For daily practice and especially regarding allergy in the diabetic patient, knowledge of type I allergy, the so-called immediate-type allergy, and type IV allergy, the so-called delayed-type allergy, is of great relevance.

Type I allergy is characterized by the rapid onset of the typical allergy symptoms (itching, reddening of the skin, wheal formation, runny nose, sneezing, itchy eyes, possibly asthma) after contact with the allergen. Immunoglobulin E (IgE) plays a central role in the mechanism by which an immediate-type allergy develops. The IgE are directed against the penetration of foreign substances into the body; this process is called sensitization. If the allergen that has become known to the immune system reappears, the immune system is "alarmed" in a chain of reactions. The defense reaction can then occur immediately, which is why it is called an immediate-type reaction. Examples are allergies to pollen, house dust (more precisely: house dust mite excrement), food, insect venom (e.g., bee venom, wasp venom), and animal hair (e.g., dog or cat hair). A type I allergy can lead to anaphylaxis (systemic immune reaction) and consequently to anaphylactic shock. Depending on the severity of the acute reaction, treatment must be topical or systemic. Allergy preparations (e.g., nasal spray, eye drops) can alleviate the symptoms of type I allergies (e.g., runny nose and sneezing). Severe type I allergies should—if possible—be treated with allergy immunotherapy (so-called hyposensitization or desensitization) [3], which serves to desensitize the immune system of those affected to the allergen, i.e., to reduce the body's sensitivity to the allergen. Desensitization is often used in patients with allergic asthma, hay fever, or insect venom allergies. Treatment consists of giving people small amounts of the allergen in the form of injections or tablets, which are gradually increased. The goal is to get the immune system to see the allergen as harmless and stop overreacting to it. Hyposensitization can significantly improve symptoms and in some cases even eliminate them completely. However, it is a lengthy treatment that can last for several years and requires high therapy adherence.

The development of a type IV allergy can be divided into two phases: the initial sensitization phase and the triggering phase (elicitation). In the sensitization phase, low-molecular haptens (still incomplete antigens) usually reach the deeper layers of the epidermis after skin contact through the *stratum corneum*, where subsequently—through biochemical processes—a full antigen is present after the hapten has fused with endogenous molecules. Then, the endogenous immune system is activated. The duration of the sensitization phase in humans after the first contact with the allergen is between 10 and 15 days. After 24–72 h, but sometimes after 3 days, renewed skin contact with the corresponding hapten to which sensitization is present triggers the allergic reaction, which is clinically characterized by the formation of erythema and eczema. In general, this reaction only becomes visible after 24–48 h, but then persists for over 72 h (and also well beyond), which is why it is referred to as a delayed-type reaction. According to current pathogenetic concepts, once a sensitization has been acquired, it persists lifelong—there is no effective causal therapy. The most important measure in the treatment of type IV allergies is the so-called allergen avoidance, which means avoiding skin contact with the causative allergen.

16.2 Allergy to Insulin Preparations

Insulin is a central hormone for the metabolism in the human body. Its primary function is to move glucose from the blood into the cells, where the sugar molecules are used for energy generation. In type I diabetes, there is an absolute deficiency of the hormone insulin, so that those affected have to inject insulin their entire lives. In type II diabetes, there is reduced sensitivity of the body's cells to insulin (insulin resistance). Various therapy modules are available for this type of diabetes. The most important measures in type II diabetes are regular exercise, an appropriate diet, and reaching a normal body weight. This improves the sensitivity of the body's cells to insulin and can thus reduce the need for insulin. At the beginning of the therapy, an attempt is therefore always made to manage with general measures such as consistent lifestyle changes. If general measures are not successful, various medications are available (e.g., metformin, sulphonylureas, gliflozine, semaglutide, liraglutide). Only if it is not possible to get the disease under control with these drugs either, insulin has to be injected for type II diabetes.

The trigger of an allergic reaction after an insulin injection can either be the pure insulin or one of the accompanying substances contained in the insulin solution, e.g., depot substances [zinc chloride, zinc acetate, protamine sulfate], preservatives (cresol, phenol, methyl 4-hydroxybenzoate), or disinfectants as well as cleaning agents used in cleaning the skin or the syringes and cannulas [4, 5]. In an allergy to

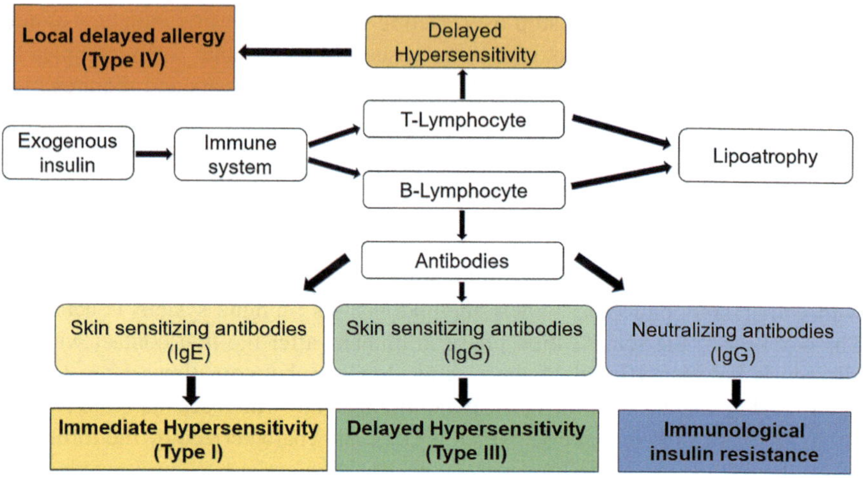

Fig. 16.1 Immunological reactions to insulin. Adapted and modified from Kahn and Rosenthal [7] and Radermecker and Scheen [9]. *IgE* immunoglobulin E, *IgG* immunoglobulin G

insulin, the immune system reacts disproportionately to insulin preparations. In the scientific literature, three types of immunological reactions to insulin have been described (Fig. 16.1) [6–8]. Mostly, insulin allergy manifests as type I allergy with immediate reactivity [4, 9]. Typical symptoms are skin changes such as redness, swelling, and itching.

The diagnosis of insulin allergy is based on a thorough allergic anamnesis in which the specific connection between the administration of insulin preparations and the occurrence of symptoms of hypersensitivity must be considered, the clinical picture, and then examination of the patients' data by the dermatologist or rather allergist [10]. Dependent on the assumed reaction type, prick testing (in type I allergy) or patch testing (in type IV allergy) can be deployed [11].

The therapy of the allergy then is based on the diagnosis. Generally, if an allergic reaction to insulin is detected in diabetic patients, an alternative to the current diabetes therapy must be found. In the case of patients with type II diabetes, it may be possible to switch to oral antidiabetics, but this is not an option for patients suffering from type I diabetes [5]. In the case of type I allergy, hyposensitization has previously been described as a feasible option [12], if no alternative preparation can be found. As reported by Fischer et al., hyposensitization in case of insulin type I allergy has been successfully conducted [13–15], favorably using the insulins lispro [15–17] or glargine [18]. It should be mentioned that treatment with lispro requires special attention (i.e., frequent blood sugar self-monitoring by the patient combined with situation-adapted injections) due to the rapid onset of treatment effects and the shorter effect duration [13]. Nowadays, also lispro preparations are available as delayed insulins; these, however, contain protamine, which must be seen critically from an allergological point of view [13]. As stated by Datz et al., for conducting hyposensitization in insulin type I allergic patients, there have been protocols published, which in these cases should be consulted (e.g., the approach by Jacquier and Chik [19] derived from Grammer [20]) [5]. In type IV allergy, there is no other option than to strictly avoid contact with the triggering allergen (allergen avoidance) [21].

It should be noted that allergic reactions to insulin have become less frequent since the introduction of human and recombinant insulins [5, 9]. The prevalence of allergic reactions to human insulin and to recombinant insulin is reported in the literature to be 0.1–3% in insulin-treated patients [5, 9, 22–24]. Nevertheless, insulin allergy continues to represent a serious phenomenon in everyday diabetology and should receive appropriate attention [5].

16.3 Allergy to Components of Glucose Sensors and Insulin Pumps

Glucose sensors and insulin pumps that stick to the skin with plasters are becoming increasingly popular [25]. This is hardly surprising, since the patch pumps in type I diabetes patients supply insulin tubeless and are worn inconspicuously; the stick-on glucose sensors save the patients the constant pricking of the finger. Some users, however, suffer from intolerance and allergies against those systems. In this, it is not always the patches that are responsible, but sometimes also plastic components [26].

For the treatment of skin reactions against glucose sensors and insulin pumps, it is of great relevance to differentiate between irritant and allergic reactions. Skin irritation can occur, for example, when the skin under the patch from glucose sensors or insulin pumps sweats; afterward it is irritated, itches, and is reddened. If an irritant skin irritation is present, the symptoms are sometimes stronger, sometimes weaker, and not necessarily with every use. Under certain circumstances, the skin under the patch can also become discolored or inflamed around the puncture site of the measuring thread or catheter. Such problems can usually be alleviated easily. Measures to prevent and treat skin irritation when using glucose sensors and insulin pumps alongside recommendations for implementation according to Kamann [26] are subsequently listed:

- Avoiding moisture and friction under the patch.
  - Not applying the sensor, patch pump, or pump cannula until the disinfectant has completely dried on the skin.
  - Choosing a spot with enough space, i.e., not under a belt, waistband, or tight pants, but rather on the upper arm.
  - Not using foil patches if the patient tends to sweat heavily.
  - After showering or bathing, the patient should gently dab the patch dry with a soft towel or facial tissue.
  - For swimming, the patient should wrap self-adhesive fixation tape around the patch pump or sensor.

- Trying out what the patients' skin tolerates well.
  - Testing of skin protection spray or a particularly skin-friendly plaster under the plaster of the sensor, patch pump, or pump cannula (the diabetes team should explain proper usage).
  - Trying other disinfectants or, if possible, pump catheters/patches.
- Taking good care of the skin.
  - Plasters and residues of the adhesive should be carefully removed, e.g., with a special plaster remover.
  - Wearing areas should be cared for after removing the patch, e.g., by using skin creams containing skin-soothing ingredients.
  - In case of severe redness and itching, a cortisone containing cream can be used (approx. 1 to 3 days, as needed).
- Recovery time for puncture sites.
  - Allowing air to reach the puncture site.
  - Not wearing tight clothes over puncture site directly after removing the device.
  - Changing puncture sites regularly.
  - Not leaving the pump cannula lying around for longer than recommended (Cave: Note manufacturer's instructions!)
  - Not placing the sensor, patch pump, or pump needle on an irritated skin area.

Paying attention to the measures for preventing skin irritation when using glucose sensors and insulin pumps is very important also in terms of allergy prevention, as in irritated, *macerated* skin, the barrier homeostasis of the *stratum corneum* is impaired. This consequently leads to potential allergens penetrating the skin easier and deeper, where they then even meet a pro-inflammatory skin milieu [27]. The risk of contact sensitization is thus increased in irritated skin, which therefore should be best prevented.

Type IV allergic reactions to components of the plaster or components of glucose sensors or insulin pumps are well described in scientific literature. In case of suspected allergic contact dermatitis due to a glucose sensor or insulin pump, patch testing must be deployed by the dermatologist or rather allergist [28]. While doing this, it must be expected that not all relevant individual substances will be available in commercial patch test preparations, which is why patch testing of "patients' own materials"—in this case components of the glucose sensor or insulin pump or the plaster used—must be conducted [29]. If a positive patch test reaction is seen against the mixture of substances or rather the full products, individual ingredients must be tested in the next step. Only this way will it be possible to identify the causative allergen and to initiate necessary allergen avoidance. To obtain individual ingredients, the testing dermatologist or allergist is often highly dependent on the willingness of the manufacturer of the patients' own material to provide those ingredients for patch testing. If the manufacturer is unwilling to disclose information, the process of diagnostics might be severely delayed to the detriment of the patient, as the testing physician then needs to acquire the respective substance on other ways (wholesaler of chemicals, etc.), for which also information on the substance is needed by the manufacturer.

Once the allergy-triggering substance has been identified, the physician and patient can look for alternative products from other manufacturers. If possible, before deciding on a glucose sensor or an insulin pump, it should be tried out whether the patient tolerates the patch and the device itself. If changing the system is not an option, in milder cases it can help to spray on a prescription nasal spray containing cortisone before inserting the sensor or pump [26]. If that is not enough, there is still the option of attaching special skin protection patches under the sensor or the pump [26]. If all of these methods fail, the system that triggers the allergy must not be used, since the type IV allergy will persist for life and there is no causal therapy.

One example of a relevant allergen in glucose monitoring systems and insulin pumps is isobornyl acrylate (IBOA) which is frequently used in glues. In the described cases, however, IBOA contained in the device itself was the trigger for allergic reactions [30–34]. Another example of a relevant allergen in plaster used for fixing glucose monitoring systems is ethyl cyanoacrylate, a glue component [35–37]. Those findings led the manufacturer to reformulate the adhesive composition [35, 38]. Other exemplary allergens in cases of allergic contact dermatitis related to medical devices in diabetic patients comprise [39]:

- Epoxy resin [40].
- Phenoxypoly(ethylenoxy) ethylacrylate [41].
- β-Carboxyethyl acrylate [41],
- Benzoylcyclohexanol [41].
- 1,6-Hexanediol diacrylate [42]
- 3-Methyl-2-buten-1-ol [43]
- γ-Butyrolactone [43],
- Dimethyl adipate [43].
- Cyanoacrylate [35].
- Colophonium [44].
- *N,N*-Dimethylacrylamide [33, 45].
- Dipropylene glycol diacrylate [46].
- 2,2′-Methylenebis(6-tert-butyl-4-methylphenol) monoacrylate [47].

If there is suspected allergic contact dermatitis in a diabetic patient using a glucose monitoring system and/or insulin pump, the allergens mentioned above should be considered. It also seems of high importance to keep not only the glue of the plaster in mind but also the components of the device itself.

References

1. Davis JE. Allergies and anaphylaxis: analyzing the spectrum of clinical manifestations. Emerg Med Pract. 2005;7(10):3.
2. Singer E, Zodda D. Allergy and anaphylaxis: principles of acute emergency management. Emerg Med Pract. 2015;17(8):1–19. quiz 20
3. Pfaar O, Ankermann T, Augustin M, Bubel P, Böing S, Brehler R, et al. Guideline on allergen immunotherapy in IgE-mediated allergic diseases: S2K Guideline of the German Society

of Allergology and Clinical Immunology (DGAKI), Society of Pediatric Allergology and Environmental Medicine (GPA), Medical Association of German Allergologists (AeDA), Austrian Society of Allergology and Immunology (ÖGAI), Swiss Society for Allergology and Immunology (SSAI), German Dermatological Society (DDG), German Society of Oto-Rhino-Laryngology, Head and Neck Surgery (DGHNO-KHC), German Society of Pediatrics and Adolescent Medicine (DGKJ), Society of Pediatric Pulmonology (GPP), German Respiratory Society (DGP), German Professional Association of Otolaryngologists (BVHNO), German Association of Paediatric and Adolescent Care Specialists (BVKJ), Federal Association of Pneumologists, Sleep and Respiratory Physicians (BdP), Professional Association of German Dermatologists (BVDD). Allergol Select. 2022;6:167–232. https://doi.org/10.5414/alx02331e.

4. Hürter P. Besonderheiten und Nebenwirkungen der Insulintherapie. In: Hürter P, editor. Diabetes bei Kindern und Jugendlichen: klinik therapie rehabilitation. Berlin, Heidelberg: Springer; 1997. p. 257–66.
5. Datz N, Arens A, Kordonouri O. Insulinallergie. Manchmal bleibt therapeutisch nur die Hyposensibilisierung. Info Diabetol. 2014;8(4):2–8.
6. deShazo RD, Boehm TM, Kumar D, Galloway JA, Dvorak HF. Dermal hypersensitivity reactions to insulin: correlations of three patterns to their histopathology. J Allergy Clin Immunol. 1982;69(2):229–37. https://doi.org/10.1016/0091-6749(82)90104-x.
7. Kahn CR, Rosenthal AS. Immunologic reactions to insulin: insulin allergy, insulin resistance, and the autoimmune insulin syndrome. Diabetes Care. 1979;2(3):283–95. https://doi.org/10.2337/diacare.2.3.283.
8. Richardson T, Kerr D. Skin-related complications of insulin therapy: epidemiology and emerging management strategies. Am J Clin Dermatol. 2003;4(10):661–7. https://doi.org/10.2165/00128071-200304100-00001.
9. Radermecker RP, Scheen AJ. Allergy reactions to insulin: effects of continuous subcutaneous insulin infusion and insulin analogues. Diabetes Metab Res Rev. 2007;23(5):348–55. https://doi.org/10.1002/dmrr.714.
10. Aberumand B, Jeimy S. The complexities of insulin allergy: a case and approach. Allergy Asthma Clin Immunol. 2021;17(1):79. https://doi.org/10.1186/s13223-021-00554-1.
11. Symanzik C, Skudlik C, John SM. Diagnostik in der dermatologie. In: Breuer J, Fritze J, Popa A, Scholtysik D, Seifert J, Wich M, editors. Die Ärztliche Begutachtung: Rechtsfragen, Diagnostik, Funktionsprüfung, Beurteilung. Berlin, Heidelberg, Springer; 2020. p. 1–11.
12. Elfekih H, Hadjkacem F, Elleuch M, Ghorbel D, Charfi N, Mnif F, et al. Successful treatment of insulin allergy with desensitization therapy: a case report and literature review. Iran J Allergy Asthma Immunol. 2019;18(5):572–83. https://doi.org/10.18502/ijaai.v18i5.1927.
13. Fischer M, Fiedler E, Marsch WC, Wohlrab J. Insulin hypersensitivity. Akt Dermatol. 2001;27:372–5.
14. Nagai T, Nagai Y, Tomizawa T, Mori M. Immediate-type human insulin allergy successfully treated by continuous subcutaneous insulin infusion. Intern Med. 1997;36(8):575–8. https://doi.org/10.2169/internalmedicine.36.575.
15. Eapen SS, Connor EL, Gern JE. Insulin desensitization with insulin lispro and an insulin pump in a 5-year-old child. Ann Allergy Asthma Immunol. 2000;85(5):395–7. https://doi.org/10.1016/s1081-1206(10)62554-9.
16. Lluch-Bernal M, Fernández M, Herrera-Pombo JL, Sastre J. Insulin lispro, an alternative in insulin hypersensitivity. Allergy. 1999;54(2):186–7. https://doi.org/10.1034/j.1398-9995.1999.00988.x.
17. Abraham MR, al-Sharafi BA, Saavedra GA, Khardori R. Lispro in the treatment of insulin allergy. Diabetes Care. 1999;22(11):1916–7. https://doi.org/10.2337/diacare.22.11.1916.
18. Moriyama H, Nagata M, Fujihira K, Yamada K, Chowdhury SA, Chakrabarty S, et al. Treatment with human analog (GlyA21, ArgB31, ArgB32) insulin glargine (HOE901) resolves a generalized allergy to human insulin in type 1 diabetes. Diabetes Care. 2001;24(2):411–2. https://doi.org/10.2337/diacare.24.2.411.

19. Jacquier J, Chik CL, Senior PA. A practical, clinical approach to the assessment and management of suspected insulin allergy. Diabet Med. 2013;30(8):977–85. https://doi.org/10.1111/dme.12194.
20. Grammer L. Immunologic reactions to high-molecular weight therapeutic agents. Patterson's allergic diseases. Baltimore, MD: Lippincott, Williams and Wilkins; 2009. p. 304–6.
21. Brans R, Skudlik C. Prevention of hand eczema. Hautarzt. 2019;70(10):797–803. https://doi.org/10.1007/s00105-019-4463-z.
22. Bodtger U, Wittrup M. A rational clinical approach to suspected insulin allergy: status after five years and 22 cases. Diabet Med. 2005;22(1):102–6. https://doi.org/10.1111/j.1464-5491.2004.01352.x.
23. Sola-Gazagnes A, Pecquet C. Allergy to insulin in 2003. J Annu Diabetol Hotel Dieu. 2004:161–79.
24. deShazo RD. Insulin allergy and insulin resistance: two immunologic reactions. Postgrad Med. 1978;63(1):85–92. https://doi.org/10.1080/00325481.1978.11714725.
25. Svedman C, Ulriksdotter J, Lejding T, Bruze M, Mowitz M. Changes in adhesive ingredients in continuous glucose monitoring systems may induce new contact allergy pattern. Contact Derm. 2021;84(6):439–46. https://doi.org/10.1111/cod.13781.
26. Kamann S. Hautprobleme durch Glukosesensoren und Insulinpumpen https://www.apotheken-umschau.de/krankheiten-symptome/diabetes/typ-1/hautprobleme-durch-glukosesensoren-und-insulinpumpen-815903.html; 2021. Accessed 10 July 2023.
27. Antonov D, Schliemann S, Elsner P. Hand dermatitis: a review of clinical features, prevention and treatment. Am J Clin Dermatol. 2015;16(4):257–70. https://doi.org/10.1007/s40257-015-0130-z.
28. Johansen JD, Aalto-Korte K, Agner T, Andersen KE, Bircher A, Bruze M, et al. European Society of Contact Dermatitis guideline for diagnostic patch testing—recommendations on best practice. Contact Derm. 2015;73(4):195–221. https://doi.org/10.1111/cod.12432.
29. Krautheim A, Lessmann H, Geier J. Patch testing with patient's own materials handled at work. In: John SM, Johansen JD, Rustemeyer T, Elsner P, Maibach HI, editors. Kanerva's occupational dermatology. Cham: Springer International Publishing; 2018. p. 1–19.
30. Kamann S, Aerts O, Heinemann L. Further evidence of severe allergic contact dermatitis from isobornyl acrylate while using a continuous glucose monitoring system. J Diabetes Sci Technol. 2018;12(3):630–3. https://doi.org/10.1177/1932296818762946.
31. Herman A, Aerts O, Baeck M, Bruze M, De Block C, Goossens A, et al. Allergic contact dermatitis caused by isobornyl acrylate in Freestyle® Libre, a newly introduced glucose sensor. Contact Derm. 2017;77(6):367–73. https://doi.org/10.1111/cod.12866.
32. Aerts O, Herman A, Mowitz M, Bruze M, Goossens A. Isobornyl acrylate. Dermatitis. 2020;31(1):4–12. https://doi.org/10.1097/der.0000000000000549.
33. Ulriksdotter J, Svedman C, Bruze M, Glimsjö J, Källberg K, Sukakul T, et al. Contact dermatitis caused by glucose sensors-15 adult patients tested with a medical device patch test series. Contact Derm. 2020;83(4):301–9. https://doi.org/10.1111/cod.13649.
34. Kamann S, Oppel E, Liu F, Reichl FX, Heinemann L, Högg C. Evaluation of isobornyl acrylate content in medical devices for diabetes treatment. Diabetes Technol Ther. 2019;21(10):533–7. https://doi.org/10.1089/dia.2019.0163.
35. Aschenbeck KA, Hylwa SA. A diabetic's allergy: ethyl cyanoacrylate in glucose sensor adhesive. Dermatitis. 2017;28(4):289–91. https://doi.org/10.1097/der.0000000000000281.
36. Peeters C, Herman A, Goossens A, Bruze M, Mowitz M, Baeck M. Allergic contact dermatitis caused by 2-ethyl cyanoacrylate contained in glucose sensor sets in two diabetic adults. Contact Derm. 2017;77(6):426–9. https://doi.org/10.1111/cod.12873.
37. Schwensen JF, Friis UF, Zachariae C, Johansen JD. Sensitization to cyanoacrylates caused by prolonged exposure to a glucose sensor set in a diabetic child. Contact Derm. 2016;74(2):124–5. https://doi.org/10.1111/cod.12503.

38. Gisin V, Chan A, Welsh JB. Manufacturing process changes and reduced skin irritations of an adhesive patch used for continuous glucose monitoring devices. J Diabetes Sci Technol. 2018;12(3):725–6. https://doi.org/10.1177/1932296817738076.
39. Herman A, de Montjoye L, Tromme I, Goossens A, Baeck M. Allergic contact dermatitis caused by medical devices for diabetes patients: A review. Contact Derm. 2018;79(6):331–5. https://doi.org/10.1111/cod.13120.
40. Boom BW, van Driel LM. Allergic contact dermatitis to epoxy resin in infusion sets of an insulin pump. Contact Derm. 1985;12(5):280. https://doi.org/10.1111/j.1600-0536.1985.tb01137.x.
41. Busschots AM, Meuleman V, Poesen N, Dooms-Goossens A. Contact allergy to components of glue in insulin pump infusion sets. Contact Derm. 1995;33(3):205–6. https://doi.org/10.1111/j.1600-0536.1995.tb00554.x.
42. Persad S, Lejding T, Svedman C, Mowitz M. The missing link: allergic contact dermatitis caused by 1,6-hexanediol diacrylate in a glucose sensor transmitter. Contact Derm. 2023; https://doi.org/10.1111/cod.14385.
43. Saccabusi S, Boatto G, Asproni B, Pau A. Sensitization to methyl methacrylate in the plastic catheter of an insulin pump infusion set. Contact Derm. 2001;45(1):47–8. https://doi.org/10.1034/j.1600-0536.2001.045001047.x.
44. Passanisi S, Lombardo F, Barbalace A, Caminiti L, Panasiti I, Crisafulli G, et al. Allergic contact dermatitis and diabetes medical devices: 2 clinical cases. Contact Derm. 2018;79(2):115–7. https://doi.org/10.1111/cod.13012.
45. Mowitz M, Herman A, Baeck M, Isaksson M, Antelmi A, Hamnerius N, et al. N,N-dimethylacrylamide—a new sensitizer in the FreeStyle Libre glucose sensor. Contact Derm. 2019;81(1):27–31. https://doi.org/10.1111/cod.13243.
46. Ulriksdotter J, Svedman C, Bruze M, Mowitz M. Allergic contact dermatitis caused by dipropylene glycol diacrylate in the Omnipod® insulin pump. Br J Dermatol. 2022;186(2):334–40. https://doi.org/10.1111/bjd.20751.
47. Oppel E, Högg C, Oschmann A, Summer B, Kamann S. Contact allergy to the Dexcom G6 glucose monitoring system-role of 2,2′-methylenebis(6-tert-butyl-4-methylphenol) monoacrylate in the new adhesive. Contact Derm. 2022;87(3):258–64. https://doi.org/10.1111/cod.14141.

Chapter 17
Diabetes and Blisters

Katharina Meier and Farzan Solimani

Abstract Development of blisters in patients with diabetes is a rare but possible clinical occurrence. Importantly, skin blistering in elderly patients might occur due to a plethora of reasons; therefore it is important for diabetic patients to accurately differentiate between blisters occurring as a sequela of diabetes and coincidently. This correct differentiation bears also relevant diagnostic and therapeutic consequences. The two single diseases that have a direct link with diabetes and/or its therapeutic management are diabetic blisters (also called bullosis diabeticorum) and the autoimmune blistering disease bullous pemphigoid.

17.1 Bullosis Diabeticorum

Diabetic bullae, also known as bullosis diabeticorum, are spontaneously occurring, noninflammatory blisters that affect patients with diabetes mellitus. Overall, diabetic bullae are a rare manifestation of diabetes and are controversially discussed as a separate entity to mechanical blisters [1].

As patients usually already have a long-standing diagnosis of diabetes with diabetic complications such as diabetic polyneuropathy, retinopathy, but also nephropathy, a microangiopathy and associated changes in cell integrity at the basement membrane zone are suspected to be etiopathogenetic. A hyaline degeneration of connective tissue and endothelia (hyalinosis) seen in diabetic nephropathy was also observed in the pancreatic cells and in the capillaries of the skin in long-term diabetics [2]. Less pertinent is the fact that the majority of diabetics do not have blisters and that diabetic blisters can also occur in rare cases as the first manifestation of impaired glucose tolerance. If one compares the development of iatrogenically produced blisters, so-called suction blisters, in patients with diabetes with age-matched

K. Meier (✉) · F. Solimani
Klinik für Dermatologie Venerologie und Allergologie der Charité—Universitätsmedizin Berlin, Berlin, Germany
e-mail: katharina.meier@charite.de; farzan.solimani@charite.de

K. Fritz, G.-S. Tiplica (eds.), *Cutaneous Manifestations in Diabetes*,
https://doi.org/10.1007/978-3-031-65300-1_17

healthy controls, the threshold for the development of blisters in diabetics is significantly lower, thus suggesting that the integrity of the dermal-epidermal junction zone in diabetic patients might be impaired. Patients often report a history of intensive UV exposure in association with the appearance of blisters [3].

Bullosis diabeticorum primarily affects the feet and ankle region, as well as the hands. The toes and the back of the foot are more frequently affected, as are the back of the hand and the fingers. Trauma plays a role in the development of blisters, particularly in the case of pronounced diabetic polyneuropathy. Often, however, no trauma can be identified in bullosis diabeticorum; the blisters occur spontaneously overnight and heal without scarring after a few days to weeks [4].

In a retrospective analysis, an incidence rate of 0.16% per year was described. Large studies are lacking [5].

Bullosis diabeticorum can occur at any age, on average between the ages of 40 and 77. Men are affected about twice as often as women are. Long-standing and inadequately treated diabetes mellitus in particular favors the development of the blisters. It does not matter whether the diabetes is insulin-dependent [3].

17.2 Clinical Presentation and Diagnostic Workup

Clinically, painless, bulging, stable bullae appear, ranging in size from a few millimeters to over 10 cm (Fig. 17.1). The toes and fingers are usually affected, but also the soles of the feet and legs, and rarely the forearms. The blisters are filled with a serous fluid and can rarely show secondary hemorrhagic symptoms. The surrounding skin is unremarkable and those affected usually describe the blisters as asymptomatic.

Histologically, there is usually a mixed picture of subepidermal bullae with partial suprabasal cleft formation without acantholysis. If a blister is older, intraepidermal clefts are usually also seen histologically. This can be explained by the onset of reepithelialization as part of the healing process. The surrounding area shows hardly any inflammatory activity and microvascular changes can occasionally be seen in

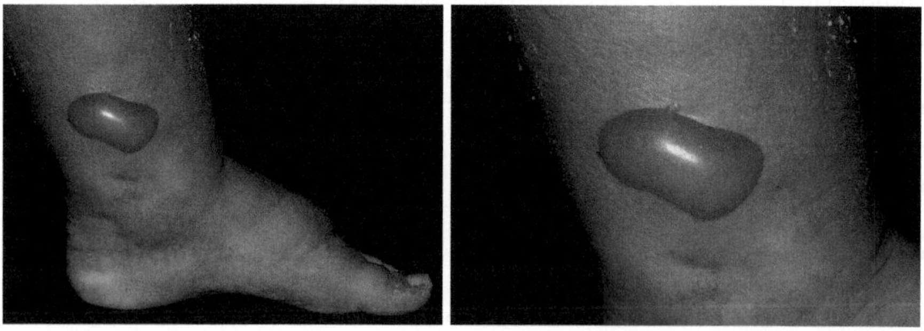

Fig. 17.1 Clinical picture of a diabetes-associated blister of the left foot

the dermis as part of the diabetes. A smaller proportion of patients show primary subepidermal clefting of the blisters. They are more frequently hemorrhagic and heal with atrophy and scarring. Electron microscopy reveals cleavage within the lamina lucida or below the lamina densa and hemidesmosomes and anchoring fibrils are reduced [3].

Direct immunofluorescence remains negative in diabetic blisters but is an important diagnostic tool in the differential diagnosis of bullous pemphigoid (Table 17.1).

Until the blisters have healed completely, meticulous wound care must be provided to prevent secondary infections and ulcerations as part of diabetic foot syndrome. Those individuals affected usually report recurrent courses at similar anatomical locations.

If there is a suspicion of bullosis diabeticorum without known diabetes, an immediate metabolic examination should be carried out. At the same time, ophthalmological and neurological checks are recommended and possible microalbuminuria should also be ruled out [4].

In the differential diagnosis of bullosis diabeticorum, traumatic blisters in the context of polyneuropathy should be considered in particular. These are usually caused by friction or burns or tension blisters from edema or infections. An incipient bullous erysipelas must be considered in the differential diagnosis, particularly in the case of blisters with hyperthermia, tenderness, and redness. Bullous drug reactions such as a fixed drug exanthema or erythema exsudativum multiforme can also occur with blisters without a clear accompanying infiltrate [1].

17.3 Management

The blisters are usually self-limiting and heal without treatment after 2–4 weeks with slight hyperpigmentation. Sterile puncturing of the blisters is only necessary if they are painful or mechanically no longer allow use, e.g., of the shoe. The blister roof should be protected. However, open blisters have an increased risk of becoming

Table 17.1 Clinical and diagnostic differences between diabetic blisters and bullous pemphigoid

	Diabetic blisters	Bullous pemphigoid
Comorbidities/medication associated	Diabetes mellitus	Association with gliptins described
Occurrence	Spontaneous	Chronic recurrent
Predilection sites	Toes and fingers	Hands and feet, axillae, torso
Symptoms	Symptomless	Pruritus
Level of cleavage	Mixed subepidermal and intraepidermal split	Subepidermal
Direct immunofluorescence	Negative	Specific depositions of IgG and C3 along the basement membrane zone
Circulating antibodies	None	Anti-BP180 and/or anti-BP230 antibodies

infected. Topical antiseptics are useful. Topical antibiotics are not recommended due to the risk of resistance and type IV sensitization. Systemic antibiotic treatment with an antibiotic that covers staphylococci and gram-negative pathogens should be considered, particularly in the case of purulent blisters, hyperthermia, and environmental erythema [1].

17.4 Bullous Pemphigoid

Bullous pemphigoid (BP) is an autoimmune skin disorder caused by the presence of circulating IgG antibodies directed against two crucial proteins of the hemidesmosome, the bullous pemphigoid (BP) antigen 180 and BP230. Hemidesmosomes are crucial skin components located at the dermal-epidermal junction zone and help to maintain the dermal/epidermal integrity. As a result of antibody attachment to BP180 and BP230, patients initially develop urticaria-like papules and erythematous lesions, which normally develop into tense pruriginous lesions. While the disease is generally limited to the skin, some patients might also develop mucosal lesions. BP is quite rare in the young and adult population, yet it becomes more frequent starting from the seventh decade. Numerous risk and triggering factors have been so far described. Especially the presence of neurological diseases (i.e., dementia, Parkinson disease, Alzheimer disease, previous strokes) seems to increase the risk of developing BP strongly. Over the years, treatment of diabetes with gliptins/dipeptidyl-peptidase-4 (DPP-4) inhibitors emerged as an important risk factor for BP. Starting from 2011 evidence that DPP-4 inhibitors might trigger BP accumulated rapidly [6]. Patients under gliptin therapy show to have a two- to tenfold higher risk of BP [7]. Importantly, not all DPP-4 inhibitors seemingly have the same capacity to trigger BP. For instance, while vildagliptin appears to be the DPP-4 inhibitor which is most commonly associated with BP, sitagliptin intake seems not to be associated with an increased risk of developing BP [8]. The pathogenesis of this BP subtype still needs to be thoroughly understood. Initial reports on the topic described the presence of distinct features, which differentiate gliptin-induced bullous pemphigoid with normal occurring BP [9]. Main differences are the presence of a noninflammatory phenotype, low IgG titers, and the presence of anti-BP180 antibodies targeting multiple epitopes rather than the non-collagenous epitope N16A, which is the main epitope in normal occurring BP [10]. Current understanding is based on the disruptive role caused by DPP-4 inhibition, which is expressed on several immune cells (B and T cells, macrophages, NK cells). It has been proposed that in certain predisposed individuals, this modulatory effect on immune cells might cause a break of tolerance, which leads to BP [7]. Importantly, in vitro results show that lisinopril, a drug belonging to the class of angiotensin-converting enzyme (ACE) inhibitors, seems to lower the risk of gliptins-induced BP through downregulation of matrix metallopeptidase 9 [11].

17.5 Diagnostic Workout and Management

Diagnostic workout of DPP-4 inhibitors-induced BP does not differentiate than that of BP. The diagnosis is based on histology, direct immunofluorescence, and enzyme-linked immunosorbent assay (ELISA). Histology normally shows the presence of a detachment and blistering along the dermal-epidermal junction zone and the presence of a rich and mixed neutrophilic/T cell infiltrate and eosinophils [12]. Direct immunofluorescence is a central diagnostic tool, since it allows detecting antibody deposition along the dermal-epidermal junction zone, which is characteristically disposed in a linear band pattern. Finally, ELISA permits antigen characterization as well as quantitative antibody measurement, which also delivers information on disease severity [6].

The treatment of DPP-4 inhibitor is similar to normally occurring BP. While DPP-4 withdrawal is recommended, this is normally insufficient to stop the disease, which is initially treated with topical (i.e., clobetasol, betamethasone) and oral (0.5–1 mg pro kg body weight) steroids. Besides this first-line treatment regimen, steroid-sparing agents (azathioprine, dapsone, methotrexate), antibiotic treatment (doxycycline), and monoclonal antibody treatment (dupilumab, anti-interleukin 4, rituximab, anti-CD20) are potential options for long-term treatment [7, 13].

17.6 Differential Diagnosis for Skin Blistering

Particularly in the adult and/or older population, blisters might also occur in other autoimmune blistering diseases such as bullous pemphigoid, epidermolysis bullosa acquisita, pemphigus vulgaris, or dermatitis herpetiformis. These disorders are often accompanied by severe itching and urticarial erythema (Fig. 17.2).

Rarely, porphyria cutanea tarda and pseudoporphyria can show a similar picture to bullosis diabeticorum. In this case, blisters usually appear on the hands and rarely

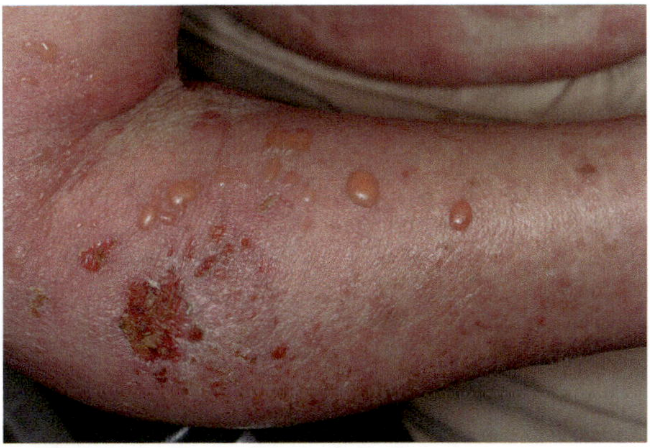

Fig. 17.2 Blisters on the arm in the context of a bullous pemphigoid with accompanying urticarial erythema

on the feet and ankles. Pseudoporphyria can occur in particular with significantly impaired kidney function and cardiovascular disease, as pseudoporphyria is frequently observed during dialysis or diuretic therapy. Other diseases which might cause skin blistering are represented by drug-associated skin reactions, such as erythema exsudativum multiforme or bullous fixed drug eruption [1].

References

1. Chouk C, Litaiem N. Bullosis diabeticorum. Treasure Island (FL): StatPearls; 2024.
2. Taylor SP, Dunn K. Bullosis diabeticorum. J Gen Intern Med. 2017;32(2):220.
3. Kurdi AT. Bullosis diabeticorum. Lancet. 2013;382(9907):e31.
4. Toonstra J, Bullosis diabeticorum. Report of a case with a review of the literature. J Am Acad Dermatol. 1985;13(5 Pt 1):799–805.
5. Ghosh SK, Bandyopadhyay D, Chatterjee G. Bullosis diabeticorum: a distinctive blistering eruption in diabetes mellitus. Int J Diabetes Dev Ctries. 2009;29(1):41–2.
6. Didona D, Schmidt MF, Maglie R, Solimani F. Pemphigus and pemphigoids: clinical presentation, diagnosis and therapy. J Dtsch Dermatol Ges. 2023;21(10):1188–209.
7. Patel PM, Jones VA, Kridin K, Amber KT. The role of dipeptidyl peptidase-4 in cutaneous disease. Exp Dermatol. 2021;30(3):304–18.
8. Harano Y, Mitamura Y, Jiang P, Fujita T, Babazono A. Risk heterogeneity of bullous pemphigoid among dipeptidyl peptidase-4 inhibitors: a population-based cohort study using Japanese latter-stage elderly healthcare database. J Diabetes Investig. 2023;14(6):756–66.
9. Tasanen K, Varpuluoma O, Nishie W. Dipeptidyl peptidase-4 inhibitor-associated bullous pemphigoid. Front Immunol. 2019;10:1238.
10. Salemme A, Fania L, Scarabello A, Caproni M, Marzano AV, Cozzani E, et al. Gliptin-associated bullous pemphigoid shows peculiar features of anti-BP180 and -BP230 humoral response: results of a multicenter study. J Am Acad Dermatol. 2022;87(1):56–63.
11. Nozawa K, Suzuki T, Kayanuma G, Yamamoto H, Nagayasu K, Shirakawa H, Kaneko S. Lisinopril prevents bullous pemphigoid induced by dipeptidyl peptidase 4 inhibitors via the Mas receptor pathway. Front Immunol. 2022;13:1084960.
12. Schmidt E, Zillikens D. Pemphigoid diseases. Lancet. 2013;381(9863):320–32.
13. Borradori L, Van Beek N, Feliciani C, Tedbirt B, Antiga E, Bergman R, et al. Updated S2 K guidelines for the management of bullous pemphigoid initiated by the European Academy of Dermatology and Venereology (EADV). J Eur Acad Dermatol Venereol. 2022;36(10):1689–704.

Chapter 18
Sclerosis in the Diabetic Patient

Andrei Tanasov and George-Sorin Tiplica

Abstract Diabetes mellitus determines the glycation of collagen fibers and the alteration of the connective tissue, resulting in various sclerodermiform manifestations in the diabetic patient. The two main clinical entities described are the scleredema and the limited joint mobility syndrome, which can significantly affect the patient's functionality and quality of life. In addition, these manifestations have been linked with numerous diabetes-related metabolic and microvascular complications and can represent a marker of uncontrolled and poor-prognosis diabetes mellitus; therefore they should be diagnosed at an early stage and managed through a multidisciplinary approach. This can be difficult due to the various presentations and the multiple differential diagnoses, the unpredictable evolution and treatment response, and the lack of validated effective therapies and rehabilitation plans.

Diabetes mellitus is a complex metabolic disorder which determines the dysregulation of multiple key cellular and molecular processes, such as the chemotaxis, phagocytosis, protein expression, antioxidant synthesis, oxygen-free-radical generation, cell proliferation, apoptosis, and extracellular matrix synthesis [1]. Prolonged hyperglycemia determines the nonenzymatic glycation of fibrillar collagen via the pathway of advanced glycation end products (AGEs) [2], similarly to the formation of glycated hemoglobin [3]. The pathogenesis of sclerotic skin changes in diabetes is still poorly understood [4], but a central role is played by the formation of these abnormal, glycated, cross-linked collagen molecules, which are significantly more resistant to mechanical and enzymatic breakdown [3]. The hyperglycemia is also causing fibroblast proliferation, which leads to the production of an abundant extracellular matrix [2], with collagen buildup and trapping of other potential damaging proteins, such as albumin, immunoglobulins, and coagulation factors [3]. Microvascular disease and hypoxia are other triggers for collagen and mucin excessive synthesis [4]. These incompletely deciphered mechanisms determine the accumulation of thickened, aberrant collagen and matrix in the skin (at first in the

A. Tanasov (✉) · G.-S. Tiplica
Dermatovenereology 2, Colentina Clinical Hospital, "Carol Davila" University of Medicine and Pharmacy, Bucharest, Romania
e-mail: George.Tiplica@umfcd.ro

K. Fritz, G.-S. Tiplica (eds.), *Cutaneous Manifestations in Diabetes*,
https://doi.org/10.1007/978-3-031-65300-1_18

papillary dermis but in time also extending to the subcutaneous tissue [2]), causing cutaneous sclerosis for a significant percentage of the diabetic patients, respectively, in the joints, restricting the joint mobility through various dysfunctions of the connective tissue [3].

Diabetes mellitus can lead to a variety of scleroderma-like manifestations, characterized by skin thickening, but differentiating themselves from scleroderma through the absence of Raynaud's phenomenon, capillaroscopic abnormalities, or scleroderma-specific autoantibodies [2]. The main clinical entities of diabetes-related sclerosis are scleredema and the syndrome of limited joint mobility. These sclerodermiform complications can significantly affect the patient's quality of life and functional status [5]; therefore they should be recognized in incipient stages in order to provide an appropriate management, through a much-needed multidisciplinary approach for the diabetic patients.

18.1 Scleredema (Scleredema Adultorum of Buschke, Scleredema Diabeticorum)

Scleredema is a relatively rare sclerodermiform fibromucinosis caused by excessive collagen and mucin accumulation in the dermis [6], mainly reported amongst obese patients with poorly controlled, long-standing diabetes mellitus [7]. The diabetic type (scleredema diabeticorum) is the most frequent, but nondiabetic scleredema also exists: idiopathic or in association with infections (usually streptococcal), monoclonal gammopathies, and other miscellaneous conditions (HIV, autoimmune disorders) [2]. Scleredema is diagnosed in 2.5–14% of the diabetics [8], and it occurs in patients of all ethnicities and ages (more than half of the cases in patients under 20 years old), with a higher prevalence in men (10:1 ratio) [2]. The analysis of 44 patients with scleredema confirms the marked association with diabetes (68%), with an important proportion of patients with poorly controlled, late-onset, insulin-dependent type 2 diabetes (type 2/type 1 diabetes ratio of 6.5) [6]. Other frequent associations are obesity, dyslipidemia, hypertension (metabolic syndrome), and complications of micro- and macroangiopathy [9].

It manifests as a symmetrical, diffuse, progressive nonpitting edema and induration with a "peau d'orange" ("orange peel") aspect of the upper back and shoulders [2], even though rare cases of unusual presentations, such as periorbital edema, have been described [10]. The edema always spares the hands and feet [6]. Patients complain of limited mobility, reduced facial expressions or difficult mastication and articulation [2], pruritus, and only rarely pain [6], while an extensive scleredema of the trunk and shoulders can even lead to restrictive lung disease [11] or an impaired cardiac function [4]. In isolated cases, the restrictive effect of the scleredema was fatal [12]. The superimposed superficial or deep infection of the affected skin can lead to cellulitis and abscess formation [13]. The main ultrasonographic features of uncomplicated scleredema adultorum of Buschke are the lack of soft tissue mass or infection, the thickening of the dermis, and multiple strong echogenic spots and/or posterior shadowing in the dermis [14].

Histology shows a normal, spared epidermis [4] and a three to four times thicker than normal dermis [2], with thickened collagen bundles separated by clefts, which usually contain mucin [8]. The overproduction of mucin may be caused by multiple factors, such as genetics or hyperinsulinism, besides the chronic hyperglycemia that leads to the accumulation of advanced glycation end products (AGEs) [9]. The subcutaneous tissue can also be affected, with fat being replaced by coarse collagen fibers [2], while the adnexal structures are typically preserved [8] but pushed upward [4]. The thickness of the dermis can also be assessed by ultrasonography, with significant differences in mean dermal thickness of the patients (7.01 ± 1.95 mm) versus controls (3.08 ± 0.87 mm) ($p = 0.001$) [14].

Dyslipidemia could be a metabolic dysfunction significantly involved in the pathogenesis of diabetic Buschke scleredema. The screening for scleredema in 113 participants with diabetes mellitus discovered important metabolic particularities in the 11 (9.7%) newly diagnosed scleredema patients: the diabetes patients with scleredema had more severe dyslipidemia (higher proportions of hypertriglyceridemia, $p < 0.05$, and increased mean levels of non-HDL cholesterol, $p < 0.01$) and more frequent vascular complications compared to those without scleredema, meaning that high non-HDL cholesterol levels could be contributing to the development of this diabetic complication [9]. There are reports of LDL apheresis and statin treatment for patients with severe diabetic scleredema, with significant improvements, which highlight once again a potential role of lipid metabolism in the pathogeny of scleredema [15]. Nonsignificant differences in HbA1c levels between the scleredema and non-scleredema groups also suggest that the condition may not be exclusively linked to uncontrolled hyperglycemia, but dyslipidemia could be another ethiopathogenic mechanism [9].

The development of scleredema is insidious and skin thickening usually does not tend to remit, following a chronic and disabling course [2]. In nine study participants who received no treatment according to a "wait and see approach," the disease remained unchanged [6]; however spontaneous remission is documented in particular case reports [4]. The treatment of scleredema is difficult and no therapy is considered specific and effective [2]. In addition, there are no guidelines on the optimal treatment of this disease because of its relative rarity, the limited number of case reports, the lack of randomized controlled trials, and the poorly understood pathogenesis [6]. For patients with debilitating manifestations, treatment with phototherapy is of first choice: UVA1, PUVA, addition of colchicine to PUVA [4], and narrowband UVB can be some of the most effective treatments [2]. Total remission has been achieved with UVA1 alone as well as with systemic steroids alone; however the use of corticoids in diabetic patients should be carefully considered due to their risk of worsening the diabetes [6]. The UVA1 phototherapy in sclerotic skin disease in general is promising due to its collagenase-stimulating effect, which leads to the degradation of the sclerotic, thickened tissue [16].

Some, but not all, patients can have a scleredema improvement with better glucose control [2]. Many other therapies including cyclophosphamide [5], cyclosporine, methotrexate, high-dose penicillin, corticosteroids (local, intralesional, or systemic), tamoxifen, and allopurinol [2] have showed variable results, while intravenous immunoglobulin, electron beam radiotherapy, and extracorporeal photopheresis have also been proposed [8]. Patients with motion or respiratory disability should be referred to physiotherapy [2]. Rehabilitation plans including ultrasonic therapy, manual lymphatic drainage, physiotherapy focused on spine mobilization, range of motion exercises, and strengthening and stretching routines have been studied for both diabetic and nondiabetic scleredema on small patient groups, with no generally appliable results [5].

18.2 Diabetic Stiff-Hand Syndrome (Diabetic Cheiroarthropathy, Syndrome of Limited Joint Mobility)

A waxy, scleroderma-like involvement of the hand with joint stiffness is frequent in both types of diabetes mellitus, affecting 25–50% of both insulin and not insulin-dependent patients, with more severe forms in long-standing disease [2]. Diabetic cheiroarthropathy is one of the most underdiagnosed diabetes mellitus complications, even though it poses an important burden on the diabetic patients [3] and ranges from mild to severe, debilitating manifestations. A symmetrical thickening of the skin on the back of the hands and on the fingers, sometimes referred to as diabetic sclerodactyly [17], is frequent in diabetic patients; however more severe cases present a progressive stiffness of the interphalangeal joints, metacarpophalangeal joints, wrists, and other peripheral flexural joints [2], which determines a restriction in wrist and finger extension and a positive "prayer sign" (failure of palmar contact when the patient is told to join his hands) [18]. A positive "prayer sign" is not specific and may also be noticed in patients with pansclerotic morphea, systemic sclerosis, or scleromyxedema [8]. Another sign observed in advanced phases of induration is the "positive tabletop test," which means that the patient is unable to place his palms flat down on a tabletop with spread fingers [19]. Other characteristic clinical findings are the Huntley's papules ("finger pebbles"), asymptomatic grouped waxy papules that can appear on the hand dorsum, knuckle, and fingers [2]. Diabetic sclerodactyly is common in diabetic children younger than 15 years old (8–50%), especially in those with moderate-severe diabetic disease [20].

The stiffness caused by the skin thickening gives one of the affection's names, and it can significantly reduce the patients' quality of life, interfering with daily activities, even in mild forms [17]. Larger joints beyond the hands, such as elbows, shoulders, and knees, can also be gradually affected in extreme cases [3]. There are even reports of feet involvement in patients with poor glycemic status, manifesting with symmetrical contractures of metatarsophalangeal and interphalangeal joints of foot, typically associating with growth failure, in pediatric patients with uncontrolled, childhood type 1 diabetes mellitus [21].

In a study on 251 type 2 diabetes patients, statistically significant differences in microvascular complications were found in patients with diabetic cheiroarthropathy, compared to the ones who did not have this sclerodermiform condition: an increased prevalence of neuropathy (34.9% vs. 14.9%), retinopathy (35.7% vs. 9.6%), and nephropathy (26.8% vs. 13%) [3]. Therefore, the presence of diabetic cheiroarthropathy could be a significant indicator of diabetic microvascular complications [19], such patients requiring a carefully controlled glycemic status in order to prevent the development of the beforementioned complications [3]. In these patients, the retinopathy risk increases 2.5 times, and, respectively, the nephropathy and neuropathy (reduced nerve velocity in the median and ulnar nerve with reduced vibratory sensation in all four limbs) risks increase 3 times, compared to diabetics without limited joint mobility [21].

Joint problems are frequent in the diabetic population, manifesting as a diversity of conditions such as Dupuytren's disease, flexor tenosynovitis, plantar fasciitis, periarthritis shoulder, Charcot's joint, and carpal tunnel syndrome [3], which can represent important differentials and, at the same time, contribute to the underdiagnosis of diabetic cheiroarthropathy [19]. The absence of pain is an important clinical finding that rules out the mentioned joint affections [21], and other signs can be used in the differential diagnosis (e.g., Tinel's and Phalen's signs for carpal tunnel syndrome) [19].

There are no specific approved treatments for the stiff-hand syndrome, but a strict glycemic control is essential for preventing disease evolution [2] and even in the resolution of some manifestations in early stages [8], while physiotherapy is essential in maintaining the joint mobility [19]. Injection of corticosteroids in the palmar flexor tendon sheath is a common symptomatic practice, and multiple treatments, such as aldose reductase inhibitors, penicillamine, aminoguanidine [2], angiotensin receptor blockers, and thiamine [19], have been tested in small patient groups with limited success [8]. Refractory cases can undergo surgical correction (excision of fibrotic adhesions or nodules) [19]. Regular checkups for joint mobility and musculoskeletal involvement in diabetic patients, which are often missed, can diagnose the cheiroarthropathy at an early stage and help the physician reconsider the patient's risks for microvascular complications [21].

References

1. Adamska O, Stolarczyk A, Gondek A, Maciąg B, Świderek J, Czuchaj P, Modzelewski K. Ligament alteration in diabetes mellitus. J Clin Med. 2022;11(19):5719. https://doi.org/10.3390/jcm11195719.
2. Ferreli C, Gasparini G, Parodi A, Cozzani E, Rongioletti F, Atzori L. Cutaneous manifestations of scleroderma and scleroderma-like disorders: a comprehensive review. Clin Rev Allergy Immunol. 2017;53(3):306–36. https://doi.org/10.1007/s12016-017-8625-4.
3. Paul A, Gnanamoorthy K. The association of diabetic cheiroarthropathy with microvascular complications of type 2 diabetes mellitus: a cross-sectional study. Cureus. 2023;15(3):e36701. https://doi.org/10.7759/cureus.36701.

4. Pereira M, Pinheiro RR, Lencastre A, Bártolo E. Scleredema diabeticorum. Dermatol Rep. 2022;14(4):9477. https://doi.org/10.4081/dr.2022.9477.
5. Mickel M, Jalili A, Gesslbauer C, Crevenna R. Implementation and evaluation of a rehabilitation concept in a patient suffering from Scleredema Adultorum Buschke: a case report. Disabil Rehabil. 2018;40(23):2833–5. https://doi.org/10.1080/09638288.2017.1355939.
6. Rongioletti F, Kaiser F, Cinotti E, Metze D, Battistella M, Calzavara-Pinton PG, Damevska K, Girolomoni G, André J, Perrot JL, Kempf W, Cavelier-Balloy B. Scleredema. A multicentre study of characteristics, comorbidities, course and therapy in 44 patients. J Eur Acad Dermatol Venereol. 2015;29(12):2399–404. https://doi.org/10.1111/jdv.13272.
7. Bustan RS, Wasim D, Yderstræde KB, Bygum A. Specific skin signs as a cutaneous marker of diabetes mellitus and the prediabetic state—a systematic review. Danish Med J. 2017;64(1):A5316.
8. Orteu CH, Ong VH, Denton CP. Scleroderma mimics—clinical features and management. Best Pract Res Clin Rheumatol. 2020;34(1):101489. https://doi.org/10.1016/j.berh.2020.101489.
9. Csonka V, Bódis B, Kovács D, Farkas N, Kálmán E, Czirják L, Varjú C. Screening for the presence of scleroedema adultorum of Buschke in patients with diabetes mellitus: newly diagnosed patients had a high prevalence of dyslipidaemia. Lipids Health Dis. 2021;20(1):47. https://doi.org/10.1186/s12944-021-01473-1.
10. Ioannidou DI, Krasagakis K, Stefanidou MP, Karampekios S, Panayiotidis J, Tosca AD. Scleredema adultorum of Buschke presenting as periorbital edema: a diagnostic challenge. J Am Acad Dermatol. 2005;52(2 Suppl. 1):41–4. https://doi.org/10.1016/j.jaad.2004.06.037.
11. García-Arpal M, Bujalance-Cabrera C, Banegas-Illescas ME, Sánchez-Caminero MP, González-Ruiz L, Villasanti-Rivas N. Scleredema diabeticorum in a patient: un uncommon etiology of restrictive lung pattern Escleredema diabeticorum en un paciente: una etiología infrecuente de patrón restrictivo pulmonar. Dermatol Online J. 2021;27(3):13030/qt71g4k3qf.
12. Miyares FJ, Kuriakose R, Deleu DT, El-Wahad NA, Al-Hail H. Scleredema diabeticorum with unusual presentation and fatal outcome. Indian J Dermatol. 2008;53(4):217–9. https://doi.org/10.4103/0019-5154.44798.
13. Shrestha B, Sharma E, Mukhtar O, Kaler J, Thapa S, Khalid M. Scleredema diabeticorum with superimposed cellulitis and abscess formation. Case Rep Endocrinol. 2018;2018:9513768. https://doi.org/10.1155/2018/9513768.
14. Ha DH, Lee MJ, Kim SJ. Ultrasonographic findings of scleredema adultorum of Buschke involving the posterior neck. Korean J Radiol. 2018;19(3):425–30. https://doi.org/10.3348/kjr.2018.19.3.425.
15. Koga N. Effects of low-density lipoprotein apheresis on coronary and carotid atherosclerosis and diabetic scleredema in patients with severe hypercholesterolemia. Therap Apheresis. 2001;5(4):244–51. https://doi.org/10.1046/j.1526-0968.2001.00341.x.
16. Kroft EB, Berkhof NJ, van de Kerkhof PC, Gerritsen RM, de Jong EM. Ultraviolet A phototherapy for sclerotic skin diseases: a systematic review. J Am Acad Dermatol. 2008;59(6):1017–30. https://doi.org/10.1016/j.jaad.2008.07.042.
17. Afzal W, Movahedian M, Singh BB, Teller K, Cervellione K, Pinsker RW. Diabetic sclerodactyly mimicking limited sclerosis: case report and review of the literature. J Endocrinol Metab. 2017;7(2):68–71. https://doi.org/10.14740/jem394e.
18. Gamage K, Bulugahapitiya U. Stiffened hands in a diabetic patient: diabetic sclerodactyly. JCEM Case Rep. 2022;1(1):luac003. https://doi.org/10.1210/jcemcr/luac003.
19. Swain J, Teli B, Sahoo A, Kasukurti L. Limited joint mobility in type 1 diabetes: diabetic cheiroarthropathy, a neglected entity. JCEM Case Rep. 2023;1(4):luad068. https://doi.org/10.1210/jcemcr/luad068.
20. Mastrangelo G, Meneghel A, Martini G, Moretti C, Zulian F. Juvenile diabetes and systemic sclerosis: just a coincidence? Pediatr Rheumatol Online J. 2022;20(1):81. https://doi.org/10.1186/s12969-022-00741-3.
21. Gerrits EG, Landman GW, Nijenhuis-Rosien L, Bilo HJ. Limited joint mobility syndrome in diabetes mellitus: a mini review. World J Diab. 2015;6(9):1108–12. https://doi.org/10.4239/wjd.v6.i9.1108.

Chapter 19
The Nail in Diabetes Mellitus

Eckart Haneke

Abstract Diabetes mellitus may affect all organ systems of the human body; however, nail changes are almost all indirect and related either to the specific biochemical action of high glucose levels, the inherent immunosuppression with increased susceptibility to mainly bacterial and fungal infections, the vascular impairment associated with diabetes, and particularly the diabetic neuropathy. All these factors act together and can damage the nail unit in many different ways.

Yellow, brittle, often opaque nails are frequent and splinter hemorrhages may be observed. Bacterial infections are commonly seen as acute paronychia, whereas *Candida* strains usually cause chronic infections. *Pseudomonas aeruginosa* may form bacterial biofilms on the nails' undersurface and stain it green. Onychomycoses, mostly co-occurring with dermatophyte foot infections, are very frequent, and their prevalence is related to the blood sugar level. Diabetic vasculopathy may cause variable nail alterations. Together with diabetic neuropathy, they lead to diabetic foot syndrome with a profound impact on the nail unit. Finally, the nail unit may also serve as a diagnostic tool giving information on the long time course of diabetes.

19.1 Introduction

The nail is both a skin as well as a musculoskeletal appendage. It consists of four different epithelial components: the nail matrix producing the nail plate, the nail bed keeping the nail plate firmly attached to the dorsal aspect of the tip of the digit, the skin of the lateral and proximal nail folds, and the epidermis of the undersurface of the proximal nail fold also called the eponychium. The proximal nail fold overlies most of the matrix, and its free margin forms the cuticle which is a firmly adhering

E. Haneke (✉)
Department of Dermatol Inselspital, Univ. Berne, Bern, Switzerland

Private Dermatol Practice Dermaticum, Freiburg, Germany

Centro Dermatol, Inst CUF, Senhora da Hora, Matosinhos, Porto, Portugal

K. Fritz, G.-S. Tiplica (eds.), *Cutaneous Manifestations in Diabetes*,
https://doi.org/10.1007/978-3-031-65300-1_19

keratin structure sealing the nail pocket against the penetration of foreign substances, potential pathogens, and dirt. Under the free margin of the nail plate is the hyponychium that is a specialized keratin structure allowing the nail plate to physiologically detach from the distal end of the nail bed; it has a similar sealing function as it prevents foreign substances to get under the nail (Fig. 19.1a, b) [1]. The subungual connective tissue is the so-called onychodermis, which is differentiated under the matrix into the onychomatricodermis [2–4]. The matrix is the sole structure to produce nail plate, which is a plaque-like sheet of hard keratin biochemically identical to hair shaft keratin. Anything that happens to the nail matrix will therefore

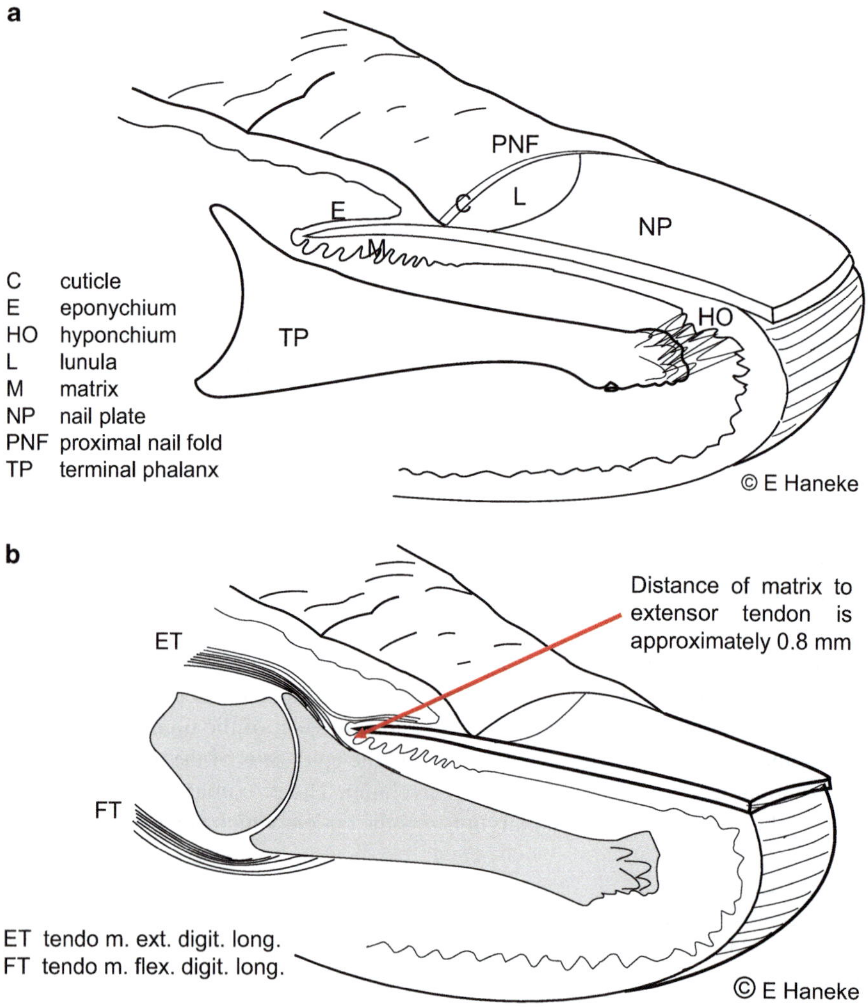

Fig. 19.1 Sagittal section through the distal phalanx (**a**). Anatomical relation of nail matrix and tendons (**b**)

result in a nail plate alteration, and anything incorporated in the nail plate comes from the matrix. The nail bed does not produce nail substance, and everything that happens in the bed remains under the nail – except when it is able to actively invade the plate, like invasive fungi.

The surgical anatomy of the nail unit is straightforward. The apex of the matrix deep in the proximal portion of the dorsal aspect of the distal phalanx is the most proximally located part of the nail unit and very close the distal interphalangeal joint; hence joint disease is often associated with nail changes, particularly in psoriasis. The matrix is also very close to the underlying bone, approximately 0.8 mm. The extensor digiti tendon inserts under the matrix in the proximal half of the distal phalanx and sends also some fibers into the connective tissue of the proximal nail fold. Together with the lateral ligaments and the very strong flexor tendon, an aponeurosis is formed for the distal joint that gives stability to it in all directions. The matrix has a white color seen as the lunula where it is not covered by the proximal nail fold. The nail bed shines through the semitransparent nail plate as a pink structure. Its capillaries run longitudinally in four to six levels one over the other; this unique arrangement is the anatomical basis for the splinter hemorrhages, 3- to 5-mm-long dark lines with a maximum diameter of 1 mm sometimes also seen in diabetes. The proximal nail fold also contains long capillaries that run longitudinally toward its end; they are seen with the dermatoscope or capillary microscope and give valuable information in a variety of metabolic and connective tissue diseases [1]. The nail was termed a "special microcirculatory region" with many arteriovenous anastomoses and blocking structures such as the glomus bodies. Computerized laser-Doppler flowmetry and infrared photo-pulse plethysmography, computerized telethermography with physical stimulations, high-performance contact thermography, and continuous registration of the skin temperature associated with pharmacological vasoactive stimulation are helpful to identify and functionally characterize the "microcirculatory regions" of the lower limbs [5].

Diabetes mellitus is a metabolic disease virtually affecting directly or indirectly all organ systems. Multiple skin lesions are seen in diabetic patients, and nail changes are also frequent. However, really specific nail alterations allowing the diagnosis of diabetes mellitus to be made right away do not exist [6]. Nail changes are almost always indirect due to metabolic disturbances, vascular disturbances, diabetic neuropathy, and associated immune deficiency including frequent infections. In addition, advanced glycosylation end products may probably be responsible for yellowing of the nails. Stiff erythrocyte membranes increase the viscosity of the blood and cause postcapillary venule engorgement. All these factors have to be considered when evaluating a patient's nails, and sometimes the nails may give a hint at diabetes of which the patient had not been aware before [7, 8]. Onychoscopy may enhance the diagnostic yield of diabetic nail changes [9]. A distinction of type 1 from type 2 diabetes by the appearance of the nails is usually not possible. Often, the nail changes are similar to those observed in old age as they are secondary to impaired blood supply. Nails are often overlooked but accessible and may serve as a window into patients' general health; they should be an integral part of all thorough clinical examinations [6].

The nail may also be used as a diagnostic tool such as the determination of C-protein (connection protein secreted by the ß cells of the pancreas) or for nail fold capillaroscopy to assess microvascular damage.

19.2 Clinical Appearance of the Nail

The nails of both the fingers and toes may be dull and lusterless, often also less transparent and more yellowish (Figs. 19.2 and 19.3). This color change of the nails is thought to be secondary to advanced glycosylation end products. Periungual erythema may develop from increased viscosity of blood caused by stiff red blood cell membranes, which results in engorgement of the postcapillary venules in the papillary dermis [7]. It is suggested that these skin changes may eventually be used as a reflection of the patient's current (as well as past) metabolic status. The nail bed may appear paler and less pink. The growth rate is often slowed down, and patients may complain of brittle or hard nails [10–12]. Some authors described virtual loss of the lunula, and disappearance of the lunula is also a characteristic sign of Terry's nails [13]. These were originally described in hepatic cirrhosis, but subsequent studies found them also in several other diseases including diabetes mellitus [14]. Terry's nails are a type of apparent leukonychia involving the fingernails of both hands just sparing the most distal part of the nail. They are similar to Lindsay's half-and-half nails in which the opacity of the nail only occupies around one half of the nail bed in contrast to the usual 80% in Terry's nails [15, 16]. Lindsay's nails may indicate the risk of chronic kidney disease [17]. Muehrcke's nails are characterized by transverse white lines running parallel to the lunula and being separated by areas of normal pink nail bed color [18]. They are actually slightly arched pale band-like zones in the nail bed thought to be a vascular phenomenon and are usually seen in association with hypoalbuminemia, e.g., from nephrotic syndrome due to chronic diabetic kidney failure but also due to liver diseases, malnutrition, and

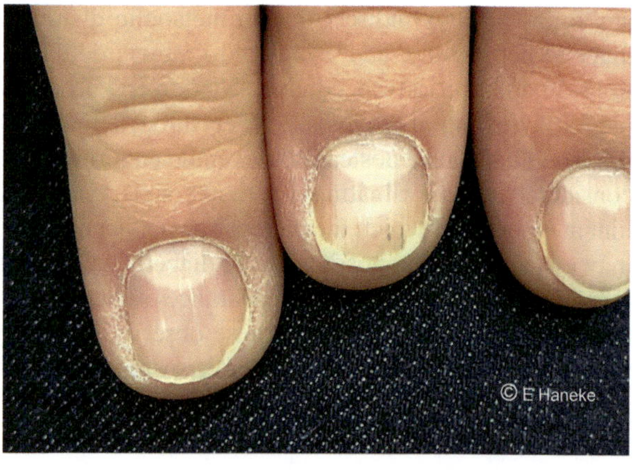

Fig. 19.2 Slightly yellowish nails with splinter hemorrhages

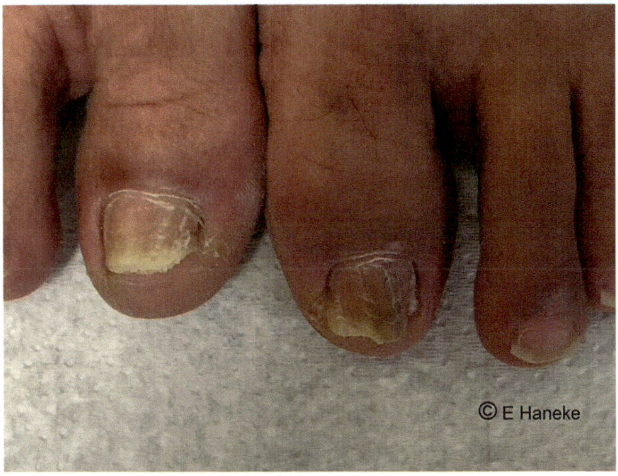

Fig. 19.3 Yellowish, thickened, and less transparent nails in a 59-year-old diabetic patient with tinea pedum and onychomycosis

chemotherapy and other diabetes mellitus comorbidities. True leukonychia is not directly related to diabetes. Beau's lines were observed in uncontrolled diabetes. Onychoscopy demonstrated nail changes in two thirds of diabetic patients revealing microhemorrhage in 24% and splinter hemorrhage in 14%. Longitudinal striations and distal subungual onychomycosis were seen in 24% each, superficial pitting in 20%, distal onycholysis in 18%, subungual hyperkeratosis in 12%, dilated vessels in 10%, and distal yellowish discoloration in 8% [8].

Onychogryposis was found to be associated with vascular disease, particularly type 2 diabetes mellitus (OR 7.89 [6.72–9.27], $p < 1E{-}6$) [19]. It may be complicated by paronychia and onychomycosis [20].

Epidermolysis bullosa acquisita was repeatedly observed in association with diabetes mellitus. This severe autoimmune disease can lead to nail dystrophy and nail loss in extreme cases, similar to dystrophic epidermolysis bullosa hereditaria [21].

About one half of the glucagonoma patients develop diabetes [22]. The most characteristic lesions around the nail are erosive skin lesion and brittle nails. These lesions are virtually identical to those of acute pellagra, acrodermatitis enteropathica, acrodermatitis acidemica, and acquired zinc deficiency.

19.3 Infections of and Around the Nail

Diabetes mellitus is notorious for the increased rate of infections of virtually all organs including the nails and periungual skin [23–25]. Infections of the nail unit in diabetes mellitus may be bacterial and fungal; viral diseases such as common warts or recurrent herpes simplex are not specifically mentioned as being more frequent [7]. Sculptured nails are artificial nails are also at higher risk to develop paronychia with subungual abscess and felon [26].

Bacterial infections may be due to staphylococci, streptococci, *Pseudomonas aeruginosa*, *Proteus vulgaris*, and *Escherichia coli*, but in principle all common pathogenic bacteria may be found. Up to one fifth of these infections are polymicrobial [27]. Infections with anaerobic and gas-producing bacteria are rare but occur predominantly in diabetics and immune-compromised individuals [28, 29]. The pyogenic cocci usually cause acute infections resulting in paronychia and bullous lesions that are also called runaround because of their specific course around the nail [30]. Involvement of deeper layers of the proximal nail fold causes a decrease in nail growth, which is later seen as a Beau's line. Severe infections necessitating amputation are mainly seen in hot climate [31, 32]. Bacterial cultures and sensitivity tests should be performed in order to allow a targeted antibiotic treatment to be instituted. "Minor" finger infections only remain minor when diagnosed and treated properly [33]. If left untreated in a diabetic subject, the matrix may irreversibly be destroyed by the infection in a relatively short period of time.

Pseudomonas aeruginosa is often found in diabetics [34]. When affecting the nail, it usually colonizes the undersurface of an onycholytic nail, more rarely its dorsal surface, coloring it dirty greenish. Although this green nail phenomenon is usually harmless for immunocompetent persons, it may pose a risk for diabetics and cancer patients and other types of immunosuppression (Fig. 19.4). As this colonization is a biofilm on the onycholytic part of the nail, systemic antibiotics are not indicated; the treatment of choice are soaks with diluted white vinegar or bleach (similar as recommended for atopic eczema) several times a day. If a subungual abscess is seen and the pus has a greenish tinge, a pseudomonas abscess has to be suspected and requires partial removal of the overlying nail plate, frequent daily soaks with a disinfective agent, and a systemic antibiotic according to the sensitivity spectrum.

Proteus vulgaris is another pathogen occasionally seen in nail infections. It stains the nail surface a dirty grey due to the generation of bacterial sulfur hydrogen,

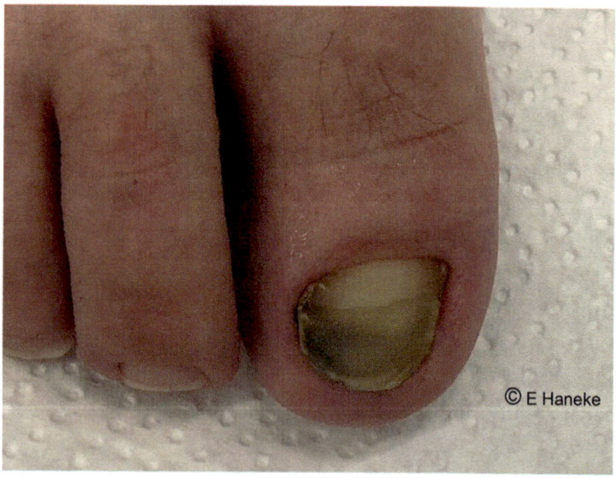

Fig. 19.4 Green nail from colonization of the undersurface of the onycholytic big toenail with *Pseudomonas aeruginosa*

which reacts with (heavy) metals from the environment to form dark metal sulfides [1].

Diabetes foot infection also involves the toes, particularly with paronychia and distal osteitis; this is often in association with diabetic neuropathy and neuropathic ulcers that may be part of the acro-osteolysis ulcero-mutilans syndrome of Bureau-Barrière although this is usually due to alcoholic neuropathy [35–38]. Here, the patients have painless hyperkeratoses of the sole of the foot including the toes, often associated with arterial hyperperfusion of the toe, macro-toe, and macro-toenail formation, which is due to autonomic neuropathy with paralysis of the arterial innervation, particularly of the arterial shunts [39]. The macro-nails in these patients tend to grow in, and as the patient has no pain, enormous granulation tissue and severe infection may be present. This often encounters enterobacteria that are frequently multiresistant. These findings are independent from the etiology of the neuropathy, whether hereditary, diabetic, or alcoholic [40–42].

Ingrown nails were seen in a diabetes clinic in almost every seventh patient with diabetes type 2 [43]. Combined with diabetic neuropathy and loss of pain sensation, enormous swelling and secondary infection may occur. Treatment may be conservative with nail braces or surgical with selective matrix horn removal by phenolization and other methods [44, 45]. The phenolization technique has the advantage that it is technically very simple, has an extremely low postoperative pain and morbidity, and does usually not require antibiotic treatment. Phenol itself is a very strong disinfective agent [46–49].

Fungal nail infections are extremely common (Figs. 19.3, 19.5, and 19.6) [50–57]. A Portuguese study cited more than 50% of the diabetes patient had an onychomycosis [58]. This was seen as extremely embarrassing in a Polish study although most patients lacked basic understanding of their disease and were not aware of prophylactic measures [59]. There is an increase in specialist treatment of onychomycoses, particularly by diabetic patients; of 7.2 million Danes, 2072 were treated in hospital for their onychomycosis, and many of them had concurrent

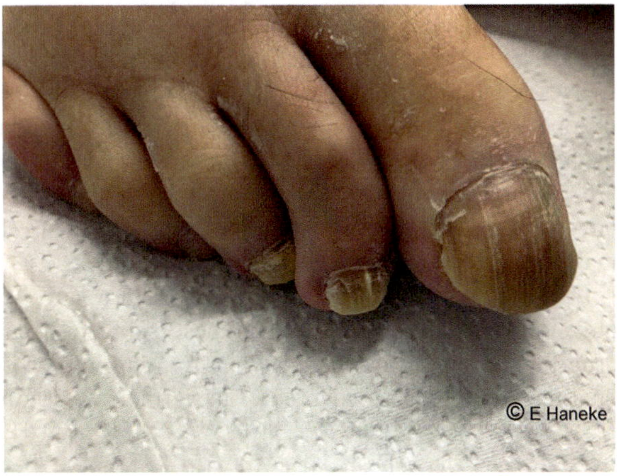

Fig. 19.5 Tinea pedum and onychomycosis in a 76-year-old male diabetic patient

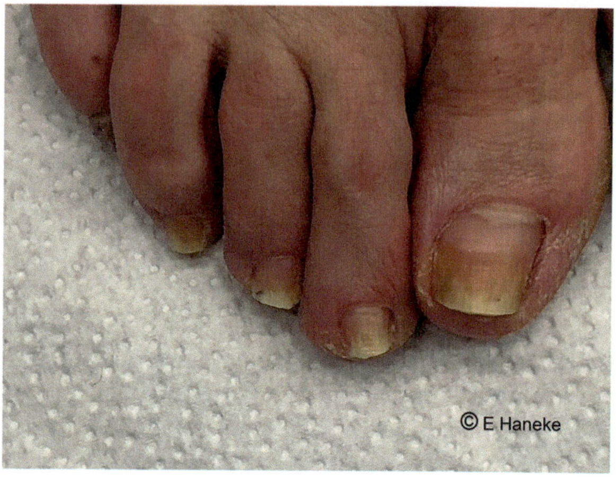

Fig. 19.6 Tinea pedum and onychomycosis in a 59-year-old male diabetic patient; the mild desquamation of the nail folds is indicative of tinea pedum

diabetes [60]. The odds ratio for diabetes in patients with onychomycosis was found to be 3.28 [61]. The predominant nail pathogens of fungal nail infections in diabetics are the dermatophytes *Trichophyton rubrum* and *Trichophyton mentagrophytes*, though yeasts and non-dermatophyte molds may also be etiologic, particularly in diabetic and immunosuppressed patients [62–65]. Fungi infect the nail plate, bed, and matrix, leading to discoloration of the nail, thickening of the subungual region, and, when advanced, onycholysis [66]. Onychomycosis may lead to secondary bacterial infections and predispose to erysipelas and cellulitis. In the diabetic population, jagged mycotic toenails may injure the adjacent tissue increasing the risk of foot ulcer, with sepsis or amputation as a potential consequence [67]. In diabetes type 1, dry moccasin type tinea pedum is often associated with onychomycosis [68, 69]. A large-scale study also found a high infection rate in almost 2500 patients where advanced age, male sex, diabetes, diabetic peripheral neuropathy, and lower limb ischemia were independent risk factors for the development of onychomycosis [70]. The longer the diabetes exists, the higher the probability to develop onychomycosis, and the frequency of onychomycosis correlates with the blood sugar level [71, 72]. Fungal infections of the nail are common and mainly due to *Trichophyton rubrum* and *Trichophyton interdigitale*, but non-dermatophyte molds like *Fusarium* species are now emergent pathogens, the latter being increasingly found since both histopathology and polymerase chain reaction (PCR) are more frequently used as diagnostic tools [73, 74]. *T. rubrum* is found in approximately 70% of the cases [75]. Wearing closed shoes increases the risk of fungal nail infection [76]. Candida onychomycosis clinically similar to dermatophyte onychomycosis may be observed in diabetics, particularly in hot climate [77, 78].

Although terbinafine and itraconazole are safe in diabetes, the treatment of onychomycosis is challenging as these subjects usually take several drugs, and drug interactions, particularly when treating with azole compounds, may render pharmacotherapy less favorable. Nevertheless, combined topical and systemic therapy is needed in most cases with terbinafine being generally the drug of choice for dermatophyte infections and itraconazole for non-dermatophytes [67, 79–81]; this is combined with atraumatic nail avulsion using 40% urea paste under occlusion for 5 days to remove all infected material and to apply either amorolfine 5% once or twice per week or ciclopirox 8% nail varnish daily [82–84]. Terbinafine is the treatment of choice in the elderly population, if there are no contraindications, as there are less associated side effects and drug interactions compared to itraconazole [85, 86].

Lasers are now more and more often recommended for the treatment of onychomycoses. Two different approaches are used: neodymium YAG laser to kill the pathogenic fungus and carbon dioxide lasers to enhance the penetration of topical antifungal drugs. It was shown that a temperature of 55 °C over a period of at least 10 min is necessary to kill *T. rubrum*; as the nail plate is not the site of primary fungal infection the laser would have to reach the nail bed keratosis where the vast majority of the fungi are located. It is impossible to apply a temperature of 55 °C or more to the nail bed without anesthesia, but it may be tolerated by patients with diabetic neuropathy who then get a severe burn [87]. Despite some appealing hypotheses, the exact mechanism of Nd-YAG laser treatment for onychomycoses is not known; nevertheless this device is now often recommended also in diabetics [88]. Neither the first controlled study nor another four-arm controlled study did find any difference in the results of Nd-YAG laser and sham treatment [89, 90]. Care has to be taken as the lack of pain sensation may pose the patient at risk for heat damage of the nail bed and distal matrix.

Particularly in fingers of middle-aged women but also in adolescents with type 1 diabetes, *Candida albicans* and some other candida strains are thought to cause chronic paronychia [91, 92]. The proximal and lateral nail folds are swollen, red, sometimes glistening, and the cuticle has disappeared [93]. This can cause a loosening of the proximal nail folds undersurface from the nail plate and a dead space develops that may trap organic material, dirt, pathogens, and potentially also sensitizing substances that keep the chronic inflammation going on. Periodic remissions and acute flares are characteristic [94]. This in turn impairs the matrix and leads to irregular transverse furrows and ridges. The diagnosis of candida paronychia should be proven by mycologic testing such as a potassium hydroxide wet mount and culture [95].

19.4 Nail Psoriasis in Diabetes Mellitus

The risk of psoriasis is doubled in persons with the metabolic syndrome that very often accompanies diabetes. However, the type and the severity of nail involvement are not significantly different [96]. The metabolic syndrome of diabetes also increases the risk for psoriatic arthritis [97].

19.5 Vascular Lesions

The normal nail unit is generously supplied with blood vessels of the paired volar and palmar/plantar proper digital arteries. However, impairment of the blood supply is a frequent cause of nail dystrophy. Both diabetic macroangiopathy and microangiopathy lead to slow nail growth with brittle nails, Beau's lines, pterygium formation, splinter hemorrhages, and yellowish nails. However, the nails may also become thicker and darker and develop surface irregularities. The thicker nails grow even slower and are prone to be infected with pathogenic fungi (Fig. 19.7) [98]. Arterial insufficiency may rarely result in a pterygium, which is a fusion of the cul-de-sac with fusion of the proximal nail fold with the underlying matrix and nail bed. Even the hyponychium may disappear and a pterygium inversum develop which is a painful obliteration of the subungual space at the level of the distal nail bed [99]. Pressure on the nail may cause nail bed ulceration. The most severe angiopathic alterations lead to digital gangrene [100]. Small arterial emboli in the nail bed may be seen as hemorrhagic spots 2–3 mm in diameter or as splinter hemorrhages, which represent capillary bleedings of the longitudinally oriented nail bed capillaries; however, splinter hemorrhages are quite common and may occur spontaneously or in association with a great variety of diseases. Some authors assume that the diabetic yellow nails have to be attributed to vascular damage. They are opaque, thickened, and excessively curved in transverse direction [101]. Coarse transverse grooves, and ridges may appear, and sometimes the cuticle disappears, and the nails may take on a greenish-yellow tinge quite like in the yellow nail syndrome. However, the co-occurrence of diabetes mellitus type 2 and yellow nail syndrome was probably coincidental [102].

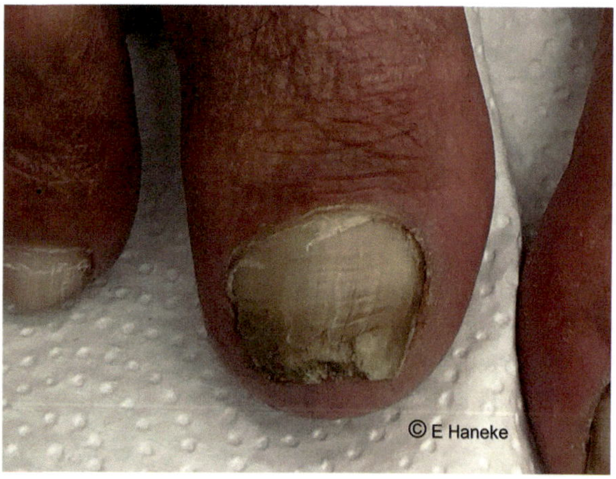

Fig. 19.7 Toenails of a 63-year-old diabetic patient with thickening of the nail, whitish discoloration, and loss of nail transparency

19.6 Diabetic Neuropathy

Typical neuropathy is the cause of most foot problems in diabetic patients. It is primarily sensory and motoric but may also involve the autonomous nerves the latter being responsible for several of the vascular phenomena of diabetes. However, in the diabetic foot and diabetic nail, none of these causes should be seen as isolated as even the microangiopathy may damage the nerves. The lack of pain, temperature, vibration, and proprioceptive sensation not only leads to the well-known thick calluses with deep-reaching plantar ulcers but may also result in ulcerations of the nail bed. The autonomic neuropathy may lead to lack of temperature adaptation and sweating. Unnoticed trauma may cause chronic repeated trauma to the matrix and nail bed with thickening of the nail and ram's horn-like nails called onychogryposis. Frostbites and burns from testing the temperature of bath water with the tip of the foot are common and have an influence on the nail organ. Bilateral little and ring finger nail dystrophy was observed in an elderly man with diabetic mononeuropathy of the ulnar nerves. He complained of tingling of these fingers and showed shortening, yellow discoloration, and fragility of these four fingernails [103].

19.7 The Nail and Periungual Tissue as a Diagnostic Tool in Diabetes Mellitus

The capillaries of the nail fold normally run almost horizontally under the epidermis and are easily observable with a capillary microscope or reflectance confocal laser scanning microscope; the latter even allows the bloodstream in the capillaries and the single erythrocytes to be evaluated [104]. It has long been a diagnostic method in rheumatology as more or less diagnostic patterns of alterations are seen in various collagen vascular diseases. This is not the place to go into details of capillaroscopy; however, the technique has proven to give valuable information in diabetic patients. It is very sensitive and correlates with the fundoscopy findings – retinopathy [105]. A deep learning model is able to give high-precision information of the presence of diabetes and predict the history of cardiovascular events [106].

Nail clippings can be examined for various substances that are associated with diabetes mellitus. Connection peptide (C-peptide) is secreted with insulin, and low insulin production is associated with low C-peptide levels in urine, hair, and nails [107].

Laser-induced breakdown spectroscopy is able to determine many metals and metalloids in solid tissues including nails and to estimate specific patterns of trace element and mineral content associated with multiple pathologies, including diabetes mellitus type 2 [108].

N-acetyl-leucine (N-Ac-Leu) is a potential biomarker of diabetes. It can be determined in the nail as it is significantly lower in diabetic patients than in prediabetics and healthy persons [109].

Confocal Raman spectroscopy is a technique that allows alterations in different biochemical components of the nails in diabetes type 2 to be determined and to detect health complications early [110].

Multi-elemental profiling of different biological samples, called ionomics, for several major types of metabolic diseases, such as diabetes mellitus, reveals distinct and dynamic patterns of ion contents and their potential benefits in the detection and prognosis of these illnesses. Each type of metabolic diseases has shown a relatively unique distribution of ions in biofluids and hair/nails from patients, potentially serving as potential indicators for the respective disease [111].

References

1. Haneke E. Histopathology of the Nail—Onychopathology. Boca Raton: CC Press; 2017.
2. Lee DY, Park JH, Shin HT, Jang KT, Kwon GY, Shim JS. Onychodermis (specialized nail mesenchyme) containing onychofibroblasts in horizontal sections of the nail unit. Br J Dermatol. 2012;166(5):1127–9. https://doi.org/10.1111/j.1365-2133.2011.10722.x.
3. Haneke E. CD10 and the nail. J Cutan Pathol. 2017;44(11):907–8. https://doi.org/10.1111/cup.13030.
4. Lee D, Abudureyimu G, Park JH, Jang KT, Kwon GY, Shim JS. Characterization of the onychomatricodermis containing onychofibroblasts of the nail unit: Histology, immunohistochemistry, and electron microscopic study. Ann Dermatol. 2021;33(2):108–15. https://doi.org/10.5021/ad.2021.33.2.108.
5. Curri SB. Anatomie microvasculaire de la peau et de ses annexes [Microvascular anatomy of the skin and its appendages]. Phlebologie. 1990;43(3):407–30. French
6. Greene RA, Scher RK. Nail changes associated with diabetes mellitus. J Am Acad Dermatol. 1987;16(5 Pt 1):1015–21. https://doi.org/10.1016/s0190-9622(87)70131-5.
7. Huntley AC. Cutaneous manifestations of diabetes mellitus. Dermatol Clin. 1989;7(3):531–46.
8. Brenner MA. Cutaneous stigmata frequently found in the diabetic limb. Clin Podiatr Med Surg. 1986;3(3):523–32.
9. Hofny ERM, Tawfik YM, Hasan MS, Salah Y, Rageh MA. Dermoscopy of subclinical nail involvement in patients with diabetes mellitus: a case-control study. Clin Exp Dermatol. 2023;48(5):490–4. https://doi.org/10.1093/ced/llad010.
10. van de Kerkhof PC, Pasch MC, Scher RK, Kerscher M, Gieler U, Haneke E, Fleckman P. Brittle nail syndrome: a pathogenesis-based approach with a proposed grading system. J Am Acad Dermatol. 2005;53(4):644–51.
11. Lee DK, Lipner SR. Optimal diagnosis and management of common nail disorders. Ann Med. 2022;54(1):694–712. https://doi.org/10.1080/07853890.2022.2044511.
12. Anees M, Butt G, Gull S, Nazeer A, Hussain I, Ibrahim M. Factors affecting dermatological manifestations in patients with end stage renal disease. J Coll Physicians Surg Pak. 2018;28(2):98–102. https://doi.org/10.29271/jcpsp.2018.02.98.
13. Terry R. White nails in hepatic cirrhosis. Lancet. 1954;266(6815):757–9. https://doi.org/10.1016/s0140-6736(54)92717-8.
14. Lin CP, Alkul M, Truitt JM, Stetson CL. Development of Terry's nails after a gastrointestinal bleed. Proc (Bayl Univ Med Cent). 2020;34(2):312–3. https://doi.org/10.1080/08998280.2020.1842078.
15. Holzberg M, Walker HK. Terry's nails: revised definition and new correlations. Lancet. 1984;1(8382):896–9. https://doi.org/10.1016/S0140-6736(84)91351-5.

16. Sharma V, Kumar V. Muehrcke lines. CMAJ. 2013;185(5):E239. https://doi.org/10.1503/cmaj.120269.
17. Raja SM. Chronic kidney disease entertained from Lindsay's nails: a case report and literature review. Clin Case Rep. 2021;9(7):e04426. https://doi.org/10.1002/ccr3.4426. PMID: 34257982
18. Witkowska AB, Jasterzbski TJ, Schwartz RA. Terry's nails: a sign of systemic disease. Indian J Dermatol. 2017;62(3):309–11. https://doi.org/10.4103/ijd.IJD_98_17.
19. Choo ZN, Lipner SR. Onychogryphosis is associated with dermatologic and vascular disease: a case-control study of the all of us research program. Skin Appendage Disord. 2023;9(4):252–7. https://doi.org/10.1159/000530096.
20. Srivastava G, Srivastava G. Onychogryphosis: ram's horn nail. J Roy Coll Phys Edinb. 2022;52(3):259. https://doi.org/10.1177/14782715221126761.
21. Xiao A, Sathe NC, Tsuchiya A. Epidermolysis bullosa acquisita. In: StatPearls. Treasure Island, FL: StatPearls Publishing; 2023.
22. Perrier M, Brugel M, Gérard L, Goichot B, Lièvre A, Lepage C, Hautefeuille V, Do Cao C, Smith D, Thuillier P, Cros J, Cadiot G, Walter T, de Mestier L. Characteristics and treatment options of glucagonomas: a national study from the French Group of Endocrine Tumors and ENDOCAN-RENATEN network. Eur J Endocrinol. 2023:lvad157. https://doi.org/10.1093/ejendo/lvad157.
23. Joshi N, Caputo GM, Weitekamp MR, et al. Infections in patients with diabetes mellitus. N Engl J Med. 1999;341:1906–12.
24. Aragón-Sánchez J, López-Valverde ME, Víquez-Molina G, Milagro-Beamonte A, Torres-Sopena L. Onychomycosis and tinea pedis in the feet of patients with diabetes. Int J Low Extrem Wounds. 2023;22(2):321–7. https://doi.org/10.1177/15347346211009409.
25. Satasia M, Sutaria AH. Nail whispers revealing dermatological and systemic secrets: An analysis of nail disorders associated with diverse dermatological and systemic conditions. Cureus. 2023;15(9):e45007. https://doi.org/10.7759/cureus.45007.
26. Roberge RJ, Weinstein D, Thimons MM. Perionychial infections associated with sculptured nails. Am J Emerg Med. 1999;17(6):581–2. https://doi.org/10.1016/s0735-6757(99)90201-2.
27. Fowler JR, Ilyas AM. Epidemiology of adult acute hand infections at an urban medical center. J Hand Surg Am. 2013;38(6):1189–93. https://doi.org/10.1016/j.jhsa.2013.03.013.
28. Brook I. Prevotella and Porphyromonas infections in children. J Med Microbiol. 1995;42(5):340–7. https://doi.org/10.1099/00222615-42-5-340.
29. Kall S, Vogt PM. Chirurgische Therapie von Infektionen der Hand--Teil I [Surgical therapy for hand infections. Part I]. Chirurg. 2005;76(6):615–25.; quiz 626-7. Germanica. https://doi.org/10.1007/s00104-005-1043-9.
30. Leggit JC. Acute and chronic paronychia. Am Fam Physician. 2017;96(1):44–51.
31. Ezeldeen K, Fahal AH, Ahmed ME. Management of hand infection in Khartoum. East Afr Med J. 1992;69(11):616–8.
32. Ahmed ME, Mahmoud SM, Mahadi SI, Widatalla AH, Shawir MA, Ahmed ME. Hand sepsis in patients with diabetes mellitus. Saudi Med J. 2009;30(11):1454–8.
33. Canales FL, Newmeyer WL 3rd, Kilgore ES Jr. The treatment of felons and paronychias. Hand Clin. 1989;5(4):515–23.
34. Molina DN, Colón M, Bermúdez RH, Ramírez-Ronda CH. Unusual presentation of Pseudomonas aeruginosa infections: a review. Bol Asoc Med P R. 1991;83(4):160–3.
35. Lipsky BA, Berendt AR, Embil J, De Lalla F. Diagnosing and treating diabetic foot infections. Diabetes Metab Res Rev. 2004;20(Suppl. 1):S56–64. https://doi.org/10.1002/dmrr.441.
36. Lipsky BA, Berendt AR, Deery HG, Embil JM, Joseph WS, Karchmer AW, LeFrock JL, Lew DP, Mader JT, Norden C, Tan JS, Infectious Diseases Society of America. Diagnosis and treatment of diabetic foot infections. Clin Infect Dis. 2004;39(7):885–910. https://doi.org/10.1086/424846.
37. Berendt AR, Lipsky B. Is this bone infected or not? Differentiating neuro-osteoarthropathy from osteomyelitis in the diabetic foot. Curr Diab Rep. 2004;4(6):424–9.

38. Mendes AL, Miot HA, Haddad V Jr. Diabetes mellitus and the skin. An Bras Dermatol. 2017;92(1):8–20. https://doi.org/10.1590/abd1806-4841.20175514.
39. Mensing H. Mit welchen dermatologischen Folgen, abgesehen von einer Akroosteopathie, ist bei Diabetespolyneuropathie zu rechnen? [What dermatologic sequelae, aside from acro-osteopathy, can be expected in diabetic polyneuropathy?]. Z Hautkr. 1986;61(18):1277–9.
40. Michel U, Hornstein OP. Akroosteopathia ulcero-mutilans der Füsse [Ulceromutilating acroosteopathy of the feet]. Dtsch Med Wochenschr. 1982;107(5):169–75. https://doi.org/10.1055/s-2008-1069893.
41. Garbe C, Vogel HP, Tebbe B, Nüssel F, Marx P, Orfanos CE. Akroosteopathia ulcero-mutilans bei hereditären Neuropathien. Differentialdiagnostische und pathogenetische Aspekte [Ulcero-mutilating acro-osteopathy in hereditary neuropathies. Differential diagnosis and pathogenesis]. Dtsch Med Wochenschr. 1989;114(16):628–32. https://doi.org/10.1055/s-2008-1066647.
42. Bühler-Singer S, Hiller D, Boateng B, Albrecht HP, Seidel C, Hornstein OP. Kutane Mikrozirkulationsstörung bei diabetischen neuropathischen Plantarulzera. Ist eine Beeinflussung durch retrograde transvenöse Perfusionstherapie möglich? [Disordered cutaneous microcirculation in diabetic neuropathic foot ulcer. Is modification by retrograde transvenous perfusion therapy possible?]. Hautarzt. 1995;46(6):400–5. https://doi.org/10.1007/s001050050273.
43. Vural S, Bostanci S, Koçyigit P, Çaliskan D, Baskal N, Aydin N. Risk factors and frequency of ingrown nails in adult diabetic patients. J Foot Ankle Surg. 2018;57(2):289–95. https://doi.org/10.1053/j.jfas.2017.10.006.
44. Erdogan FG, Erdogan G. Long-term results of nail brace application in diabetic patients with ingrown nails. Dermatologic Surg. 2008;34(1):84–6.; discussion 86-87. https://doi.org/10.1111/j.1524-4725.2007.34013.x.
45. Misiak P, Terlecki A, Rzepkowska-Misiak B, Wcisło S, Brocki M. Comparison of effectiveness of electrocautery and phenol application in partial matricectomy after partial nail extraction in the treatment of ingrown nails. Pol Przegl Chir. 2014;86(2):89–93. https://doi.org/10.2478/pjs-2014-0016.
46. Haneke E. Surgical treatment of ingrowing toenails. Cutis. 1986;37(4):251–6.
47. Baran R, Haneke E. Matricectomy and nail ablation. Hand Clin. 2002;18(4):693–6., viii; discussion 697. https://doi.org/10.1016/s0749-0712(02)00038-0.
48. Haneke E. Controversies in the treatment of ingrown nails. Dermatol Res Pract. 2012;2012:783924. https://doi.org/10.1155/2012/783924.
49. Thakur V, Vinay K, Haneke E. Onychocryptosis—decrypting the controversies. Int J Dermatol. 2020;59(6):656–69. https://doi.org/10.1111/ijd.14769.
50. Lugo-Somolinos A, Sanchez JL. Prevalence of dermatophytosis in patients with diabetes. J Am Acad Dermatol. 1992;26:408–10.
51. Buxton PK, Milne LJ, Prescott RJ, Proudfoot MC, Stuart FM. The prevalence of dermatophyte infection in well-controlled diabetics and the response to Trichophyton antigen. Br J Dermatol. 1996;134:900–3.
52. Romano C, Massai L, Asta F, Signorini AM. Prevalence of dermatophytic skin and nail infections in diabetic patients. Mycoses. 2001;44(3–4):83–6.
53. Dogra S, Kumar B, Bhansali A, Chakrabarty A. Epidemiology of onychomycosis in patients with diabetes mellitus in India. Int J Dermatol. 2002;41(10):647–51. https://doi.org/10.1046/j.1365-4362.2002.01528.x.
54. Piérard GE, Piérard-Franchimont C. The nail under fungal siege in patients with type II diabetes mellitus. Mycoses. 2005;48:339–42.
55. Gupta AK, Konnikov N, MacDonald P, Rich P, Rodger NW, Edmonds MW, McManus R, Summerbell RC. Prevalence and epidemiology of toenail onychomycosis in diabetic subjects: a multicentre survey. Br J Dermatol. 1998;139(4):665–71. https://doi.org/10.1046/j.1365-2133.1998.02464.x.
56. Saunte DM, Holgersen JB, Haedersdal M, Strauss G, Bitsch M, Svendsen OL, Arendrup MC, Svejgaard EL. Prevalence of toe nail onychomycosis in diabetic patients. Acta Dermatol Venereol. 2006;86(5):425–8. https://doi.org/10.2340/00015555-0113.

57. Manzano-Gayosso P, Hernández-Hernández F, Méndez-Tovar LJ, Palacios-Morales Y, Córdova-Martínez E, Bazán-Mora E, López-Martinez R. Onychomycosis incidence in type 2 diabetes mellitus patients. Mycopathologia. 2008;166(1):41–5. https://doi.org/10.1007/s11046-008-9112-5.
58. Sanches MM, Roda Â, Pimenta R, Filipe PL, Freitas JP. Cutaneous manifestations of diabetes mellitus and prediabetes. Acta Medica Port. 2019;32(6):459–65. https://doi.org/10.20344/amp.10738.
59. Korpowska K, Majchrzycka M, Adamski Z. The assessment of prophylactic and therapeutic methods for nail infections in patients with diabetes. Postepy Dermatol Alergol. 2022;39(6):1048–52. https://doi.org/10.5114/ada.2022.113585.
60. Lindsø Andersen P, Jørgensen IF, Saunte DML, Jemec GB, Pedersen OB, Brunak S. An increase in specialist treatment for onychomycosis: an unexplained tendency. A retrospective study of patients treated for onychomycosis in Danish hospitals from 1994 to 2018. J Fungi (Basel). 2022;9(1):33. https://doi.org/10.3390/jof9010033.
61. Albucker SJ, Falotico JM, Choo ZN, Matushansky JT, Lipner SR. Risk factors and treatment trends for onychomycosis: a case-control study of onychomycosis patients in the all of US Research Program. J Fungi (Basel). 2023;9(7):712. https://doi.org/10.3390/jof9070712.
62. Rich P, Hare A. Onychomycosis in a special patient population: focus on the diabetic. Int J Dermatol. 1999;38:17–9.
63. Borba OSM, Ogawa MM, Kirsztajn GM, Tomimori J. Onychomycosis in immunocompromised population: phenotypic and molecular identification. Mycoses. 2023;66(11):1018–24. https://doi.org/10.1111/myc.13634.
64. Khalifa A, Alreshidi IG, Alaradi LA, Alrashidi YM. Tinea unguium and tinea pedis and their correlation with diabetes mellitus in the general population in the Hail region, Saudi Arabia: a cross-sectional study. Cureus. 2023;15(6):e40116. https://doi.org/10.7759/cureus.40116.
65. Vazheva GZ, Zisova LG, Becheva EA, Chonov VR, Dichev VD, Miteva-Katrandzhieva TM, Rachkovska ZV, Orbetzova MM, Belovezhdov VT. In search of dermatophytes—frequency and etiology of fungal infections in patients with and without diabetes mellitus. Folia Med (Plovdiv). 2022;64(6):922–31. https://doi.org/10.3897/folmed.64.e85486.
66. Gupta AK, Humke S. The prevalence and management of onychomycosis in diabetic patients. Eur J Dermatol. 2000;10:379–84.
67. Liddell LT, Rosen T. Laser therapy for onychomycosis: fact or fiction? J Fungi (Basel). 2015;1(1):44–54. https://doi.org/10.3390/jof1010044.
68. Mayser P, Hensel J, Thoma W, Podobinska M, Geiger M, Ulbricht H, Haak T. Prevalence of fungal foot infections in patients with diabetes mellitus type 1: underestimation of moccasin-type tinea. Exp Clin Endocrinol Diabetes. 2004;112(5):264–8. https://doi.org/10.1055/s-2004-817974.
69. Szepietowski JC, Reich A, Garlowska E. Factors influencing coexistence of toenail onychomycosis with tinea pedis and other dermatomycoses: a survey of 2761 patients. Arch Dermatol. 2006;142:1279–84.
70. Ogawa T, Matsuda A, Ogawa Y, Tanaka R. Risk factors for the development of tinea pedis and onychomycosis: Real-world evidence from a single-podiatry center, large-scale database in Japan. J Dermatol. 2023; https://doi.org/10.1111/1346-8138.16991.
71. Alteras I, Saryt E. Prevalence of pathogenic fungi in the toe-webs and toe-nails of diabetic patients. Mycopathologia. 1979;67(3):157–9. https://doi.org/10.1007/BF00470749.
72. Boyko EJ, Ahroni JH, Cohen V, Nelson KM, Heagerty PJ. Prediction of diabetic foot ulcer occurrence using commonly available clinical information: the Seattle Diabetic Foot Study. Diabetes Care. 2006;29(6):1202–7. https://doi.org/10.2337/dc05-2031.
73. Rammlmaier A, Mühlethaler K, Haneke E. Fusarium onychomycoses in Switzerland—a mycological and histopathological study. Mycoses. 2019;62:928–31.
74. Navarro-Pérez D, García-Oreja S, Tardáguila-García A, León-Herce D, Álvaro-Afonso FJ, Lázaro-Martínez JL. Microbiological culture combined with PCR for the diagnosis of onychomycosis: descriptive analysis of 121 patients. Mycoses. 2023;66(12):1045–9. https://doi.org/10.1111/myc.13648.

75. Lipner SR, Scher RK. Onychomycosis: clinical overview and diagnosis. J Am Acad Dermatol. 2019;80(4):835–51.
76. Ilkit M, Durdu M. Tinea pedis: the etiology and global epidemiology of a common fungal infection. Crit Rev Microbiol. 2015;41(3):374–88.
77. Aljehani FH, Alluhaibi R, Alhothali OS, Fageeh SM, Al Ahmadi GA, Malyani RZ. An unusual presentation of candidal onychomycosis: a case report. Cureus. 2023;15(8):e43222. https://doi.org/10.7759/cureus.43222.
78. Jayatilake JA, Tilakaratne WM, Panagoda GJ. Candidal onychomycosis: a mini-review. Mycopathologia. 2009;168(4):165–73. https://doi.org/10.1007/s11046-009-9212-x.
79. Cribier B, Bakshi R. Terbinafine in the treatment of onychomycosis: a review of its efficacy in the high-risk populations and in patients with nondermatophyte infections. Br J Dermatol. 2004;150:414–20.
80. Gupta AK, Ryder JE, Lynch LE, Tavakkol A. The use of terbinafine in the treatment of onychomycosis in adults and special populations: a review of the evidence. J Drugs Dermatol. 2005;4(3):302–8.
81. Cathcart S, Cantrell W, Elewski B. Onychomycosis and diabetes. J Eur Acad Dermatol Venereol. 2009;23(10):1119–22.
82. Haneke E. General aspects of onychomycoses. In: Torres-Rodiguez JM, editor. Proceedings of the X congress of the international society for human and animal mycology—ISHAM. Barcelona: JR Prous Sci Publ; 1988. p. 235–9.
83. Shemer A, Eshel Y, Gupta AK, Farhi R, Haneke E, Daniel R, Foley K, Quinlan EM. Once weekly application of urea 40% and bifonazole 1% leads to earlier nail removal in onychomycosis. Skin Appendage Disord. 2020;6:304–8.
84. Baran R, Hay R, Haneke E, Tosti A. Onychomycosis. 2nd ed. Oxon: Taylor & Francis; 2006.
85. Farkas B, Paul C, Dobozy A, Hunyadi J, Horváth A, Fekete G. Terbinafine (Lamisil) treatment of toenail onychomycosis in patients with insulin-dependent and non-insulindependent diabetes mellitus: a multicentre trial. Br J Dermatol. 2002;146:254–60.
86. Loo DS. Onychomycosis in the elderly: drug treatment options. Drugs Aging. 2007;24(4):293–302.
87. Helou J, Korkomaz J, Haber R, Habre M, Tomb R. Laser treatment of onychomycosis: beware of ring block anesthesia! Lasers Med Sci. 2015;30(9):2399–400. https://doi.org/10.1007/s10103-015-1744-3.
88. Ramzy B, Emily AH, Jiryis B, Ziad K. Nd:YAG 1064 nm laser treatment for onychomycosis—is it really effective? A prospective assessment for efficiency and factors contributing to response. Mycoses. 2023; https://doi.org/10.1111/myc.13657.
89. Hollmig ST, Rahman Z, Henderson MT, Rotatori RM, Gladstone H, Tang JY. Lack of efficacy with 1064-nm neodymium:yttrium-aluminum-garnet laser for the treatment of onychomycosis: a randomized, controlled trial. J Am Acad Dermatol. 2014;70(5):911–7. https://doi.org/10.1016/j.jaad.2013.12.024.
90. Nijenhuis-Rosien L, Kleefstra N, van Dijk PR, Wolfhagen MJHM, Groenier KH, Bilo HJG, Landman GWD. Laser therapy for onychomycosis in patients with diabetes at risk for foot ulcers: a randomized, quadruple-blind, sham-controlled trial (LASER-1). J Eur Acad Dermatol Venereol. 2019;33(11):2143–50. https://doi.org/10.1111/jdv.15601.
91. Chabasse D. Peut-on chiffrer la fréquence des onychomycoses? [Can we evaluate the frequency of onychomycosis?]. Ann Dermatol Venereol. 2003;130(12 Pt 2):1222–30. French
92. Kapellen TM, Galler A, Kiess W. Higher frequency of paronychia (nail bed infections) in pediatric and adolescent patients with type 1 diabetes mellitus than in non-diabetic peers. J Pediatr Endocrinol Metab. 2003;16(5):751–8. https://doi.org/10.1515/jpem.2003.16.5.751.
93. Haneke E. Fungal infections of the nail. Semin Dermatol. 1991;10(1):41–53.
94. Dorko E, Baranová Z, Jenca A, Kizek P, Pilipcinec E, Tkáciková L. Diabetes mellitus and candidiases. Folia Microbiol (Praha). 2005;50(3):255–61. https://doi.org/10.1007/BF02931574.
95. Chi CC, Wang SH, Chou MC. The causative pathogens of onychomycosis in southern Taiwan. Mycoses. 2005;48(6):413–20. https://doi.org/10.1111/j.1439-0507.2005.01152.x.

96. Agarwal K, Das S, Kumar R, De A. Psoriasis and its association with metabolic syndrome. Indian J Dermatol. 2023;68(3):274–7. https://doi.org/10.4103/ijd.ijd_418_23.
97. Makos A, Kuiper JH, Kehoe O, Amarasena R. Psoriatic arthritis: review of potential biomarkers predicting response to TNF inhibitors. Inflammopharmacology. 2023;31(1):77–87. https://doi.org/10.1007/s10787-022-01092-x.
98. Levin C. Medical evaluation and treatment. In: Levin ME, O'Neal LW, editors. The diabetic foot. 3rd ed. CV Mosby; 1983. p. 16.
99. Domonkos AN, Arnold HL Jr, Odom RB. Andrews' diseases of the skin: clinical dermatology. 7th ed. Philadelphia: WB Saunders; 1982. p. 978.
100. Zaias N. The Nail in Health and Disease. Jamaica NY: SP Medical and Scientific Books; 1980. p. 207.
101. Lithner F. Purpura, pigmentation and yellow nails of the lower extremities in diabetics. Acta Med Scand. 1976;199(3):203–8. https://doi.org/10.1111/j.0954-6820.1976.tb06717.x.
102. Gorguner M, Kaynar H, Karaoglanoglu N. Yellow nail syndrome in association with protein-losing enteropathy in a diabetic patient. Ann Saudi Med. 2002;22(3–4):207–9. https://doi.org/10.5144/0256-4947.2002.207.
103. Mann RJ, Burton JL. Nail dystrophy due to diabetic neuropathy. Br Med J (Clin Res Ed). 1982;284(6327):1445. https://doi.org/10.1136/bmj.284.6327.1445.
104. Hegyi J, Hegyi V, Messer G, Arenberger P, Ruzicka T, Berking C. Confocal laser-scanning capillaroscopy: a novel approach to the analysis of skin capillaries in vivo. Skin Res Technol. 2009;15(4):476–81. https://doi.org/10.1111/j.1600-0846.2009.00393.x.
105. Bogusz-Górna K, Polańska A, Dańczak-Pazdrowska A, Żaba R, Sumińska M, Fichna P, Kędzia A. Non-invasive detection of early microvascular changes in juveniles with type 1 diabetes. Cardiovasc Diabetol. 2023;22(1):285. https://doi.org/10.1186/s12933-023-02031-y.
106. Shah R, Petch J, Nelson W, Roth K, Noseworthy MD, Ghassemi M, Gerstein HC. Nailfold capillaroscopy and deep learning in diabetes. J Diabetes. 2023;15(2):145–51. https://doi.org/10.1111/1753-0407.13354.
107. Salih JM, Abdulateef DS. Detection of C-peptide in human hair and nail: a comparison between healthy persons and persons with type 1 diabetes. BMJ Open Diabetes Res Care. 2020;8(1):e001297. https://doi.org/10.1136/bmjdrc-2020-001297.
108. Skalny AV, Korobeinikova TV, Aschner M, Baranova OV, Barbounis EG, Tsatsakis A, Tinkov AA. Medical application of laser-induced breakdown spectroscopy (LIBS) for assessment of trace element and mineral in biosamples: laboratory and clinical validity of the method. J Trace Elem Med Biol. 2023;79:127241. https://doi.org/10.1016/j.jtemb.2023.127241.
109. Li J, Zhou X, Takashi M, Todoroki K, Toyo'oka T, Shi Q, Jin T, Zhe MJ. Development of a novel method for analysing N-acetyl-DL-leucine enantiomers in human fingernail by UPLC-ESI-MS/MS and the evaluation in diabetes mellitus. Clin Chim Acta. 2023;545:117367. https://doi.org/10.1016/j.cca.2023.117367.
110. Veras JMMF, Coelho LS, Neto LPM, Almeida RM, Silva GCD, Santana FB, Garcia LA, Martin AA, Favero PP. Identification of biomarkers in diabetic nails by Raman spectroscopy. Clin Chim Acta. 2023;544:117363. https://doi.org/10.1016/j.cca.2023.117363.
111. Zhang Y, Huang B, Jin J, Xiao Y, Ying H. Recent advances in the application of ionomics in metabolic diseases. Front Nutr. 2023;9:1111933. https://doi.org/10.3389/fnut.2022.1111933.

Chapter 20
Acne Inversa and Diabetes

Evgenia Makrantonaki and Christos C. Zouboulis

Abstract Diabetes has been clearly associated with hidradenitis suppurativa (HS) in the last years. HS is a chronic inflammatory skin disease that has a significant impact on patients' quality of life. It is characterized by recurrent painful nodules, abscesses and draining tunnels in predominantly intertriginous areas. The average prevalence of HS ranges from 0.4% to 1%, with familial and sporadic forms of the disease. HS is mostly diagnosed by clinical observation and history. An emerging tool for the assessment of deep-seated lesions is ultrasound imaging. Severity grading is still enormously based on the Hurley staging system, whereas a new validated, dynamic classification, severity grading and outcome measure, the International Hidradenitis Suppurativa Severity Score System (IHS4), has been developed. Chronic symptoms or consequences of uncontrolled disease include pain, drainage, pruritus, odour, low self-esteem, sleep and sexual dysfunction, and poor mental health. The pathogenesis of HS is thought to involve follicular dyskeratosis, hyperkeratosis and dilatation, follicular rupture and chronic inflammation with architectural tissue changes. Apart from diabetes, HS is in general associated with metabolic syndrome and other cardiovascular risk factors, polycystic ovary syndrome and depression. It has also been mainly associated with other immune-mediated diseases, such as inflammatory bowel disease and spondyloarthropathy.

E. Makrantonaki (✉)
Departments of Dermatology, Venereology, Allergology and Immunology, Staedtisches Klinikum Dessau, Brandenburg Medical School Theodor Fontane and Faculty of Health Sciences Brandenburg, Dessau, Germany

Derma Center Wildeshausen, Wildeshausen, Germany

Department of Dermatology and Allergology, Ulm University, James Franck Ring/Meyerhoffstraße, Ulm, Germany

C. C. Zouboulis
Departments of Dermatology, Venereology, Allergology and Immunology, Staedtisches Klinikum Dessau, Brandenburg Medical School Theodor Fontane and Faculty of Health Sciences Brandenburg, Dessau, Germany

European Hidradenitis Suppurativa Foundation e.V., Auenweg, Dessau, Germany
e-mail: christos.zouboulis@klinikum-dessau.de

K. Fritz, G.-S. Tiplica (eds.), *Cutaneous Manifestations in Diabetes*,
https://doi.org/10.1007/978-3-031-65300-1_20

HS has a profound negative impact on patients' quality of life and is an under-diagnosed and under-treated disease. A multidisciplinary management approach may be required to ensure the best outcomes, given the associated comorbid disorders. Few isolated lesions (mild disease according to IHS4) might be treated by topically applied preparations, and locally limited lesions (moderate disease) can be treated by conventional surgery or laser, whereas widespread lesions (severe disease) may be better treated with systemic therapy alone or in combination with radical surgery, if scarring is prominent. Systemic therapy may include antibiotics (clindamycin and rifampicin, tetracyclines), acitretin and biologic agents (adalimumab, secukinumab – registered biologics – but also infliximab, bimekizumab, anakinra (off label)). Adjuvant measures such as pain management, treatment of superinfections, weight loss and tobacco cessation must be taken into account.

20.1 Introduction

Hidradenitis suppurativa (HS)/acne inversa is a chronic, inflammatory, recurrent, debilitating skin disease of the hair follicles. It usually presents post-pubertally with painful, deep, inflamed lesions in the apocrine gland-bearing areas of the body, most commonly the axillary, inguinal and anogenital regions [1]. HS is a disease of the terminal hair follicle. It is associated with lymphohistiocytic inflammation, granulomatous reaction, sinus tract formation and scarring. It appears that the deep part of the follicle is involved. A consistent finding regardless of disease duration is follicular occlusion due to dyskeratosis and hyperkeratosis. This leads to occlusion of the apocrine gland with subsequent follicular rupture, inflammation and rarely secondary infection [1] (Fig. 20.1). HS has been associated with overweight, cardiovascular diseases, active smoking, high triglycerides and low high-density lipoprotein (HDL) [2, 3]. In particular, an association with diabetes and metabolic syndrome has been recently documented [4, 5]. HS has a profound negative impact on patients' quality of life and is an under-diagnosed and under-treated disease [6].

20.2 Epidemiology

The prevalence of HS in epidemiological studies shows a significant variability owing to heterogeneous measurement methods and populations being studied. On average, it ranges from 0.4 to 1%, with familial and sporadic forms of the disease [7]. Numerous studies have shown that HS occurs more frequently in women than in men. In a US cohort, 73.8% of those affected were female. The peak incidence was found to be in the third decade of life [8]. In contrast, a Korean secondary data analysis showed a higher incidence of HS in male patients (61.3%) [9]. Genetic factors could play a role here. In this sense, patients of Caucasian origin in the USA had a lower prevalence of HS than African-American patients [8]. Asians, on the

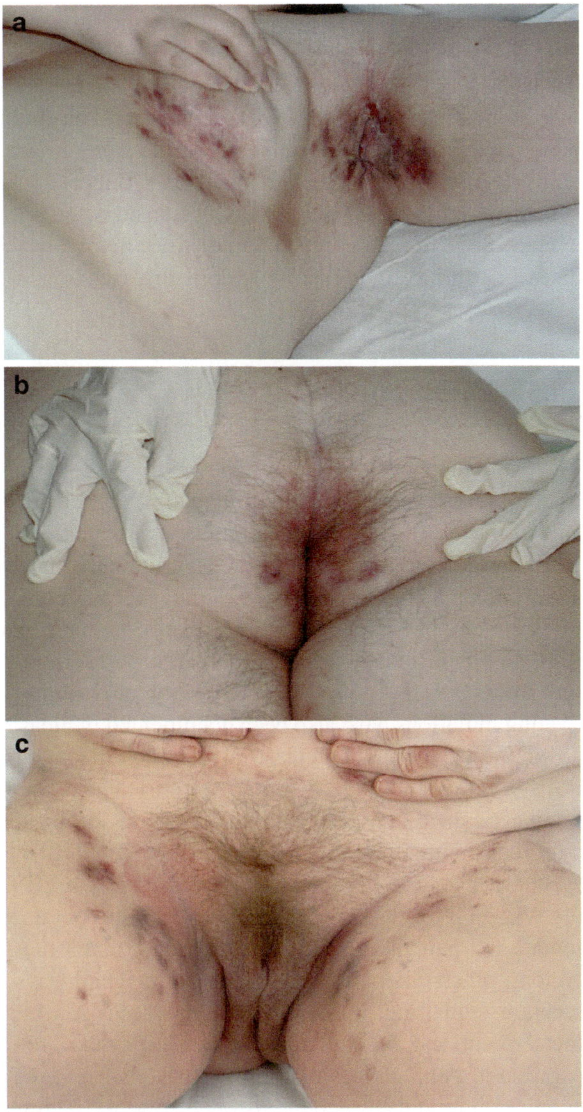

Fig. 20.1 Clinical manifestation of moderate to severe hidradenitis suppurativa in the axillary and submammary region (**a**), in the anal (**b**) and genital (**c**) regions of a female diabetes patient

other hand, appeared to be less frequently affected [9]. An association between HS and metabolic syndrome has been reported in several studies [5, 10]. Truncal obesity, high blood pressure, type 2 diabetes mellitus and dyslipoproteinemia, which are characteristics of the metabolic syndrome, are frequently found in patients with HS. A metabolic syndrome is present in 32.4% of patients with HS [11, 12]. In a recent meta-analysis, the pool ratio for the metabolic syndrome in HS was estimated to be 2.66 (95% CI, 1.90–3.72) [13]. There has also been a clear association between HS and diabetes mellitus [9]. A meta-analysis showed that there is a 1.69-fold increase in the risk of developing diabetes mellitus with HS [14]. The overall prevalence of type 2 diabetes mellitus in HS was 24.8% in a cross-sectional analysis in the USA [15]. The prevalence of type 2 diabetes mellitus in non-HS patients was 15.6% in the same cohort. Further common comorbidities in HS are considered to be the pyoderma gangrenosum; pyoderma gangrenosum, acne, suppurative hidradenitis (PASH) syndrome; Adamantiades-Behçet's disease; spondyloarthropathy, synovitis, acne, pustulosis, hyperostosis and osteitis (SAPHO) syndrome, pachyonychia congenita, systemic amyloidosis, inflammatory bowel disease, e.g., Crohn's disease; arthritis; and other hyperergic diseases reviewed in [5].

20.3 Pathogenesis

The pathogenic event in HS is believed to be the occlusion of the upper part of the hair follicle leading to a perifollicular lymphohistiocytic inflammation. Several studies have suggested that immune dysregulation [16], bacterial growth [17], genetic predisposition [18–21] and environmental factors such as smoking and lifestyle habits including obesity [2] may be some of the initiating factors. First, Fitzsimmons et al. identified autosomal dominant inheritance in 11 UK families [22], and later linkage analysis in a large 4-generation Chinese HS family showed linkage to 1p21.1–1q25.3, a 73-Mb region of chromosome 1 [23]. In addition, inactivating mutations have also been documented in nicastrin (NCSTN), a gene located at 1 q22-23 and encoding nicastrin, as well as in two other c-secretase subunit genes, PSEN1 and PSENEN [24]. With regard to the European HS population, Pink et al. sequenced the c-secretase genes of seven HS families and identified two additional c-secretase mutations in NCSTN and PSENEN [18].

In order to decipher the mechanisms underlying HS, whole-genome gene profiling was employed in lesional and healthy skin obtained from European Caucasian female HS patients (mean age 37.4 years) using the Agilent array platform [21]. Among others alterations to key regulatory pathways involving aryl hydrocarbon receptor signalling, retinoid signalling, oestrogen receptor signalling, xenobiotic metabolism and NF-kB transcription factors which are key regulators of gene expression culminating in response to stress, and the development of innate and acquired immunity was demonstrated. Further pathways including glucocorticoid receptor, atherosclerosis, HIF1alpha and IL17A signalling as well as inhibition of matrix metalloproteases were detected. From a functional standpoint, cellular assembly, maintenance and movement, haematological system development and function, immune cell trafficking and antimicrobial response were key processes probably being affected in HS [21]. These findings highlighted a panel of immune-related drivers in HS, which influence innate immunity and cell differentiation in follicular and epidermal keratinocytes as well as skin glands [21].

Inflammation plays an important role in the pathogenesis of HS. In HS lesional skin, a number of cytokines have been found to be highly upregulated, such as toll-like receptor 2 (TLR2), interleukin 12 (IL-12) and interleukin-23 (IL-23) [25, 26].

Especially IL-23 has been shown to induce the IL-17-producing T helper cells (Th17), which infiltrate the dermis in HS lesions. Therapy with anti-TNF (tumour necrosis factor)-alpha agent adalimumab suppresses the expression of most of these cytokines [27]. Kelly et al. have recently illustrated the primary role for the immune system in driving HS pathogenesis and provided evidence that CD45 + CD4+ T cells are responsible for IL-17 production and dendritic cells (DCs) CD11c + CD1a-CD14+ cells are the main producers of IL-1β in HS lesional skin. The last finding correlated with activation of caspase-1 and expression of the NALP-3 inflammasome (nlrp3) [28].

Hormones also seem to play a pivotal role in the pathogenesis of HS. Although data on sex hormones in HS are controversial, androgens have been suggested to be involved in pathogenesis of female HS patients [29, 30]. In men, it seems that androgens play a subordinate role in HS. Peripubertal onset of HS, premenstrual deterioration and postpartum deterioration supported the role of sex hormones in HS [31, 32]. Thyroid disease and PCOS are also more commonly associated with HS. Both hyperthyroidism and hypothyroidism have been described. The frequent occurrence of thyroid diseases in HS could be related to the smoking behaviour of HS patients [33]. Furthermore, in HS there is a shift towards pro-inflammatory adipokines. Adiponectin is decreased in HS [34]. The pro-inflammatory adipokines visfatin, resistin, omentin-1 and RBP4 are all increased in HS. An imbalance in adipokines could lead to an impairment in the regulation of fat storage, glucose tolerance and the release of insulin.

Insulin resistance (IR) is present in between 43.4% and 45.9% of patients with HS, which is higher than in healthy control subjects [11, 35]. A cross-sectional case-control study showed significantly increased IR in HS patients compared to healthy controls (43.4% vs. 16.4%, $p = 0.001$) [35]. Almost half of the patients showed IR. Therefore, for early detection of possible diabetes mellitus, testing for IR in HS patients is useful. Secondary diseases of diabetes mellitus and metabolic syndrome could thus be prevented. Cardiovascular risk factors, as indicated by a significant increase in systemic immune-inflammation-based biomarkers [5], are significantly more common in HS patients. For this reason, screening for typical cardiovascular risk factors should be a priority. In order to better understand HS, the exact mechanism of IR should be investigated in future studies.

20.4 Clinical Diagnosis

The diagnosis of HS is mostly based on the disease narrative, topography, clinical (Fig. 20.1) and histological features (Fig. 20.2). Based on the Dessauer definition, three diagnostic criteria should be met: presence of typical lesions, typical locations and chronicity. The clinical picture of HS can be very diverse including superficial abscesses (furuncles, carbuncles; "boils"), abscesses that are subcutaneous and suprafascial, cysts, painful erythematous papules and plaques, folliculitis, open ulcerations, pyogenic granulomas, chronic tunnels (fistules and sinuses, i.e.,

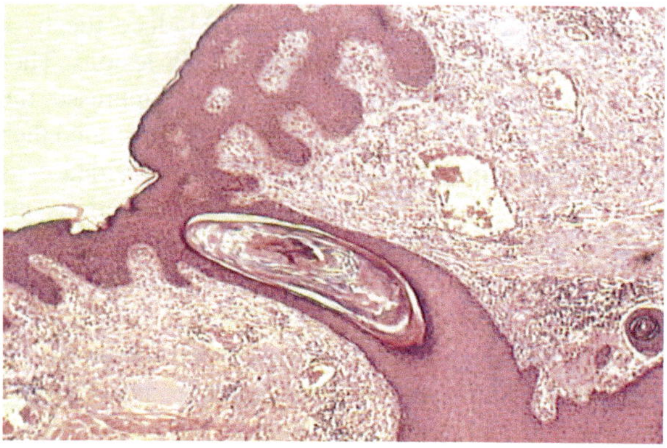

Fig. 20.2 Common histological features of hidradenitis suppurativa illustrated by haematoxylin eosin staining. Pathogenesis of HS involves follicular hyperkeratosis and dilatation, follicular rupture and chronic inflammation with architectural tissue changes [1]

Table 20.1 Hurley grading [38]

Hurley stage I	Abscess formation, single or multiple, without sinus tracts and cicatrization
Hurley stage II	Recurrent abscesses with tract formation and cicatrization, single or multiple, widely separated lesions
Hurley stage III	Diffuse or near-diffuse involvement, or multiple interconnected tracts and abscesses across the entire area

circinate, linear, arcuate), scrotal and genital lymphedema, dermal contractures, keloid scars, skin tags, fibrosis, anal fissures, scarring folliculitis of the buttocks (from mild to cigarette paper-like scarring), condyloma-like lesions, fishmouth scars and morphea-like plaques [36, 37]. Further HS accompanying follicular diseases are pilonidal cysts, acne conglobate, dissecting folliculitis (folliculitis and perifolliculitis capitis abscedens and suffodiens) and acanthosis nigricans. HS can be also associated with pyoderma gangrenosum or Crohn's disease and other inflammatory follicular skin diseases. Common skin regions of HS manifestation are the intertriginous areas, the buttocks and the scalp. Chronic symptoms or consequences of uncontrolled disease include pain, drainage, pruritus, odour, low self-esteem, sleep and sexual dysfunction, and poor mental health. Disease activity has long been assessed with the Hurley grading [38] (Table 20.1), the modified Sartorius score [39], the International Hidradenitis Suppurativa Severity Score System (IHS4) and its dichotomous variant IHS4-55 [40, 41] (Fig. 20.3) and the HS physician's global assessment (HS-PGA) [40]. Disease burden can be measured by, e.g., the numeric rating scale for pain [42], the Dermatology Life Quality Index (DLQI) and the Hospital Anxiety and Depression Scale (HADS), which are validated scores, and by the number of days of inability to work [36]. A more reliable classification of skin inflammation and severity of active disease also results from ultrasound sonography. Long-wave medical infrared thermography (MIT) may further offer an inflammation and blood flow lesional evaluation based on the temperature-associated differential assessment in inflammatory lesions [43].

Active, inflammatory lesions	Dynamic score
• Nodule (raised, 3D, round, infiltrated lesion >10 mm)	1 point
• Abscess (tender but fluctuating mass >10 mm surrounded by an erythematous area)	2 points
• Draining tunnel (sinus/fistula; raised, tender but fluctuating longitudinal mass of variable length and depth, ending at the skin surface, and sometimes oozing a fluid)	4 points

Classification score	
• Mild	1–3 points
• Moderate	4–10 points
• Severe	≥11 points

Dichotomous IHS4 (IHS4-55)

- Outcome: 55% reduction of IHS4 score vs baseline

Fig. 20.3 International Hidradenitis Suppurativa Severity Score System (IHS4) and dichotomous IHS4 (IHS4-55). A nodule (inflammatory nodule) is a raised, three-dimensional, round, infiltrated lesion with a diameter of >10 mm. An abscess is a tender but fluctuating mass with a diameter of >10 mm, surrounded by an erythematous area; the middle of an abscess contains pus. A draining tunnel is a raised, tender but fluctuating longitudinal mass of variable length and depth, ending at the skin surface and sometimes oozing a fluid. Fistulae and sinuses are examples of tunnels [40, 41]

20.5 Treatment of HS in Diabetes Patients

Treatment of HS in diabetes patients is challenging, and despite the beneficial effects of certain agents, the majority of patients have a partial response with subsequent relapses. To address the large unmet therapeutic need, elucidation of the disease-driving mechanisms is still required. Studies that characterize the genomic, transcriptomic and proteomic profiles of HS will therefore be invaluable [21, 44].

Antidiabetic drugs have shown a beneficial effect on HS progression. A therapeutic response to metformin, an insulin sensitizer, in HS patients has been described in the literature. In a prospective study ($n = 25$) with metformin, a clinical improvement of HS was observed in 72% of the patients [45]. In 64% of patients, the DLQI also improved. In a retrospective study of children with HS, the response to treatment was observed in 50% of the patients [46]. The Jennings study has so far analysed the largest number of patients treated with metformin [47]. The response rate was 68% in this study. The use of metformin led to complete HS remission in 19% of patients. It was interesting to note that 75% of the patients were found to have insulin resistance [47]. Metformin was well tolerated by the patients. The most common side effect was gastrointestinal symptoms.

Liraglutide is another antidiabetic drug. There is only one case report of clinical experience with the use of liraglutide in HS [48, 49]. Liraglutide is a GLP-1 agonist and acts by direct stimulation of the GLP-1 receptor. Stimulation of GLP-1 leads to glucose-dependent insulin secretion and inhibits glucagon secretion. As is the case with metformin, the most common side effect of liraglutide is gastrointestinal symptoms, but genitoanal fungal infections might also manifest. Pancreatitis and pancreatic carcinoma may occur in rare cases. An obese patient who was not insulin-resistant showed clinical improvement in HS and DLQI after 4 weeks of liraglutide therapy [48]. There was a reduction in HS-PGA from 4 to 1 and in DLQI from 24 to 14 under liraglutide treatment.

Further medical therapy may include antibiotics (clindamycin and rifampicin, tetracyclines), acitretin and the registered biologic agents adalimumab, a tumour necrosis factor-α (TNF-α) inhibitor, and secukinumab, an IL-17A inhibitor infliximab [50–52, 53]. The highly elevated levels of TNF-α in HS have been the driving force behind the therapeutic use of TNF-α antagonists. Both biologics have been associated with decreased pain and depressive symptoms compared to baseline [52–54]. Despite the significant short- and long-term efficacy of adalimumab, a percentage of patients do not have an adequate response to adalimumab, and a proportion of primary responders experience progressive loss of response [55]. Dose intensification significantly improved IHS4 score, pain index, HS-physician global assessment, pain and Cardiff Dermatology Life Quality Index [55]. Off-label biologics, such as infliximab, bimekizumab and anakinra can also be considered in selected cases [50, 56].

Since metabolic syndrome and HS are closely linked, weight loss represents a key lifestyle alteration that can improve HS symptoms, of which both exercise and diet are important aspects. Fasting is well-known to be a dietary intervention with the potential to improve insulin sensitivity [57, 58]. A significant improvement in IHS4 was seen in a multicentre, observational, cross-over pilot study of the so-called Ramadan fasting in HS [59].

Single lesions (mild disease according to IHS4) can be treated by topical means, and localized lesions (moderate disease) can be treated with systemic therapy if the lesions are mostly inflammatory and by conventional surgery or laser techniques, if the lesions are apparently noninflammatory, whereas widespread lesions (severe disease) may be better treated with systemic therapy alone or in combination with radical surgery. Adjuvant measures such as pain management, treatment of superinfections and tobacco cessation must be taken into account [49].

References

1. Zouboulis CC, Del Marmol V, Mrowietz U, Prens EP, Tzellos T, Jemec GB. Hidradenitis suppurativa/acne inversa: criteria for diagnosis, severity assessment, classification and disease evaluation. Dermatology. 2015;231(2):184–90.
2. Dessinioti C, Katsambas A, Antoniou C. Hidradenitis suppurrativa (acne inversa) as a systemic disease. Clin Dermatol. 2014;32(3):397–408.
3. Dessinioti C, Zisimou C, Tzanetakou V, Ntritsos G, Kontochristopoulos G, Antoniou C. A retrospective institutional study of the association of smoking with the severity of hidradenitis suppurativa. J Dermatol Sci. 2017;87(2):206–7.
4. Tzellos T, Zouboulis CC, Gulliver W, Cohen AD, Wolkenstein P, Jemec GB. Cardiovascular disease risk factors in patients with hidradenitis suppurativa: a systematic review and meta-analysis of observational studies. Br J Dermatol. 2015;173(5):1142–55.
5. Tzellos T, Zouboulis CC. Which hidradenitis suppurativa comorbidities should I take into account? Exp Dermatol. 2022;31(Suppl. 1):29–32.

6. Garg A, Rawal S, Akilov O, Alavi A, Ardon C, Bechara FG, et al. Factors associated with disease-specific life impact in patients with hidradenitis suppurativa: results from the Global VOICE project. Br J Dermatol. 2023;188(6):808–10.
7. Jfri A, Nassim D, O'Brien E, Gulliver W, Nikolakis G, Zouboulis CC. Prevalence of hidradenitis suppurativa: a systematic review and meta-regression analysis. JAMA Dermatol. 2021;157(8):924–31.
8. Garg A, Kirby JS, Lavian J, Lin G, Strunk A. Sex- and age-adjusted population analysis of prevalence estimates for hidradenitis suppurativa in the United States. JAMA Dermatol. 2017;153(8):760–4.
9. Lee JH, Kwon HS, Jung HM, Kim GM, Bae JM. Prevalence and comorbidities associated with hidradenitis suppurativa in Korea: a nationwide population-based study. J Eur Acad Dermatol Venereol. 2018;32(10):1784–90.
10. Goldburg SR, Strober BE, Payette MJ. Hidradenitis suppurativa: epidemiology, clinical presentation, and pathogenesis. J Am Acad Dermatol. 2020;82(5):1045–58.
11. Ozkur E, Erdem Y, Altunay IK, Demir D, Dolu NC, Serin E, et al. Serum irisin level, insulin resistance, and lipid profiles in patients with hidradenitis suppurativa: a case-control study. An Bras Dermatol. 2020;95(6):708–13.
12. Ozkur E, Karadag AS, Ustuner P, Aksoy B, Esme P, Caliskan E, et al. Clinical and demographic features of hidradenitis suppurativa: a multicentre study of 1221 patients with an analysis of risk factors associated with disease severity. Clin Exp Dermatol. 2021;46(3):532–40.
13. Mintoff D, Benhadou F, Pace NP, Frew JW. Metabolic syndrome and hidradenitis suppurativa: epidemiological, molecular, and therapeutic aspects. Int J Dermatol. 2022;61(10):1175–86.
14. Phan K, Charlton O, Smith SD. Hidradenitis suppurativa and diabetes mellitus: updated systematic review and adjusted meta-analysis. Clin Exp Dermatol. 2019;44(4):e126–e32.
15. Garg A, Birabaharan M, Strunk A. Prevalence of type 2 diabetes mellitus among patients with hidradenitis suppurativa in the United States. J Am Acad Dermatol. 2018;79(1):71–6.
16. Dreno B, Khammari A, Brocard A, Moyse D, Blouin E, Guillet G, et al. Hidradenitis suppurativa: the role of deficient cutaneous innate immunity. Arch Dermatol. 2012;148(2):182–6.
17. Matusiak L, Bieniek A, Szepietowski JC. Bacteriology of hidradenitis suppurativa—which antibiotics are the treatment of choice? Acta Derm Venereol. 2014;94(6):699–702.
18. Pink AE, Simpson MA, Desai N, Dafou D, Hills A, Mortimer P, et al. Mutations in the gamma-secretase genes NCSTN, PSENEN, and PSEN1 underlie rare forms of hidradenitis suppurativa (acne inversa). J Invest Dermatol. 2012;132(10):2459–61.
19. Pink AE, Simpson MA, Desai N, Trembath RC, Barker JNW. gamma-Secretase mutations in hidradenitis suppurativa: new insights into disease pathogenesis. J Invest Dermatol. 2013;133(3):601–7.
20. Kelleher RJ 3rd, Shen J. Genetics. Gamma-secretase and human disease. Science. 2010;330(6007):1055–6.
21. Zouboulis CC, Nogueira da Costa A, Makrantonaki E, Hou XX, Almansouri D, Dudley JT, et al. Alterations in innate immunity and epithelial cell differentiation are the molecular pillars of hidradenitis suppurativa. J Eur Acad Dermatol Venereol. 2020;34(4):846–61.
22. Fitzsimmons JS, Guilbert PR. A family study of hidradenitis suppurativa. J Med Genet. 1985;22(5):367–73.
23. Gao M, Wang PG, Cui Y, Yang S, Zhang YH, Lin D, et al. Inversa acne (hidradenitis suppurativa): a case report and identification of the locus at chromosome 1p21.1–1q25.3. J Invest Dermatol. 2006;126(6):1302–6.
24. Liu Y, Gao M, Lv YM, Yang X, Ren YQ, Jiang T, et al. Confirmation by exome sequencing of the pathogenic role of NCSTN mutations in acne inversa (hidradenitis suppurativa). J Invest Dermatol. 2011;131(7):1570–2.
25. Seyed Jafari SM, Hunger RE, Schlapbach C. Hidradenitis suppurativa: current understanding of pathogenic mechanisms and suggestion for treatment algorithm. Front Med (Lausanne). 2020;7:68.

26. Schlapbach C, Hanni T, Yawalkar N, Hunger RE. Expression of the IL-23/Th17 pathway in lesions of hidradenitis suppurativa. J Am Acad Dermatol. 2011;65(4):790–8.
27. van der Zee HH, Laman JD, de Ruiter L, Dik WA, Prens EP. Adalimumab (antitumour necrosis factor-alpha) treatment of hidradenitis suppurativa ameliorates skin inflammation: an in situ and ex vivo study. Br J Dermatol. 2012;166(2):298–305.
28. Kelly G, Hughes R, McGarry T, van den Born M, Adamzik K, Fitzgerald R, et al. Dysregulated cytokine expression in lesional and nonlesional skin in hidradenitis suppurativa. Br J Dermatol. 2015;173(6):1431–9.
29. Yu W, Barrett J, Liu P, Parameswaran A, Chiu ES, Lu CP. Novel evidence of androgen receptor immunoreactivity in skin tunnels of hidradenitis suppurativa: assessment of sex and individual variability. Br J Dermatol. 2021;185(4):855–8.
30. Zouboulis CC, Nogueira da Costa A, Fimmel S, Zouboulis KC. Apocrine glands are bystanders in hidradenitis suppurativa and their involvement is gender specific. J Eur Acad Dermatol Venereol. 2020;34(7):1555–63.
31. Collier EK, Price KN, Grogan T, Fernandez JM, Seivright JR, Alhusayen R, et al. Provider perspectives on the management of hidradenitis suppurativa in pregnancy—a survey study. Int J Womens Dermatol. 2021;7(3):346–8.
32. Fernandez JM, Hendricks AJ, Thompson AM, Mata EM, Collier EK, Grogan TR, et al. Menses, pregnancy, delivery, and menopause in hidradenitis suppurativa: a patient survey. Int J Womens Dermatol. 2020;6(5):368–71.
33. Liakou AI, Kontochristopoulos G, Marnelakis I, Tsantes AG, Papadakis M, Alevizou A, et al. Thyroid disease and active smoking may be associated with more severe hidradenitis suppurativa: data from a prospective cross sectional single-center study. Dermatology. 2021;237(1):125–30.
34. Malara A, Hughes R, Jennings L, Sweeney C, Lynch M, Awdeh F, et al. Adipokines are dysregulated in patients with hidradenitis suppurativa. Br J Dermatol. 2018;178(3):792–3.
35. Vilanova I, Hernandez JL, Mata C, Duran C, Garcia-Unzueta MT, Portilla V, et al. Insulin resistance in hidradenitis suppurativa: a case-control study. J Eur Acad Dermatol Venereol. 2018;32(5):820–4.
36. Schultheis M, Grabbe S, Staubach P, Hennig K, Mauch M, Burckhardt M, et al. Clinical features of persons suffering from acne inversa. Dtsch Arztebl Int. 2023;120(19):345–6.
37. Scheinfeld N. An atlas of the morphological manifestations of hidradenitis suppurativa. Dermatol Online J. 2014;20(4):22373.
38. Hurley HJ. Axillary hyperhidrosis, apocrine bromhidrosis, hidradenitis suppurativa, and familial benign pemphigus:surgical approach. In: Roenigk RK, Roenigk HH, editors. Dermatologic surgery. New York: Marcel Dekker; 1989. p. 729–39.
39. Sartorius K, Emtestam L, Jemec G, Lapins J. Objective scoring of hidradenitis suppurativa reflecting the role of tobacco smoking and obesity. Br J Dermatol. 2009;161(4):831–9.
40. Zouboulis CC, Tzellos T, Kyrgidis A, Jemec GBE, Bechara FG, Giamarellos-Bourboulis EJ, et al. Development and validation of the International Hidradenitis Suppurativa Severity Score System (IHS4), a novel dynamic scoring system to assess HS severity. Br J Dermatol. 2017;177(5):1401–9.
41. Tzellos T, van Straalen KR, Kyrgidis A, Alavi A, Goldfarb N, Gulliver G, et al. Development and validation of IHS4-55, an IHS4 dichotomous outcome to assess treatment effect for hidradenitis suppurativa. J Eur Acad Dermatol Venereol. 2023;37(2):395–401.
42. Jemec GB. Hidradenitis suppurativa. J Cutan Med Surg. 2003;7(1):47–56.
43. Zouboulis CC, Nogueira da Costa A, Jemec GBE, Trebing D. Long-wave medical infrared thermography: a clinical biomarker of inflammation in hidradenitis suppurativa/acne inversa. Dermatology. 2019;235(2):144–9.
44. Zouboulis CC, Nogueira da Costa A. Drug repurposing through drug-gene interaction profiles for hidradenitis suppurativa/acne inversa treatment. J Eur Acad Dermatol Venereol. 2021;35(4):e251–e4.

45. Verdolini R, Clayton N, Smith A, Alwash N, Mannello B. Metformin for the treatment of hidradenitis suppurativa: a little help along the way. J Eur Acad Dermatol Venereol. 2013;27(9):1101–8.
46. Moussa C, Wadowski L, Price H, Mirea L, O'Haver J. Metformin as adjunctive therapy for pediatric patients with hidradenitis suppurativa. J Drugs Dermatol. 2020;19(12):1231–4.
47. Jennings L, Hambly R, Hughes R, Moriarty B, Kirby B. Metformin use in hidradenitis suppurativa. J Dermatol Treat. 2020;31(3):261–3.
48. Jennings L, Nestor L, Molloy O, Hughes R, Moriarty B, Kirby B. The treatment of hidradenitis suppurativa with the glucagon-like peptide-1 agonist liraglutide. Br J Dermatol. 2017;177(3):858–9.
49. Emtestam L, Sartorius K. Glucagon-like peptide-1 agonists for treatment of hidradenitis suppurativa. Br J Dermatol. 2017;177(3):625–7.
50. Zouboulis CC, Desai N, Emtestam L, Hunger RE, Ioannides D, Juhasz I, et al. European S1 guideline for the treatment of hidradenitis suppurativa/acne inversa. J Eur Acad Dermatol Venereol. 2015;29(4):619–44.
51. Kimball AB, Okun MM, Williams DA, Gottlieb AB, Papp KA, Zouboulis CC, et al. Two phase 3 trials of adalimumab for hidradenitis suppurativa. N Engl J Med. 2016;375(5):422–34.
52. Kimball AB, Jemec GBE, Alavi A, Reguiai Z, Gottlieb AB, Bechara FG, et al. Secukinumab in moderate-to-severe hidradenitis suppurativa (SUNSHINE and SUNRISE): week 16 and week 52 results of two identical, multicentre, randomised, placebo-controlled, double-blind phase 3 trials. Lancet. 2023;401(10378):747–61.
53. Scheinfeld N, Sundaram M, Teixeira H, Gu Y, Okun M. Reduction in pain scores and improvement in depressive symptoms in patients with hidradenitis suppurativa treated with adalimumab in a phase 2, randomized, placebo-controlled trial. Dermatol Online J. 2016;22(3):13030/qt38x5922j.
54. Tchernev G. Loss of efficacy of adalimumab in hidradenitis suppurativa: focus on alternatives. Georgian Med News. 2023;340–341:297–300.
55. Zouboulis CC, Hansen H, Caposiena Caro RD, Damiani G, Delorme I, Pascual JC, et al. Adalimumab dose intensification in recalcitrant hidradenitis suppurativa/acne inversa. Dermatology. 2020;236(1):25–30.
56. Kimball AB, Jemec GBE, Sayed CJ, Kirby JS, Prens EP, Ingram JR, et al. Efficacy and safety of bimekizumab in patients with moderate to severe hidradenitis suppurativa: two 48-week, randomised, double-blind, placebo-controlled, multicentre phase 3 trials (BE HEARD I and II). Lancet. 2024;403(10443):2504–2519.
57. Prasetya G, Sapwarobol S. Intermittent fasting during Ramadan improves insulin sensitivity and anthropometric parameters in healthy young Muslim men. Am J Lifestyle Med. 2021;15(2):200–6.
58. Gnanou JV, Caszo BA, Khalil KM, Abdullah SL, Knight VF, Bidin MZ. Effects of Ramadan fasting on glucose homeostasis and adiponectin levels in healthy adult males. J Diabetes Metab Disord. 2015;14:1–6.
59. Damiani G, Mahroum N, Pigatto PDM, Pacifico A, Malagoli P, Tiodorovic D, et al. The safety and impact of a model of intermittent, time-restricted circadian fasting ("ramadan fasting") on hidradenitis suppurativa: Insights from a multicenter, observational, cross-over, pilot, exploratory study. Nutrients. 2019;11(8):1781.

Part III
Influence of Diabetes on Skin Diseases

Chapter 21
Psoriasis and Diabetes

David A. De Luca and Diamant Thaçi

Abstract There is a complex interplay between psoriasis, a chronic immune-mediated skin condition, and its association with various co-occurring health concerns on a global scale. Psoriasis, which extends beyond just visible scaly red patches, reveals complex ties with conditions such as atherogenesis, insulin resistance, obesity, hypertension, dyslipidemia, metabolic syndrome, and diabetes mellitus. Psoriasis and diabetes have a significant correlation supported by epidemiological evidence. This chapter delves into the distinctive features of psoriasis and meticulously explores the intricate relationship it shares with diabetes. Uncovering potential connections and shared mechanisms, this exploration not only enriches our understanding of these conditions but also opens avenues for redefining diagnostic and treatment approaches to address both psoriasis and diabetes concurrently.

21.1 Psoriasis

21.1.1 Introduction

Psoriasis, an immune-mediated chronic skin condition, is a significant global health concern, affecting millions of individuals. Beyond its prominent scaly, red patches, psoriasis highlights its intricate relationship with various co-occurring conditions like atherogenesis, atherosclerosis, insulin resistance, obesity, hypertension, dyslipidemia, metabolic syndrome (MetS), and diabetes mellitus. Epidemiological findings highlight the association between psoriasis and type 2 diabetes mellitus (T2DM), suggesting an increased risk for patients with psoriasis to develop T2DM,

D. A. De Luca (✉) · D. Thaçi
Institute for Inflammation Medicine, University Medical Center Schleswig-Holstein, Lübeck, Germany
e-mail: davidaldo.delucalaredo@uksh.de; diamant.thaci@uksh.de

K. Fritz, G.-S. Tiplica (eds.), *Cutaneous Manifestations in Diabetes*,
https://doi.org/10.1007/978-3-031-65300-1_21

with prevalence rates reported at 11.6% in psoriatic cohorts [1]. This chapter aims to outline the characteristics of psoriasis and explore the relationship between psoriasis and diabetes, uncovering potential connections and shared mechanisms that could influence approaches in diagnosis and treatment for both conditions.

21.1.2 Epidemiology

Psoriasis is a frequent skin disease that affects about 2–4% of the population in western countries. The prevalence of psoriasis varies across the world, with the highest prevalence in Western and Central Europe, as well as North America [2]. The prevalence of psoriasis was computed to range from 0.14% in East Asia to 1.10–1.50% in southern Latin and North America, 1.83–92% in Oceania, and 2.10–2.30% in Asia Pacific [3]. Psoriasis prevalence in African Americans is 1.5% compared to 3.6% of Caucasians [4].

The incidence of psoriasis in children demonstrated an age-related increase, rising from 13.5 per 100,000 person-years among those aged 0–3 years to 53.1 per 100,000 person-years for those aged 14–18 years. The UK and the USA consistently showed a trend of increasing psoriasis incidence up to 39 years of age, followed by a decline at 40–49 years and a subsequent increase with a second peak around 50–59 years (in the UK) or 60–69 years (both in the UK and the USA) [5, 6]. Psoriasis incidence generally decreases toward the later stages of life. While some variability existed in reported incidence rates by sex, girls had a slightly higher overall incidence than boys among those under 18 years (43.9 and 37.9 per 100,000 person-years, respectively) [7]. However, this pattern was not consistent across all age groups. Women tended to experience onset peaks around 18–29 and 50–59 years, while men exhibited peaks more commonly in the age ranges of 30–39 and 60–69 or 70–79 years [2].

21.1.3 Pathogenesis

21.1.3.1 Immunopathogenesis

Psoriasis is a systemic chronic inflammatory skin condition influenced by genetic and environmental factors, leading to an epidermal thickening and immune cell infiltration in the skin. It is well characterized by disturbances in both innate and adaptive cutaneous immune responses, where autoimmune-like and autoinflammatory responses co-occur, and the delicate equilibrium between these two elements plays a pivotal role in defining its clinical manifestations [8]. The psoriasis complexity arises from intricate interactions among keratinocytes, immune cells, and other resident skin cells. Traditionally, psoriasis has been viewed as primarily

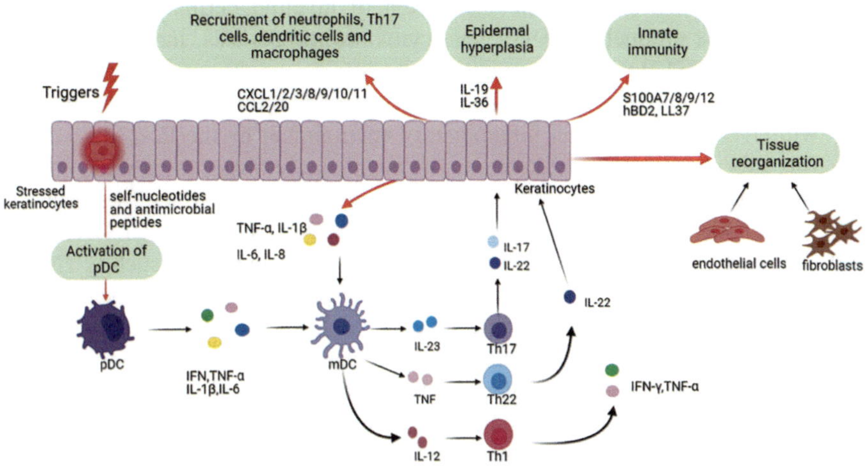

Fig. 21.1 Pathogenesis of psoriasis: The pathogenesis of psoriasis involves external triggers leading to the release of self-nucleotides, forming complexes with cathelicidin antimicrobial peptides. These complexes bind to Toll-like receptors on the surface of plasmacytoid dendritic cells (pDC) and prompt the activation and clonal expansion of CD8+ T cells (not shown), resulting in local inflammation and keratinocyte proliferation. Activated pDC and keratinocytes release cytokines, including IFN, IL-1β, IL-6 and TNF-α, activating myeloid dendritic cells (mDC). Subsequently, mDC releases pro-inflammatory mediators, such as IL-12, IL-23, and TNF-α. These cytokines stimulate CD4+ Th1, Th17, and Th22 cells, which release INFγ, TNF-α, IL-17, and IL-22. In response, keratinocytes produce chemokines, attracting neutrophils, lymphocytes CD4 Th17, dendritic cells, and macrophages, amplifying the local inflammation. Additionally, keratinocytes express IL-19 and IL-36, which act autocrinally, amplifying epidermis proliferation and also activating the innate immune response. Finally, there is a tissue reorganization by angiogenic factors such as angiopoietin, vascular endothelial growth factor (VEGF), TNF-α, IL-8, IL-17, and hypoxia-inducible factor 1 (HIF1), which are released from activated keratinocytes, guiding to vascular proliferation and tortuous papillary dermal vessels. Image from Zhou et al. [10]

immune cell-driven, with keratinocytes serving as executors of immune cell functions during the disease, where the interleukin (IL)-23/IL-17 pathogenic axis plays a pivotal role [9]. The immunopathogenesis of psoriasis is depicted in Fig. 21.1.

One of the most well-investigated initiation mechanisms, leading to dysregulated skin immune responses, involves keratinocytes releasing the cationic antimicrobial peptide LL-37 following physical trauma (Koebner phenomenon) or infection. LL-37 binds to self-DNA/RNA fragments released by damaged skin cells, forming LL-37/self-DNA/RNA complexes commonly found in psoriasis lesions [11]. Plasmacytoid dendritic cells play a crucial role in the initial stages of the disease, and their activation is triggered by LL-37/self-DNA/RNA complexes through Toll-like receptors TLR9, TLR7, and TLR8 [12]. Consequently, the activation of plasmacytoid dendritic cells (pDCs) results in the secretion of type I interferons (IFN). Furthermore, in conjunction with the pro-inflammatory cytokines released by activated keratinocytes such as interleukin-1β (IL-1β), IL-6, and tumor necrosis factor

(TNF), this process prompts the maturation of myeloid dermal dendritic cells (mDCs) and the production of essential cytokines in psoriasis, including TNF-α, IL-12, and IL-23 [13].

The development of psoriatic plaques relies on pDC activation and their interaction with T cells, fostering an inflammatory environment by the IL-23/IL-17 axis [9]. This axis plays a crucial role during the maintenance phase of psoriatic inflammation through the adaptive immune response mediated by distinct T-cell subsets [11]. The mDCs as well as macrophage-derived IL-23 activate T-helper Th1, Th17, and Th22 cells, resulting in the secretion of inflammatory cytokines such as TNF-α, IL-17, IL-19, IL-21, IL-22, and IL-36 [10, 14]. In particular, Th17 cells are abundant in psoriatic skin and contribute to IL-17A, IL-17F, and IL-22 production. IL-17A and IL-17F activate keratinocytes to release chemokines and antimicrobial peptides, establishing a pathogenic loop between T cells and keratinocytes [15]. Additionally, IL-17C induces an autocrine pro-inflammatory loop in keratinocytes, and IL-22 plays a significant role in epidermal hyperplasia. IL-19, also expressed in the skin and regulated by IL-17, leads to increased IL-19 and IL-22 production in response to IL-17, stimulating epidermal hyperproliferation and the upregulation of pro-inflammatory signals, including antimicrobial peptides [16]. Subsequently, keratinocytes are stimulated by these cytokines, especially IL-17, to produce antimicrobial peptides, cytokines, and chemokines, intensifying the inflammatory response. IL-36 can activate DC subsets and promote the differentiation of IL-17-producing T cells through the increased production of keratinocyte-derived cytokines or chemokines [17]. *Streptococcus pyogenes* and *Candida albicans* were shown to activate IL-36 cytokines, and infection with this pathogen has been associated with psoriasis flares [18, 19]. IL-36, together with IL-17-induced IL-19 and IL-22 produced by keratinocytes, contributes to epidermal hyperplasia and altered terminal differentiation, which leads to the characteristic thickening of the skin seen in patients with chronic psoriasis.

21.1.3.2 Genetics

The genetic landscape of psoriasis is characterized by a combination of skin-specific and immune-related genes. Genetic studies have uncovered 15 psoriasis susceptibility regions, named psoriasis susceptibility 1–15 (PSORS1–15), representing the primary factors in the genetic basis of psoriasis (Table 21.1) [20]. Skin-specific genes, particularly those within the late cornified envelope (LCE) family, are crucial in psoriasis susceptibility due to their involvement in skin barrier formation. Furthermore, there is a genetic interaction between LCE deletions and HLA-C [21]. In the realm of immune genes, four key immunological processes and pathways contribute significantly to psoriasis susceptibility: antigen presentation, NF-κB signaling, the IL-23/IL-17 axis, and the type I IFN pathway. Antigen presentation through HLA-C is of great importance, demonstrating the strongest association in genome-wide association studies in psoriasis. The NF-κB pathway, vital for sustaining inflammation, includes genes downstream from TNF and IL-17 regulation, such

Table 21.1 Key features of the well-explored psoriasis susceptibility regions [11]

PSORS	Feature
PSORS1	Located on chromosome 6p21.3 within the major histocompatibility complex region. HLA-C06:02 is the most significant risk allele within PSORS1 and is implicated in the immune response and skin autoimmune reactions in psoriasis. HLA-C06:02 is associated with psoriasis in various populations and defines disease severity, onset, and inheritance
PSORS2	Located on chromosome 17q25 and primarily involves mutations in the CARD14 gene, which activates the NF-κB pathway. CARD14 mutations may lead to inflammatory responses and psoriasis-like lesions. Association with psoriasis vulgaris and generalized pustular psoriasis
PSORS3	Located on chromosome 4q and contains the IRF2. IRF2 synthesizes interferon regulatory factor 2, which blocks the activation of interferons alpha and beta by competing with IRF1
PSORS4	Located on 1q21, encompasses the epidermal differentiation complex (EDC). Some genes of EDC were identified as a genetic risk factor for psoriasis in Caucasian and Asian populations for a possible effect in skin barrier function. For example, in German patients it was found that LCE3C-LCE3B-del was only associated with psoriasis vulgaris, but not psoriatic arthritis
PSORS5	Found in 3q21 and includes SLC12A8 and CSTA genes. SLC12A8 in PSORS5 has been described as having an association with psoriasis vulgaris in the Swedish population
PSORS6	PSORS6 is located on chromosome 19p13. The risk factor associated with PSORS6, which contributes to the development of psoriasis at a younger age, has been confirmed to interact with PSORS1

as TNFAIP3, TNIP1, and TRAF3IP2. Rare and common gene variants in CARD14, predominantly expressed in the skin epidermis, highlight intrinsic defects in skin keratinocytes as potential drivers of psoriasis [22]. Genes associated with the type I IFN pathway, such as IL-28RA and RNF114, underscore the role of innate antiviral responses in psoriasis [23]. Finally, the IL-23/IL-17 pathway, comprising genes such as IL-23, IL-12B, and IL-23R, is well-established in psoriasis pathogenesis. The protective Arg381Gln IL-23R allele is supported by functional evidence, showing reduced IL-17 responses in carriers [24].

21.1.3.3 Epigenetics

In psoriasis, genetics and environmental factors contribute to the development of the disease. Epigenetics plays a crucial role in modulating gene expression and influencing the likelihood of developing psoriasis [25]. The significance of epigenetics in psoriasis is underscored by the relatively low concordance (35–72%) of the disease in monozygotic twins who share an identical DNA sequence [26].

DNA methylation involves the addition of a methyl group to CpG dinucleotides, influencing chromatin structure and gene transcription by inhibiting or promoting gene expression. Distinct patterns of DNA methylation are observed in psoriasis when comparing affected skin to adjacent normal skin. These differential methylation patterns encompass various genes, including known PSORS genes like S100A9,

PTPN22, SELENBP1, CARD14, and KAZN, some of which are located at gene promoters [27]. Furthermore, differential methylation patterns are also evident in psoriatic scales, with hypomethylation of CpG sites associated with increased disease severity. An example is the MGRN1 gene, which encodes a protein involved in the degradation of misfolded proteins. Alterations in DNA methylation have been also identified in peripheral blood mononuclear cells (PBMCs) of psoriatic patients, with increased expression of DNMT1 and decreased expression of methyl-CpG binding domain protein 2 and methyl-CpG binding protein 2, which are key regulators of DNA methylation [28].

Histone modifications play a critical role in psoriasis pathogenesis, influencing the transcriptional activity of key genes [25]. Methylation of the histone H3K9 can impact IL-23 expression in keratinocytes, while H3K4 methylation is detected in PBMCs from psoriasis patients [29]. Additionally, changes in histone acetylation levels, particularly reduced histone H4 acetylation in PBMCs of psoriasis patients, suggest an open chromatin state and active transcription. Lesional psoriasis skin exhibits dysregulated histone acetyltransferases and histone deacetylases (HDACs), with elevated HDAC-1 potentially contributing to vascular endothelial growth factor (VEGF) overexpression, endothelial cell proliferation, and keratinocyte survival. Furthermore, elevated H3K9 and H3K27 acetylation in the IL-17A promoter region in immune cells of psoriatic patients promotes Th17 differentiation and psoriasis development [30].

Noncoding RNAs (ncRNAs), particularly microRNAs (miRNAs), influence the gene expression through mRNA degradation, DNA methylation, and histone modification. miR-125b, one of the downregulated miRNAs in psoriasis, affects keratinocyte proliferation and differentiation, while other dysregulated miRNAs contribute to the immune response, skin inflammation, and epithelial processes [31]. In particular, miR-230, mir-383, miR-214-3p, and miR-125a-5p showed downregulation in psoriasis, while miR-378a, miR-31, miR-210, miR-200c, and miR-155 are upregulated [25]. Long noncoding RNAs (lncRNAs), involved in immunological and epidermal functions, also exhibit differential expression in psoriasis, with lncRNA-RP6-65G23.1 promoting keratinocyte proliferation and suppressing apoptosis [32]. Moreover, circular RNAs (circRNAs) impact gene expression, skin inflammation, and keratinocyte hyperproliferation in psoriasis, with various circRNAs being upregulated or downregulated, indicating their role in the disease pathogenesis [33].

21.1.3.4 Environmental Triggers

While a significant progress in identifying psoriasis susceptibility genes has been achieved, the environmental factors contributing to the onset of the disease remain largely undefined. Known environmental triggers for psoriasis include drugs, infections, physical trauma, smoking, alcohol consumption, and stress [11].

Medications

Certain medications, including imiquimod, antidepressants (e.g., lithium), antihypertensives (e.g., beta blockers), interferons (IFNs), and anti-cytokine therapies (e.g., anti-TNF antibodies), have been clinically linked to psoriasis initiation, exacerbation, or worsening. Lithium is known to trigger or worsen psoriasis. It may interfere with intracellular calcium channels, affecting keratinocyte proliferation and differentiation. Inhibition of glycogen synthase kinase-3 (GSK-3) can induce keratinocyte proliferation [34]. TNF inhibitors, including adalimumab, etanercept, certolizumab pegol, golimumab, and infliximab, used for inflammatory diseases such as psoriasis, have been linked to psoriasis induction or exacerbation, as a form of paradoxical reaction. The pathogenesis of this phenomenon is not fully understood but may involve the IL-23/helper T-cell 17 (Th17) axis and IFN-α dysregulation alongside TNF suppression. It tends to occur more frequently with infliximab, especially in the first year of treatment for conditions like Crohn's disease (CD) and rheumatoid arthritis [35].

Infections

Infections, particularly *Streptococcus* and human immunodeficiency virus (HIV), have been linked to the onset and exacerbation of psoriasis. Streptococcal infections, in various forms, can trigger psoriasis, and throat infections may worsen existing psoriatic symptoms. The mechanism involves cross-reactivity between streptococcal M surface antigen and human keratinocytes, potentially influenced by genetic factors [36]. Tonsillectomy has been explored as a potential treatment, but it may benefit only patients with recurrent tonsillitis-associated exacerbations. HIV infection can lead to new-onset psoriasis or worsen existing cases, with severity often correlating with declining immune function. The most common clinical subtypes in HIV-associated psoriasis include guttate, inverse, and erythrodermic. The mechanisms behind this paradoxical relationship between HIV (Th2 cytokine-mediated) and psoriasis (Th1 cytokine-mediated) are not fully understood, but CD8+ memory T-cell expansion is considered a key factor [37]. Other infections, including bacteria such as *Staphylococcus aureus* and *Helicobacter pylori*, fungi (e.g., *Malassezia*, *Candida*), and various viruses (e.g., papillomaviruses, retroviruses), have also been suggested as potential triggers or exacerbators of psoriasis [38].

Smoking

Zhou et al. [39] examined the association between smoking and psoriasis, finding an increased risk of psoriasis among ever smokers compared to never smokers, including current and former smokers. There was a potential link between heavier smoking and psoriasis severity. The impact of quitting smoking on psoriasis showed potential benefits. Furthermore, passive smoking was also considered a risk factor for psoriasis [40]. Regarding psoriasis treatment, smoking negatively affected the efficacy of treatment, particularly biologic agents [39].

Alcohol Consumption

Alcohol consumption may have complex effects on psoriasis. Studies indicate an association between alcohol use and psoriasis, with a positive correlation between alcohol intake and the extent of psoriasis in women, though some studies have shown it as a risk factor for young and middle-aged men [41, 42]. Alcohol abuse is linked to more severe inflammation and distinctive disease distribution, with minimal scale, distribution in the face, groin, and flexures, or typically hyperkeratotic lesions with a predominant acral distribution [43]. While alcohol intake has been suggested to induce pruritus, evidence is inconclusive. Psychological factors, such as anxiety and depression, are more prevalent among psoriasis patients with alcohol problems [44]. Additionally, alcohol-related mortality, particularly alcoholic liver disease, is higher in patients with psoriasis, potentially contributing to their increased risk of premature death [45].

21.1.4 Clinical Picture

21.1.4.1 Psoriasis Vulgaris

Psoriasis vulgaris, also referred to as chronic plaque-type psoriasis, presents as a common clinical manifestation within the realm of psoriasis, affecting 90% of individuals with this condition. The clinical manifestations are erythematous plaques with sharp boundaries and are covered with white scale, which vary in size from pinpoint papules to large plaques (Fig. 21.2). Lesions tend to be symmetrically distributed and are commonly found on the knees, elbows, scalp (Fig. 21.3), and the sacral region. The preference for these particular areas may be attributed to prior traumatic events, a phenomenon referred to as Koebnerization or the isomorphic response [46].

Brocq's methodical maneuver or scratching with a blunt scalpel highlights the whitening and fragmentation of the scales, adopting a candle wax aspect. The wax spot phenomenon makes evident the presence of hyperparakeratosis. Deeper scraping of the plaques can uncover a moist, smooth layer, known as the last membrane phenomenon. The detachment of the deeper layer of scales can result in pinpoint bleeding, known as the Auspitz sign, attributed to the occurrence of dermal papillomatosis [47]. Furthermore, the Woronoff ring is a hypopigmented macular ring around treated psoriatic plaques. Historically, psoriasis vulgaris has been

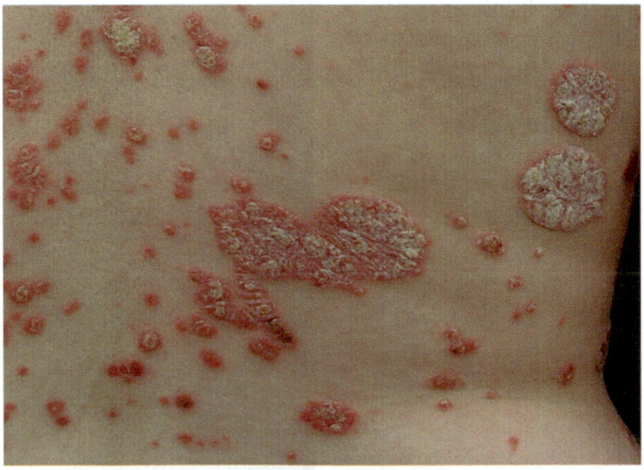

Fig. 21.2 Psoriasis vulgaris: well-demarcated, raised, red papules and plaques of skin covered with silvery-white scales and crusts. (Foto: Institute for Inflammation Medicine, Lübeck)

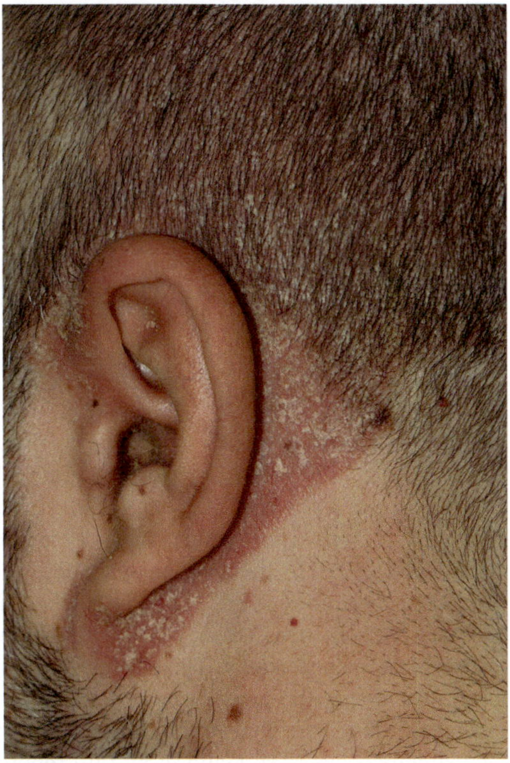

Fig. 21.3 Scalp psoriasis: Red, thickened, well-demarcated plaques with overlying silvery-white scales, affecting the temporal region of the scalp and the periauricular skin

subclassified by the shape and scale of the plaques. Terms such as psoriasis geographica (Fig. 21.4), psoriasis gyrata, rupioid lesions, ostraceous plaques, and elephantine psoriasis have in the present little clinical significance [46].

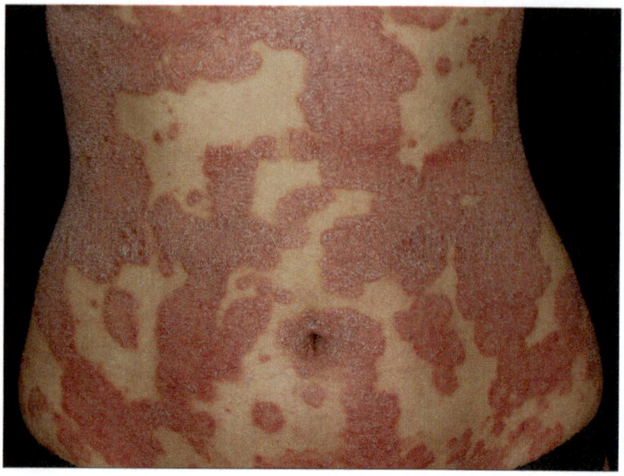

Fig. 21.4 Psoriasis vulgaris var. geographica: clinical variant of psoriasis characterized by well-demarcated, map-like erythematous patches with a scaly border on the skin, leaving areas of healthy skin

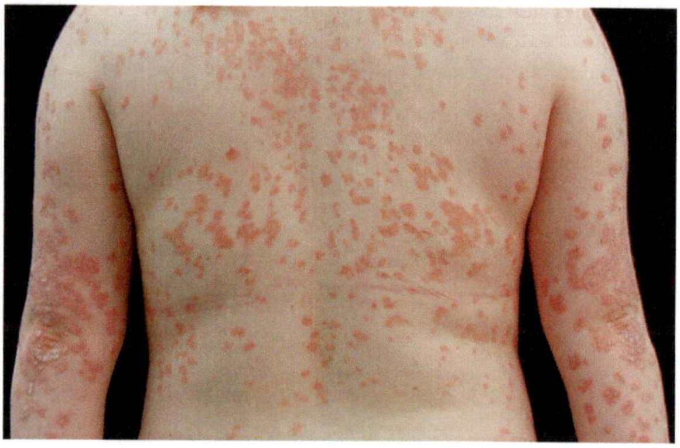

Fig. 21.5 Guttate psoriasis. Multiple small, eruptive light red papules and plaques covered with scales are scattered across the upper trunk. Simultaneously, there are erythematosquamous plaques on the elbows consistent with psoriasis vulgaris

21.1.4.2 Guttate Psoriasis

Guttate psoriasis presents as multiple, small, scattered papules and plaques, often described as drops. These lesions typically measure 2–6 mm in size. Guttate psoriasis is characterized by the eruption of small psoriatic papules on the upper trunk and proximal extremities (Fig. 21.5). They also display an isomorphic response or Koebner phenomenon. This type of psoriasis commonly appears in children, adolescents, and young adults. The evaluation of potential risk factors plays a major role in the diagnostic procedure. It is noteworthy that guttate psoriasis frequently emerges from a preceding streptococcal infection, classically a pharyngitis or perianal streptococcus [48]. Galili et al. [49] reported that after an average follow-up period of 6.2 years, 49.1% of patients initially diagnosed with guttate psoriasis continued to experience persistent and active psoriasis. Additionally, within the study cohort, a notable transition to the psoriasis vulgaris phenotype was observed in 17.5% of cases.

21.1.4.3 Inverse Psoriasis

Inverse, intertriginous, or flexural psoriasis is defined by the presence of smooth, moist, and scale-free dark-red patches. These distinctive patches manifest in regions susceptible to friction and direct skin-to-skin contact, encompassing the inguinal folds, axillae, inframammary folds, anogenital areas, umbilicus, and retro-auricular regions (Fig. 21.6). The demarcated limits and shiny texture of these lesions serve as distinguishing features to differentiate from other skin conditions in skin folds [50]. Affected areas often exhibit reduced perspiration, and localized fungal or bacterial infections can serve as potential triggers [46]. In addition, psoriasis frequently impacts the genital area, and around 63% of individuals with psoriasis will experience lesions in the genital region as the disease progresses [51]. Genital psoriasis, although it involves a relatively limited body surface area (BSA), is associated with a significant decline in quality of life and heightened stress levels [52].

21.1.4.4 Pustular Psoriasis

Generalized Pustular Psoriasis

The clinical course of generalized pustular psoriasis (GPP) exhibits significant variability. GPP can manifest as a relapsing condition marked by recurrent flares without pustulation in between, or it may present as a persistent ailment with constant pustulation and occasional, more severe flares. Patients also present with systemic symptoms. High fever has been documented in a range of 24–96% of patients during a GPP flare. Additional commonly linked symptoms include arthritis in one third of the patients as well as an extensive sense of malaise and fatigue. GPP often displays associations with trigger factors, as well as a history of prior plaque psoriasis [53].

There are four recognized forms distinguished by the onset of flares and the morphology of the lesions [54]. von Zumbusch GPP represents the most severe presentation, potentially posing life-threatening risks, such as hypocalcemia, acute

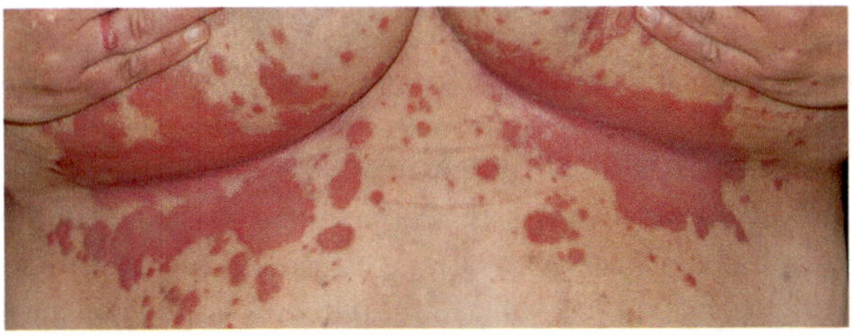

Fig. 21.6 Inverse psoriasis: Red, shiny, and smooth elevated patches on the submammary fold, accompanied by small satellite papules. Inverse psoriasis lacks the thick, scaly plaques typical of other types of psoriasis

respiratory distress syndrome, bacterial superinfection that can progress to sepsis, and dehydration [55]. This acute form of GPP is characterized by a rapid onset, occurring in 7 days or fewer, of a widespread pustular flare experienced by up to 90% of GPP patients. The sudden eruption of sterile pustules that manifest across the face, trunk, extremities, nail beds, palms, and soles is often accompanied by skin pain. Clinical examination reveals a background of erythematous skin, which initially appears as patches but eventually coalesces into erythroderma. Over time, chronic disease may lead to the development of fingertip atrophy [46].

Annular GPP or Lapière-Millian variant is characterized by the occurrence of a generalized flare marked by circinate or annular lesions displaying peripheral pustules, distinct from the classic plaque psoriasis manifestations. This form develops between 7 days and 3 months and is often accompanied by relatively mild symptoms and often exhibits comparatively mild symptoms [54]. Most reported cases have been observed in childhood, characterized by a relatively benign course, and they tend to experience rapid and sustained remission following treatment [56]. Chronic acral GPP is defined by the emergence of lesions starting in acral regions and gradually spreading to form a generalized pustular flare. The fourth category is a mixed GPP that encompasses features associated with more than one subtype [57].

Impetigo herpetiformis (IH), now referred to as pustular psoriasis of pregnancy (PPG), is a variant observed during pregnancy, presenting clinical and histological similarities to generalized pustular psoriasis. While its exact cause remains unknown, factors such as hormonal changes, stress, bacterial infections, and certain medications have been suggested. Clinical examination reveals lesions originating in skin folds and spreading centrifugally that can extend to the entire skin, accompanied by symptoms like poor general condition, fever, diarrhea, dehydration, tachycardia, and seizures. Laboratory findings include leukocytosis, elevated erythrocyte sedimentation rate, negative bacterial cultures in pustules, and peripheral blood, along with potential reductions in calcium, phosphate, and albumin levels. During pregnancy, the preferred treatment for pustular psoriasis involves systemic corticosteroids, typically 30–60 mg of prednisone daily, while refractory cases may consider the use of cyclosporine (CsA). While maternal deaths have significantly reduced with current steroid and antibiotic therapy, there remains a high risk of stillbirth and perinatal mortality due to various complications [58].

Localized Pustular Psoriasis

Palmoplantar pustulosis is a localized pustular subtype of palmar and plantar psoriasis. It is a chronic form of psoriasis accompanied by the formation of pustules with a well-known association with psoriatic arthritis (PsA) [59]. The pustular type is characterized by repeated crops of painful white to yellowish sterile pustules on well-defined erythema or red, non-scaly plaques (Fig. 21.7). The mixed pustular-hyperkeratotic type exhibits a polymorphic combination of erythema, dyshidrotic vesicles, pustules, and scaly papules or plaques [60, 61].

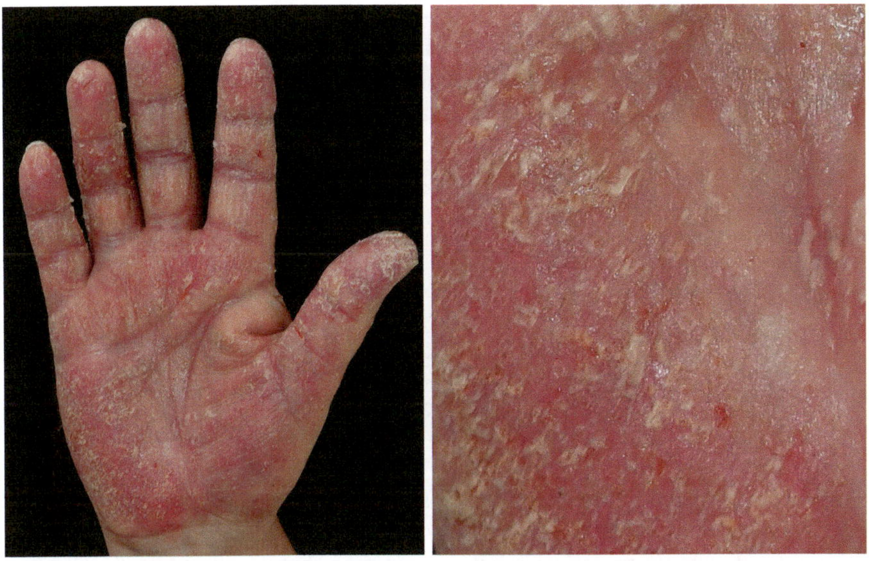

Fig. 21.7 Palmoplantar pustulosis: Sterile confluent pustules on the palms, varying in size from small to large, containing a yellow turbid liquid. These pustules are situated atop thickened, scaly, red skin, accompanied by painful fissures

Acrodermatitis continua of hallopeau (ACH) is a recurring, chronic inflammatory pustular condition that primarily affects the nails and is often preceded by minor trauma [62]. Characterized by tender, sterile pustules at the tip of digits, more commonly on fingers than toes, ACH leads to onychodystrophy and, in severe cases, osteolytic changes in the phalanges [63]. While usually localized to affected digits, it can sometimes spread to the dorsal areas of the hand and foot or evolve into GPP. It predominantly affects middle-aged females and often presents a chronic, relapsing, or persistent course. PsA occurs in a significant percentage of ACH patients [64, 65].

21.1.4.5 Nail Psoriasis

Nail psoriasis is a relatively common condition, affecting approximately half of individuals with psoriasis, and occurring in 80–90% of cases over a lifetime [66]. Nail psoriasis is also considered a risk factor for the development of PsA [67]. The extent of nail involvement varies with a higher prevalence in adults compared to children. Nail psoriasis typically manifests in various ways depending on the specific site of the nail affected, such as the nail matrix, nail bed, proximal nail fold, or hyponychium [68]. It may affect all nails or only a few, resulting in distinctive symptoms (Fig. 21.8). For instance, nail matrix involvement often leads to characteristic signs such as pitting, lunulae red spots, and nail plate crumbling. Pitting is a hallmark feature of nail psoriasis, characterized by small depressions on the nail

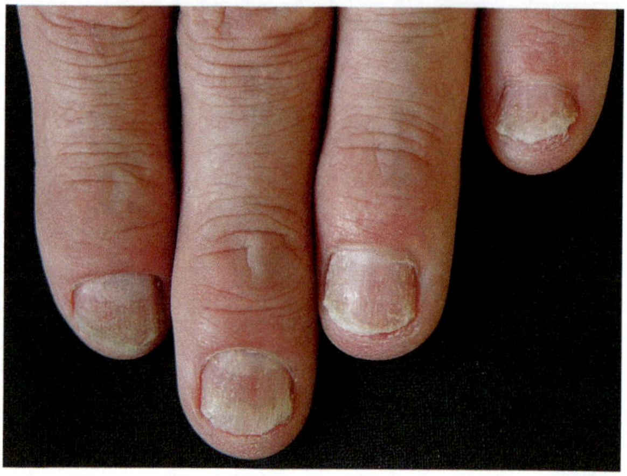

Fig. 21.8 Nail psoriasis: Nail matrix involvement consists of small depressions on the nail plate surface (pitting) and nail plate crumbling. Nail bed alterations include onycholysis, distal subungual hyperkeratosis, oil-drop or salmon spots, and splinter hemorrhages

plate surface. Nail bed alterations due to psoriasis can result in onycholysis, subungual hyperkeratosis, oil-drop or salmon spots, and splinter hemorrhages. These features are not specific to psoriasis but are common manifestations of the disease. Onycholysis, in particular, is marked by an erythematous border surrounding the areas of nail detachment [69].

21.1.4.6 Psoriatic Arthritis

PsA presents with two major types of musculoskeletal features: peripheral and axial manifestations. PsA affects both males and females equally and typically manifests in middle age. The presence of psoriasis on the scalp and intergluteal regions or nail psoriasis is often associated with PsA. The disease exhibits heterogeneity, with subtypes including polyarticular, oligoarticular, distal, arthritis mutilans, and axial or spondyloarthritis. These patterns can change and overlap throughout the disease course [70].

Peripheral manifestations encompass peripheral arthritis, dactylitis, and enthesitis. The distal subtype primarily affects distal interphalangeal joints (DIP), often involving the fingers and toes closest to the nails, frequently accompanied by nail changes. The oligoarticular subtype affects fewer than four joints, often asymmetrically distributed, while the polyarticular subtype involves five or more joints, potentially resembling rheumatoid arthritis. Arthritis mutilans, the most severe subtype, is rare but leads to destructive joint damage and deformities [70]. Enthesitis affects 30–50% of patients, commonly involving the plantar fascia and Achilles tendon insertion sites [71]. Dactylitis, characterized by diffuse swelling of an entire finger or toe (often termed a "sausage digit"), affects 40–50% of patients, particularly in the polyarthritis subtype [72].

The axial type of PsA shares genetic and clinical features with other spondyloarthritis forms and is grouped accordingly. Axial PsA primarily involves the spine and sacroiliac joints, with occasional peripheral involvement. It affects 25–70% of PsA patients, and exclusive axial involvement occurs in 5% of cases [73]. Axial PsA differs from ankylosing spondylitis AS but still significantly impacts quality of life. Symptoms of the axial subtype include back or neck pain, affecting various spinal regions. Detailed anamnesis, considering inflammatory features such as morning stiffness and pain that improves with activity but worsens with rest, can help differentiate axial PsA from other causes. However, existing criteria for inflammatory back pain are less suitable for axial PsA [74].

21.1.5 Comorbidities and Associated Conditions

21.1.5.1 Autoimmunity

Autoimmune diseases share common characteristics, such as their association with other autoimmune conditions, genetic factors, and immune system activity leading to organ damage. Psoriasis has been linked to several autoimmune diseases, including Hashimoto's and Graves' disease, Crohn's disease, celiac disease, type 1 diabetes mellitus (T1DM), vitiligo, and alopecia areata, although precise correlations and epidemiological data remain scarce [75]. Furthermore, large-scale studies have associated psoriasis with various immune-related rheumatic diseases such as ankylosing spondylitis, rheumatoid arthritis, Behçet disease, and systemic lupus erythematosus, particularly higher in male patients [76]. Interestingly, a small subset of individuals treated with TNF-α inhibitors for psoriasis has exhibited lupus-like symptoms, labeled as anti-TNF-induced LE (ATIL), particularly prominent in rheumatoid arthritis patients [77]. Moreover, psoriasis has been associated with autoimmune bullous skin diseases such as bullous pemphigoid (BP) and pemphigus disease, potentially due to shared skin antigens. BP, characterized by antibodies against skin proteins, often manifests in older individuals and may have connections to chronic inflammation from psoriasis or its treatments [78].

21.1.5.2 Metabolic Syndrome

Individuals with psoriasis commonly exhibit a higher prevalence of MetS, a cluster of interconnected conditions such as abdominal obesity, hypertension, atherogenic dyslipidemia, T2DM, insulin resistance, and nonalcoholic fatty liver disease [79]. In particular, obesity stands as an independent risk factor for psoriasis, showing a direct relationship between psoriasis severity and body mass index (BMI) [80]. Furthermore, psoriasis not only increases the risk of diabetes but also escalates the likelihood of insulin resistance and diabetic complications, particularly in more severe cases. MetS is more prevalent in both adult and pediatric populations with psoriasis [81]. Psoriasis is associated with altered cholesterol levels, including decreased high-density lipoprotein (HDL) levels and increased low-density lipoprotein (LDL), very low-density lipoprotein (VLDL), and triglycerides. HDL, known for its role in cholesterol transport and anti-inflammatory properties, experiences reduced function during chronic inflammation such as psoriasis [82]. Conversely, treatments for psoriasis can restore the composition and function of HDL [83]. On the other hand, LDL levels rise with increased TNF-α in severe psoriasis, contributing to vascular diseases [84]. The relation between psoriasis and diabetes will be further explained in the next section.

21.1.5.3 Obesity

Obesity, a pervasive and multifaceted metabolic condition, is linked to various health issues, from cardiovascular to immune system diseases. Furthermore, obesity leads to insulin resistance and chronic inflammation, including skin conditions such as psoriasis [85]. A clear association between increased BMI and a higher prevalence and severity of psoriasis is widely known. Importantly, interventions focusing on weight reduction and physical activity have shown improvement in psoriatic symptoms, emphasizing the importance of managing the obese phenotype during psoriasis management [86]. The relationship between obesity, high-fat diets, and psoriasis lies in their impact on inflammation and immunity. The development of psoriasis involves genetic factors playing a crucial role, and high-fat diets and obesity can foster an inflammatory environment that contributes to psoriasis development [85]. For instance, high-fat diets may increase palmitic acid levels, which is related to endoplasmic reticulum stress in keratinocytes and adipocytes, leading to the secretion of IL-6, TNF-α, and IL-1β as well as to the activation of NF-κB pathway [87]. Moreover, palmitic acid has been shown to aid in the activation of keratinocytes by IL-17, while a strong correlation has been found between the levels of palmitic or oleic acid in the blood and the severity of skin inflammation in high-fat diet-triggered worsening psoriasis [88]. The cytokine imbalance not only induces stress in specific cells, but they can also impact the gut microbiota, potentially leading to increased intestinal permeability, allowing the passage of inflammatory substances into the bloodstream. Psoriasis showcases a dysfunctional gut microbiota, identified by specific bacterial imbalances that contribute to chronic inflammation, affecting metabolic enzymes and potentially exacerbating the condition [89]. These processes collectively contribute to the damage of tissues and activation of immune cells, such as dendritic cells and T-helper lymphocytes (Th1, Th17, and Th22), ultimately leading to the manifestation of psoriasis lesions. While the body typically resolves these mechanisms through natural inflammatory mediators, such as resolvins, maresins, protectins (derived from ω-3 polyunsaturated fatty acids), and lipoxins (produced from ω-6 PUFAs), their production and signaling are disrupted under conditions of obesity and high-fat diets, potentially contributing to the persistence of psoriasis [90].

21.1.5.4 Cardiovascular Disease

Psoriasis sets the stage for cardiovascular disease by promoting inflammation, potentially leading to severe heart conditions. The cascade of inflammatory responses and physiological changes in psoriasis appears to significantly impact cardiovascular health, elevating the risk of heart attacks and strokes in affected individuals. Gelfand et al. [91] confirmed a notable link between severe psoriasis and heart attacks. Since then, various studies have consistently supported the connection between psoriasis and cardiovascular issues, such as heart attacks, strokes, and cardiovascular-related deaths, especially in younger patients with severe forms of the condition, and this risk remains even after considering traditional cardiovascular risk factors. Notably, the severity and duration of psoriasis seem to heighten these risks. As it was mentioned, psoriasis is often accompanied by an increased prevalence of cardiovascular risk factors like hypertension, diabetes, dyslipidemia, and obesity, exacerbating its impact. Boehncke et al. [92] have proposed a model known as the psoriatic march, to explain how psoriasis triggers cardiovascular problems, suggesting that inflammation in psoriasis could lead to insulin resistance and endothelial dysfunction, fostering conditions for heart disease. This chronic inflammation not only connects psoriasis and atherosclerosis but also prompts the production of substances that promote artery hardening and inflammation, increasing the risk of heart disease. Specific molecules such as TNF-α and IL-17 have been identified as contributors to vascular inflammation and atherosclerosis and coronary artery calcification in individuals with psoriasis [93]. Furthermore, increased levels of leptin and resistin can trigger the production of pro-inflammatory cytokines, including MCP-1, IL-6, IL-2, and TNF-α, known to encourage atherogenesis and inflame blood vessels by attracting monocytes and stimulating macrophages [94].

21.1.5.5 Nonalcoholic Fatty Liver Disease

Nonalcoholic fatty liver disease (NAFLD) involves the accumulation of liver fat without significant alcohol consumption or specific medication. Rhuan et al. [95] confirmed an association between psoriasis and nonalcoholic fatty liver disease (NAFLD), particularly pronounced in those with psoriasis and diabetes. Although NAFLD shares pathogenic similarities with MetS, the two pathologies are distinguished histologically in the liver [96]. Patients with NAFLD, regardless of the variant, face higher mortality rates, primarily due to cardiovascular disease. Physiopathologically, the involvement of IL-17 in both psoriasis and NAFLD suggests a potential link accelerating the progression of liver inflammation. Neutralizing IL-17 reduces in mouse model liver injury, suggesting that rebalancing Th17 cells and regulatory T cells might prevent NAFLD progression to severe liver conditions [97]. The bidirectional relationship between these conditions also involves cytokines such as TNF-α and IL-23, exacerbating insulin resistance and impacting T-cell balance, exacerbating NAFLD [98].

21.1.5.6 Inflammatory Bowel Diseases

Inflammatory bowel diseases (IBDs), encompassing ulcerative colitis (UC) and Crohn's disease (CD), are significant gastrointestinal-associated diseases of psoriasis. Studies revealed a strong bidirectional relationship between psoriasis and these conditions, highlighting associated gastrointestinal symptoms and varied risks based on psoriasis type and joint involvement [99]. The prevalence of psoriasis in patients with IBD is between 3% and 4%, with the prevalence slightly higher in patients with CD. Shared mechanisms include lifestyle factors, genetic overlap, and potential epigenetic links. Both diseases result from a combination of genetic/epigenetic and environmental factors, leading to immune activation. Both diseases result from a combination of genetic/epigenetic and environmental factors, leading to immune activation. TNF-α and IL-23 play crucial roles in promoting inflammation among these conditions, but the roles of IL-17 and IL-22 differ between psoriasis and IBD, affecting responses to targeted treatments [100].

21.1.5.7 Mental Health Conditions

Psoriasis patients show a significantly higher risk of various mental disorders compared to the general population. Increased prevalence of anxiety and depression among psoriasis patients, along with a connection between severe psoriasis and mental health issues, impacts quality of life. The prevalence of anxiety/depression among psoriasis patients reaches 27% [101]. The presence of psoriasis is significantly associated with depression, and this association is linked to elevated risks of psoriatic arthritis, cardiovascular events, and complications related to atherosclerosis. Moreover, psoriasis and depression are linked to chronic inflammation, raising the risk of cardiovascular issues [81]. Furthermore, psoriasis is associated with anxiety and an increased likelihood of suicidal thoughts and behaviors. Patients with severe psoriasis and younger age are identified as having higher rates of suicidal ideation and attempts [102]. The association between dementia and psoriatic disease displays mixed results, with some studies supporting a link and others showing contradictory outcomes [103]. Additionally, psoriasis appears to have links to sleep disorders like obstructive sleep apnea and restless legs syndrome and chronic fatigue syndrome, the latter of which may be related to factors like smoking, pain, and depression [104]. Further comorbidities associated with psoriasis include Parkinson's disease, migraines with aura, schizophrenia, alexithymia, and impulse control issues [103].

21.1.5.8 Ocular Manifestations

Ocular manifestations in psoriasis patients are more prevalent than previously recognized, reported in 10% of these patients, impacting various eye structures [105]. The findings affect the conjunctiva, eyelids, or the cornea, resulting in blepharitis, conjunctival hyperemia, and conjunctivitis, tear film changes, meibomian dysfunction, symblepharon, xerosis, ectropion, trichiasis, madarosis, punctate keratitis, corneal scar, corneal melting, and dry eye [106]. Notably, psoriasis often coexists with uveitis, an inflammatory eye condition affecting 2–3% of the global population, potentially leading to severe vision impairment if untreated [107]. Furthermore, there's a higher incidence and prevalence of uveitis among psoriasis patients, especially those with PsA. The severity of psoriasis seems linked to an increased risk of uveitis. The immune mechanisms underlying both conditions appear interlinked, involving cell types and cytokines such as Th1/Th17 cells, IL-17, IL-23, TNF-α, and IL-6 [108]. Genetic factors such as HLA-B27 and IL-23 receptor gene polymorphisms potentially contribute to the co-occurrence of psoriasis and uveitis [24]. Clinical observations highlight that psoriasis-associated uveitis predominantly affects males and often presents bilaterally with chronic, severe symptoms. The most common type of uveitis in psoriasis patients is anterior uveitis, characterized by red and painful eyes. Recurrence rates are high, and uveitis typically appears after the onset of psoriasis, sometimes preceding psoriatic arthritis [109].

21.1.5.9 Malignancies

Assessing malignancies in psoriasis patients is complex; however, studies suggest an increased risk of lymphoproliferative malignancies and nonmelanoma skin cancers in patients with severe psoriasis [110]. Lymphomas show consistency in increased risk, especially in severe psoriasis, with specific associations observed with Hodgkin's lymphoma and cutaneous T-cell lymphoma. Evidence of increased risk for solid tumors is inconsistent. However, a higher risk for colorectal cancer and urological malignancies was confirmed in psoriasis patients in Japan [111]. Chiesa Fuxench et al. [112] revealed a 60% increased risk of lung cancer in patients with moderate-to-severe psoriasis compared to those without, suggesting a complex relationship between psoriasis, smoking, and lung cancer. The association between phototherapy and an increased risk of skin cancer, especially nonmelanoma skin cancers, is evident. Psoralen and ultraviolet A (PUVA) treatment, particularly with higher doses, showed an elevated risk, whereas narrowband or broadband UVB treatments displayed lower risks, especially at lower exposure levels [113]. Among systemic non-biologic therapies, methotrexate (MTX) and cyclosporine (CsA) have been associated with an increased risk of malignancies, particularly lymphoproliferative disorders [113]. MTX has shown an association with skin cancers, particularly squamous cell carcinoma, especially in patients with prior PUVA exposure [114]. CsA exhibited an increased risk of skin malignancies, predominantly squamous cell carcinoma, related to longer treatment duration and prior therapies [115]. For TNF-α inhibitors, particularly in psoriasis, there have been varying results. Early findings of increased cancer risk were not consistently supported by subsequent data. TNF-α inhibitors do not seem to significantly increase the overall risk of systemic malignancies, although an elevated risk of squamous cell carcinoma has been observed [113, 116]. The emergence of newer treatments such as biologics targeting IL-12, IL-23, IL-17, Janus kinase, and phosphodiesterase-4 has expanded therapeutic options. Safety data from clinical trials for these agents have been promising, especially in terms of malignancy rates similar to the general population [113].

21.1.6 Diagnosis

The diagnosis of psoriasis relies primarily on clinical examination rather than specific tests. This recognition leads to various classifications of psoriasis based on factors like age of onset, severity, distribution patterns, morphology, anatomical site, and stage of development. These classifications help in understanding and diagnosing this condition more effectively [117].

21.1.6.1 Severity Assessment

Assessing psoriasis severity involves subjective and objective evaluations, considering physical aspects, symptoms, disease impact, and treatment response history. The challenge lies in accurately measuring disease severity and the limitations of current clinical scores, impacting treatment selection and assessing therapeutic effectiveness. Additionally, the lack of consensus on severity classification and the distinction between moderate and severe disease types delays treatment decisions. The most common assessment tools in psoriasis are described in Table 21.2 [118].

21.1.6.2 Histology

Skin biopsy is usually not needed to diagnose psoriasis; however, certain distinctive histopathological features can aid in its identification [119]. In plaque psoriasis, classic findings include hyperkeratosis, parakeratosis, loss of the granular cell layer, epidermal thickening (acanthosis), dilated and tortuous vasculature, and a leukocytic infiltrate (Fig. 21.9). The histopathological features vary depending on the lesion stage (Table 21.3). Key histological markers of psoriasis stem from hyperproliferation and impaired differentiation of keratinocytes [120]. Erythrodermic psoriasis is characterized by the absence of the stratum corneum and pronounced dilation of dermal vasculature, more prominent than in plaque psoriasis. Early plaque psoriasis features may also be observed in erythrodermic psoriasis. The diagnosis can be challenging due to nonspecific histological findings, often necessitating multiple biopsies [120]. Palmoplantar psoriasis is marked by multiple foci with alternating parakeratosis and orthokeratosis and an inflammatory infiltrate. Palmoplantar pustulosis shares similarities with generalized pustular psoriasis, including epidermal sterile pustules, while also exhibiting mild acanthosis and parakeratosis seen in plaque psoriasis [121].

Table 21.2 Psoriasis severity assessment tools

Assessment tool	Description
Body surface area (BSA)	Measures psoriasis extent based on body surface involvement, utilizing the "palm method" where each patient's palm accounts for 1% BSA. BSA classifies psoriasis as mild (<3% BSA), moderate (3–10% BSA), and severe (>10% BSA)
Physician's Global Assessment (PGA)	Rates psoriasis severity on a seven-item scale from clear to severe, used for both localized and extensive disease assessment. Differentiates between static and dynamic disease assessments. The static PGA, capturing the disease's severity at a specific point, is commonly employed for practical use
Psoriasis Area and Severity Index (PASI)	Evaluates severity and treatment response by scoring scaling, redness, induration, and plaque extent per body region. PASI is recommended as being a more accurate measurement for daily practice: PASI <1 (minimal), PASI <3 (very mild), PASI <5 (mild), PASI 5–10 (moderate), and PASI >10 (severe)
Investigator Global Assessment (IGA)	IGA uses a scale of 0 (clear) to 4 (severe) for visual assessment, requiring a score of 0 or 1 and a two-point improvement from baseline for treatment success
Dermatology Life Quality Index (DLQI)	A patient-reported questionnaire assessing life quality affected by psoriasis, but it may undervalue disease severity due to limitations in addressing psychological impacts. The DLQI comprises questions rated on a 4-point scale: 0 for "not at all/not relevant," 1 for "a little," 2 for "a lot," and 3 for "very much," resulting in a total DLQI score ranging from 0 to 30. DLQI score of ≥10 is used for defining severe psoriasis
Psoriasis Scalp Severity Index (PSSI)	Measures scalp psoriasis severity, excluding face and neck areas, using scores from 0 (absence of psoriasis) to 72 (most severe involvement). Scalp lesions' visibility and associated pruritus impact the patient's quality of life
Nail Psoriasis Severity Index (NAPSI)	An objective assessment tool for nail psoriasis, grading nail bed and matrix involvement in four quadrants of each nail for nail psoriasis features. Each nail receives a matrix and nail bed score (0–4), culminating in a total NAPSI score (0–80)
Erythema, Scaling, Induration, and Fissuring (ESIF)	Assesses palm and sole psoriasis severity using a 4-point scale (0 = clear to 3 = severe), with a total score from 0 (absence of disease) to 24 (most severe involvement)

21.1.7 Management

21.1.7.1 Topical Medication

Topical medications emerge as primary agents in managing mild to moderate psoriasis, or frequently complementing phototherapy, systemic, or biologic treatments. A list of topical treatments in psoriasis is listed in Table 21.4 [122].

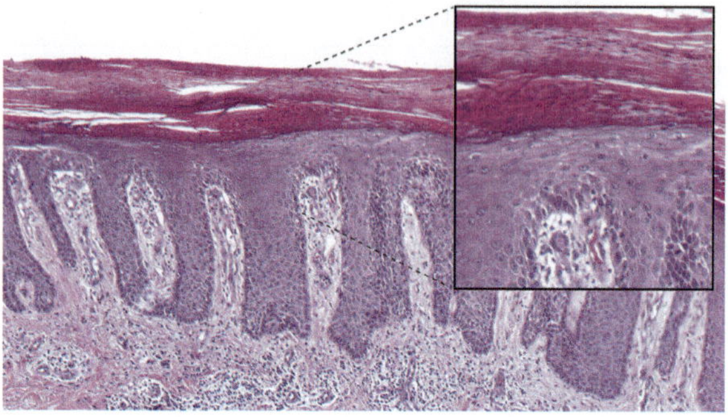

Fig. 21.9 Histopathology of psoriasis (H&E 10×): The epidermis exhibits hyperparakeratosis, along with regular epidermal acanthosis featuring elongated rete ridges, papillomatosis, and dilated, tortuous capillaries within the dermal papillae accompanied by a leukocytic infiltrate. A magnified view reveals parakeratosis with aberrant retention of nuclei in the stratum corneum, loss of the granular cell layer, acanthosis, dilated capillaries, and a mononuclear leukocytic infiltrate in the dermal papillae

Table 21.3 Histopathological features of psoriasis vulgaris [120]

Histopathological features of psoriasis vulgaris
– Hyperkeratosis
– Parakeratosis
– Loss of granular cell layer
– Epidermal acanthosis
– Dilated and tortuous vasculature
– Leukocytic infiltrate
– Epidermal thickening with elongated rete ridges
– Dilated and tortuous capillaries in dermal papillae
– Fine fibrillary collagen bundles in papillae
– Parakeratosis with aberrant retention of nuclei in stratum corneum
– Alternating areas of orthokeratosis and parakeratosis
– Increased mitoses in basal and suprabasal layer
– Mononuclear leukocytic infiltrate of lymphocytes
– Munro's microabscesses (neutrophil foci in parakeratotic stratum corneum)
– Spongiform neutrophilic micropustules of Kogoj (in spinous layer)

21.1.7.2 Phototherapy

Psoriasis has been treated with various forms of phototherapies over the years. These include narrowband ultraviolet B (NB-UVB), psoralen ultraviolet A (PUVA), pulsed dye laser (PDL), photodynamic therapy, intense pulsed light, and light-emitting diodes. Excimer laser/lamp and NB-UVB are first-line therapies. UV light and PDL are effective for stable plaque psoriasis, while PUVA is recommended for refractory cases if side effects are managed. Furthermore, PDL is preferred for nail psoriasis. Low-level light/laser therapy shows promise due to its strong penetration and photobiomodulation [123].

Table 21.4 Topical treatments in psoriasis

Treatment	Efficacy	Risks/harms	General comments
Topical corticosteroids	High efficacy, potency-based variation for localized disease Anti-inflammatory, antiproliferative, immunosuppressive, and vasoconstrictive effects	Skin atrophy, striae, folliculitis, telangiectasia, and purpura. Face, intertriginous areas, and chronically treated areas are at greater risk for adverse effects Exacerbation of acne, rosacea, perioral dermatitis, and tinea infections is possible Rebound effect upon abrupt withdrawal Rare: Cushing syndrome, osteonecrosis of the femoral head, and type 2 diabetes	Classified into seven categories; appropriate selection based on severity, location, and patient factors. "Proactive treatment" twice weekly of clinically quiescent areas to reduce flare frequency Tachyphylaxis: loss of effectiveness with prolonged corticosteroid use (>12 weeks)
Calcineurin inhibitors	Effective for intertriginous psoriasis. Block phosphorylation of calcineurin, inhibiting T-cell activation. Used as steroid-sparing agents for prolonged use (≥4 weeks)	Burning, pruritus, flushing with alcohol ingestion; boxed warning for potential lymphoma risk. No evidence of increased malignancy risk	Off-label use for up to 8 weeks; long-term use considered; combination with salicylic acid for plaque psoriasis
Vitamin D analogues	Bind to vitamin D receptors, inhibit keratinocyte proliferation, and enhance differentiation	Burning, pruritus, edema, peeling, dryness, and erythema; hypercalcemia with systemic use	Can be used in combination with topical corticosteroids; safe during pregnancy with low doses
Tazarotene	Acts on keratinocyte differentiation and proliferation Downregulates expression of pro-inflammatory genes Effective for mild to moderate psoriasis	Erythema, burning, and pruritus; side effects reduced in combination with corticosteroids and phototherapy; avoid in pregnant women	8–12 weeks recommended; combination with corticosteroids and phototherapy for enhanced efficacy

(continued)

Table 21.4 (continued)

Treatment	Efficacy	Risks/harms	General comments
Salicylic acid	Topical keratolytic agent in psoriasis treatment Reduces binding between keratinocytes, minimizing scaling, and softening psoriatic plaques	Caution in renal or hepatic disease due to systemic absorption and potential salicylate toxicity, especially for large body surface areas Avoid concomitant UVB phototherapy to maintain efficacy	Combination therapy, especially with corticosteroids, enhances efficacy by improving skin penetrationAlone or combined with corticosteroids and immunomodulators
Dithranol	Polycyclic aromatic hydrocarbon derivative Prevention of T-lymphocyte activation and promoting keratinocyte differentiation	Perilesional erythema, burning, and mild-to-severe staining of the skin. Short-contact application to avoid side effects No evidence of toxicities related to prolonged use	Avoid application to the face or other highly visible areas and flexures to prevent staining
Coal tar/LCD	Polyaromatic hydrocarbons in coal tar bind to the aryl hydrocarbon receptor Decreases keratinocyte proliferation by suppressing DNA synthesis Suppresses inflammation and may affect immunologic function	Local irritation, folliculitis, contact dermatitis, and phototoxicity Controversial evidence regarding possible carcinogenicity. Advisable to avoid coal tar preparations during pregnancy and lactation. Coal tar products can stain clothes	Coal tar preparations are frequently used with phototherapy

UV phototherapy, particularly NB-UVB, is a widely used and effective treatment for psoriasis. NB-UVB uses wavelengths between 311 and 313 nm [124]. Typical NB-UVB regimens involve three sessions per week for at least 3 months. The underlying mechanisms of UV therapy in psoriasis involve apoptosis of pathogenic T cells and keratinocytes, leading to local and systemic immunosuppression [125]. NB-UVB downregulates the Th17 pathway, increases Treg cells, and suppresses interferon signaling, contributing to psoriasis alleviation [126].

PUVA, utilizing psoralen and UVA, is considered the gold standard for topical therapy in psoriatic plaques [123]. It induces apoptosis and has shown better efficacy than UVB in palmoplantar pustular psoriasis [61]. Psoralens are available in various forms such as oral treatment, cream, or bath. However, the use of systemic psoralens is limited due to gastrointestinal symptoms and long-term carcinogenic risk [127]. Despite PUVA being more effective, NB-UVB is favored due to its superior safety profile, simplicity, and cost-effectiveness.

21.1.7.3 Systemic Medication

Cyclosporine A

CsA is a highly effective systemic therapy for psoriasis. CsA is used in psoriasis due to its potent inhibitory effect on T lymphocytes, suppressing their response to antigens by inhibiting cytokine secretion and proliferation. Marsili et al. [128] found that 39.3% of patients showed partial or suboptimal responses to CsA. The mean reduction in PASI score was 71.15%, indicating partial response. The most significant proportion of patients achieved a PASI 90 response. In psoriasis, a low-dose CsA therapy, meaning 2.5–3 mg/kg body weight daily, is preferred. CsA demonstrates dose-dependent adverse effects, particularly on kidney function, which may become irreversible with long-term use. Further adverse effects include an increased risk of infection, hypertension, arrhythmia, dyslipidemia, hypomagnesemia, hyperkalemia, gynecomastia, and hypertrichosis. Additionally, CsA poses an elevated risk of malignancies, including skin cancers, and increases susceptibility to various infections [129], due to low benefit/risk not suitable for the long-term management especially in patients with diabetes, due to increased risk for skin infection as well as risk for hypertension and renal impairment. Cyclosporine was reported to cause posttransplant diabetes mellitus by a number of mechanisms, including decreased insulin secretion, increased insulin resistance, or a direct toxic effect on the beta cell [130].

Methotrexate

MTX is a prodrug that is polyglutaminated in its active in vivo form. MTX exerts its impact on psoriasis through various mechanisms, including DNA synthesis blockade by the inhibitory effect on 5-aminoimidazole-4-carboxamide ribonucleotide transformylase. As a consequence, MTX induces apoptosis in keratinocytes and modulates immune responses, including the inhibition of chemotaxis in neutrophils and monocytes, the modulation of TNF-α by macrophages, and the proliferation of lymphocytes [131]. MTX should preferably be administered subcutaneously once a week to improve bioavailability [129]. The recommended initial and maintenance dose is usually 15 mg of MTX once a week, followed by the administration of 5 mg of folic acid 24 h after MTX application. The two most significant adverse events associated with MTX therapy are myelosuppression and hepatotoxicity. Factors such as alcohol consumption, obesity, hepatitis, and diabetes increase the risk of hepatotoxicity. Nausea, abdominal discomfort, and alopecia as well as infections are common adverse reactions of MTX. Treatment with MTX of psoriasis may have a positive effect on reducing the risk for T2DM in patients with moderate to severe psoriasis [129].

Acitretin

Acitretin, particularly in combination therapies, demonstrates modest efficacy in treating various psoriasis subtypes, such as palmoplantar pustulosis. Initial daily dosages between 10 and 25 mg, with stepwise escalation, demonstrated higher clinical efficacy and lower adverse event incidence compared to higher doses. Combination regimens, such as retinoids with PUVA or UVB, were more effective than monotherapy [132]. It is advisable to monitor the growth regularly in children undergoing treatment with acitretin. Hypertriglyceridemia and hypercholesterolemia are common adverse effects during the treatment. Dietary and lifestyle changes, including reducing alcohol consumption and adopting a low-fat, low-carbohydrate diet, represent an effective first-line management for lowering triglyceride levels. Other typical side effects include dry skin, cheilitis, epistaxis, xerophthalmia, retinoid-induced alopecia, hepatotoxicity, paronychia, dysglycemia, and pruritus [129]. Acitretin is not an ideal systemic medication for managing psoriasis in patients with diabetes, as it can lead to an increase in blood lipid levels.

Fumarates

Fumaric acid esters (FAEs), approved in Germany for psoriasis treatment since 1994, comprise diverse FAE, including the active drug dimethyl fumarate (DMF). The pure form of DMF, without other fumarate salts, has been available in Europe since 2017 and targets moderate-to-severe plaque psoriasis requiring systemic treatment [133]. While the mechanisms of action of DMF are not fully understood, its key roles in psoriasis involve anti-inflammatory, antioxidant, and immunomodulatory effects. DMF interacts through several pathways, including intracellular glutathione, inhibition of NF-κB activity, activation of the hydroxycarboxylic acid receptor 2, and degradation of hypoxia-inducible factor HIF-1α. Additionally, DMF promotes apoptosis in IL-12-producing dendritic cells by inactivating JAK/STAT [134]. The suggested starting dose is 30 mg/day, gradually increasing until clinical improvement is observed. If such improvement occurs before reaching the daily limit of 720 mg, that dosage can be maintained without the need for further increases. Side effects often include fatigue, asthenia, and flushing. Additionally, diarrhea, nausea, and abdominal pain, along with reduced appetite and elevated liver enzymes, are commonly reported. Hematological effects often manifest as very common leukopenia and lymphopenia, while neurological symptoms include common headaches and paresthesias, with occasional dizziness [135]. Treatment with FAE was shown to have a positive effect on insulin resistance [92].

Small Molecules

Apremilast

Apremilast, an oral phosphodiesterase 4 (PDE4) inhibitor, regulates the inflammatory response by elevating cyclic adenosine monophosphate levels. While approved for moderate-to-severe plaque psoriasis, apremilast inhibits PDE4, reducing inflammatory cytokines and promoting anti-inflammatory mediators [136]. The oral dosage of apremilast comprises 30 mg taken twice a day. It has an acceptable safety profile, without an increased incidence of cardiac events and malignancies. Common side effects such as diarrhea, nausea, and upper respiratory tract infections often self-resolve. Mental health-related events, such as depression and increased suicidality, were reported. Apremilast offers an oral alternative for psoriasis treatment, demonstrating efficacy and long-term tolerability [137].

JAK Inhibitors

JAK inhibitors have shown promise in the treatment of moderate-to-severe psoriasis and PsA, offering a new approach to managing these conditions. Several JAK inhibitors have been approved for various indications. Tofacitinib in combination with MTX is indicated for the treatment of active PsA in adult patients who have inadequately responded to other therapies [138]. Deucravacitinib 6 mg oral once daily is the only JAK inhibitor approved for the treatment of moderate-to-severe plaque psoriasis. Deucravacitinib inhibits tyrosine kinase 2 (TYK2), which facilitates immune signaling for IL-12, IL-23, and type I interferons without disrupting essential systemic functions [139]. Common side effects of JAK inhibitors for skin conditions include the common infections, headache, and nausea, while more serious side effects such as pneumonia or tuberculosis (TB) have also been reported. JAK inhibitors are linked to off-target effects, such as alterations in laboratory parameters such as hemoglobin, platelets, neutrophils, lipid panel, and creatine phosphokinase. Additionally, their use is associated with an increased risk of infections, malignancies, and thromboembolic events. For individuals with prominent risk factors such as advanced age and increased risks for malignancies or cardiovascular events including smoking, thromboses, and severe infections, medications from other drug classes should be recommended [140].

Biologics

Advancements in clinical trial data on biologics, in particular monoclonal antibodies, have significantly expanded therapeutic options for addressing moderate-to-severe psoriasis. Currently approved biologics for psoriasis encompass TNF alpha inhibitors (anti-TNFs), interleukin IL-17 inhibitors, ustekinumab (an IL-12/23 inhibitor), and IL-23 inhibitors. A summary of biologic treatments in psoriasis are listed in Table 21.5 [141]. Biologic therapies for moderate-to-severe psoriasis in the presence of comorbid conditions are a multifaceted process that demands meticulous consideration of various factors, including costs, patient preferences, and the severity of the disease. The selection of biologics should be especially considered

Table 21.5 Summary of biologic therapies in psoriasis vulgaris

Biologic	Structure	Target	Standard dosing	Average half-life	Efficacy (PASI-75)
Adalimumab	Human IgG1κ	TNF-α	Loading dose 80 mg; 40 mg every 2 weeks	14 days	71% at week 16
Certolizumab pegol	PEGylated fab fragment of humanized IgG1	TNF-α	400 mg weeks 0, 2, and 4, then 200 mg every 2 weeks	14 days	76.7% at week 16
Etanercept	TNF receptor and IgG Fc fusion protein	TNF-α	50 mg weekly	3 days	34% at week 12
Infliximab	Human-murine chimeric IgG1	TNF-α	5 mg/kg at weeks 0, 2, and 6, then every 8 weeks	8–9.5 days	89% at week 10
Secukinumab	Human IgG1κ	IL-17A	300 mg weeks 1–5, then 300 mg monthly	27 days	81.6% at week 12
Ixekizumab	Humanized IgG4	IL-17A	160 mg week 0, 80 mg at weeks 2, 4, 6, 8, 10, and 12, then 80 mg every 4 weeks	13 days	82.6% at week 12
Brodalumab	Human IgG2	IL-17RA	210 mg weeks 0, 1, and 2, then every 2 weeks	11 days	86% at week 12
Bimekizumab	Humanized IgG1	IL-17A, IL-17F, IL-17AF	320 mg weeks 0, 4, 8, 12, and 16, then every 8 weeks	23 days	91% at week 16
Ustekinumab	Human IgG1κ	p40 subunit of IL-12 and IL-23	45 mg weeks 0 and 4, then every 12 weeks	21 days	67% at week 12
Guselkumab	Human IgG1λ	p19 subunit of IL-23	100 mg weeks 0 and 4, then every 8 weeks	15–18 days	70% at week 16
Risankizumab	Humanized IgG1	p19 subunit of IL-23	150 mg weeks 0 and 4, then every 12 weeks	28–29 days	75% at week 16
Tildrakizumab	Humanized IgG1κ	p19 subunit of IL-23	100 mg weeks 0 and 4, then every 12 weeks	23.4 days	64% at week 12

when managing comorbid conditions such as PsA, multiple sclerosis, congestive heart failure, inflammatory bowel disease (IBD), hepatitis B, latent tuberculosis infection, and neoplasms [142]. For instance, anti-TNFs pose a risk of HBV reactivation, especially in HBsAg-positive psoriasis patients, with higher risks in the absence of antiviral prophylaxis [143]. Table 21.6 outlines the most common adverse events and guidelines regarding breastfeeding and pregnancy [141, 144, 145].

Table 21.6 Adverse events and recommendations in biologics for psoriasis

Adverse event/ conditions	Summary
Infections	– Serious infections show increased risk with anti-TNF infliximab, while ustekinumab demonstrates lower risk – Risk of candida infection with all anti-IL17 agents, particularly bimekizumab – Increased odds of developing tuberculosis (TB) with anti-TNFs. Screening for TB with interferon gamma release assay before initiating biologic therapy. Treat latent TB before biologic initiation
Postoperative infections	Lack of data on postoperative risk in psoriasis patients. Consider pausing biologic therapy on a case-by-case basis or timing surgery prior to the next dose if the risk of psoriasis flare is high
COVID-19 infection and vaccine response	– Anti-TNFs may be associated with a better prognosis in COVID-19 compared with conventional systemic agents – Reduced seroconversion following the first dose of certain vaccines in immunomodulator-treated psoriasis patients
Neoplasms	Observational studies do not demonstrate an increased cancer risk with biologic therapies. It should be considered risks and benefits of treatment discontinuation on a case-by-case basis
Cardiovascular	– Anti-TNFs may increase the risk of heart failure, and they are relatively contraindicated in this condition – Little data supporting biologics contributing to major adverse cardiovascular events (MACE). No evidence to influence biologic selection in those at high risk of MACE
Central nervous system	Anti-TNFs are not recommended for individuals with multiple sclerosis or with a first-degree relative with MS
Pregnancy	Certolizumab pegol does not cross the placenta, making it a consideration for women planning conception. Limited data on other biologics; no increases in prematurity, fetal death, or teratogenicity observed
Breastfeeding	Biologics are protein molecules unlikely to be absorbed systemically from breast milk. Breastfeeding should be theoretically safe, but evidence is lacking
Mental health	Biologic initiation is associated with an improvement in psychiatric symptoms. Psychiatric comorbidity should not influence the choice of biologic
Cutaneous adverse events	A range of potential adverse events reported, including paradoxical psoriasis and eczema, in particular with anti-TNFs and anti-IL-17 agents, respectively
IBD exacerbations	Anti-IL-17 s associated with new onset or exacerbation of existing IBD. Avoid anti-IL17s in patients with comorbid IBD

21.2 Psoriasis and Diabetes

21.2.1 Type 1 Diabetes Mellitus and Psoriasis

T1DM is a chronic autoimmune disease characterized by the destruction of insulin-producing β cells in the pancreas, resulting in disrupted glucose homeostasis. The well-established connection between psoriasis vulgaris and autoimmune disorders includes a finding that 1.3% of psoriasis patients in the study had T1DM [146]. Key mechanisms involve CD8+ and CD4+ T lymphocytes, along with pro-inflammatory cytokines, contributing to the destruction of approximately 90% of insulin-secreting β cells. T1DM onset is triggered by the breakdown of tolerance toward islet cell antigens in the pancreas, a result of the abrogation of CD4+ CD25+ FoxP3+ Treg cells [147]. Recent research emphasizes the involvement of Th17-dependent immunity in autoimmune diabetes, and inhibiting Th17 cells has shown to alleviate T1DM [148]. Although the role of Th17-dependent immunity in human T1DM is not fully elucidated, evidence links the upregulation of the IL-17 response to other immune-mediated diseases [149]. As established, individuals with T1D are more susceptible to other autoimmune diseases, including psoriasis [147]. In psoriasis, T-cell populations in lesions include Th1, Th22, and Th17 cells, with cytokines like TGFβ, IL-6, IL-1, IL-21, and IL-23 playing roles in Th17 cell differentiation and potentially perpetuating inflammatory processes. The pro-inflammatory cytokine IL-17 is a key player in psoriasis, contributing to inflammatory processes [150]. Additionally, cytokines such as IL-1β, IFN-γ, and TNF-α, implicated in T1DM, contribute to pancreatic β cell apoptosis [151].

21.2.2 Type 2 Diabetes Mellitus and Psoriasis

T2DM represents a persistent metabolic disorder marked by insulin resistance and compromised insulin secretion, frequently associated with lifestyle factors, including obesity and sedentarism. The chronic inflammation associated with psoriasis can give rise to concurrent disorders, including atherogenesis, atherosclerosis, insulin resistance, hypertension, obesity, dyslipidemia, MetS, and T2DM. Epidemiological studies have reported an average T2DM prevalence of 11.6% in psoriatic cohorts compared to controls [152]. Furthermore, late-onset psoriasis patients have a greater risk of T2DM compared to the early ones [153]. Nevertheless, it appears to be no correlation between the prevalence of T2DM and the severity of psoriasis and no discernible distinction in the risk or prevalence of T2DM among patients with both PsA and psoriasis vulgaris in comparison to those with psoriasis vulgaris alone [154]. Psoriasis shares a common pathogenic link with T2DM, primarily through the upregulation of pro-inflammatory cytokines, such as TNF-α, and the involvement of the IL-23/Th17 axis [155]. Systemic inflammation in psoriasis induces insulin resistance, an independent risk factor for T2DM

[156]. For instance, individuals with normal glucose tolerance and moderate to severe psoriasis exhibit higher insulin resistance compared to controls, suggesting that psoriasis may signify a prediabetic state [157]. Additionally, homeostatic model assessment for insulin resistance (HOMA-IR) values are elevated in psoriatic patients compared to control subjects, and a reduction in the PASI corresponds to a decrease in HOMA-IR values [158]. Insulin resistance is also linked to inflammatory cytokines and adipocytokines secreted by adipocytes, with comparable levels observed between psoriasis and prediabetic individuals [159].

21.2.3 Shared Pathogenesis

21.2.3.1 Genetics

The intricate genetic landscapes unravel their roles in autoimmune disorders, glucose metabolism, and immune response. The interplay of multiple genetic factors (Table 21.7) and their variants unfolds a complex tapestry underlying diabetes and psoriasis, providing insights into the intricate mechanisms governing these multifaceted biologic processes.

21.2.3.2 Epigenetics

MicroRNAs (miRNAs) are short, noncoding RNAs that regulate gene expression. Particularly, miR-21 was significantly upregulated in psoriasis skin lesions and correlated with disease activity and also plays an important role in diabetes and obesity (Table 21.8).

21.2.3.3 Inflammation

Psoriasis is characterized by sustained inflammation, driven by intricate interactions among diverse cell types and cytokines, in particular IL-17, TNF-α, IL-22, and IL-18 [183]. Tissue inflammation is a critical factor in insulin resistance, a primary defect in T2DM development, and a central component of MetS [184]. IL-17 plays a crucial role in inflammation, insulin resistance, and T2DM, suggesting it as a potential mediator connecting MetS and psoriasis. Elevated serum IL-17 levels are observed in MetS and T1DM patients [185]. IL-17 promotes a vascular inflammatory response and plays a critical role in angiotensin II-induced hypertension and vascular dysfunction. Secukinumab shows efficacy in treating plaque psoriasis, reduces fasting glucose levels, and improves hyperglycemia in psoriasis patients, mean body weight, waist circumference, and BMI consistently decreased with potential benefits on body weight and metabolic parameters [186]. Moreover, TNF is closely associated with psoriasis pathogenesis. TNF-α inhibitors improve

Table 21.7 Genes implicated in psoriasis and diabetes

PTPN22	– PTPN22 encodes the lysine tyrosine phosphatase (Lyp) protein that prevents spontaneous T-cell activation and inactivating T-cell receptor-associated kinases [160, 161] – The Lyp R620W variant in type 1 diabetes mellitus (T1DM) increases autoreactive B cells, contributing to autoimmune diseases by presenting autoantigens to T lymphocytes [162] – In T1DM patients, this variant leads to reduced B-cell receptor signaling and resistance to cell death in transitional and naïve B cells, irrespective of the PTPN22 genotype [163] – The PTPN22 C1858T variant disrupts the balance of B cells and Toll-like receptor (TLR)-9-mediated responses in T1DM patients, impacting both innate and adaptive immunity [164] The Lyp variant may influence cytokine production, with some Caucasian T1DM patients exhibiting a defect in IL-2 production [161, 165] – Specific genetic variants within PTPN22 are associated with psoriatic arthritis (PsA), particularly the coding variant R620W, highlighting the gene's role in this autoimmune disease [166] – PTPN22 may influence various cells and pathways in PsA, potentially contributing to differential phenotypes of Th17 in PsA, psoriasis vulgaris, or ankylosing spondylitis [167]
MTHFR	– MTHFR gene encodes methylenetetrahydrofolate reductase, a crucial enzyme for methionine conversion, vital for DNA methylation [168] – MTHFR C667T polymorphism is related to hyperhomocysteinemia, psoriasis, and diabetes – Homozygous MTHFR 677TT genotype in psoriasis may exhibit altered demethylation levels of the SHP-1 promoter II, impacting keratinocyte terminal differentiation and epidermal differentiation [169] – MTHFR is crucial in folate metabolism and plays a vital role in diabetes The C667T polymorphism is associated with insulin resistance, inflammation, and hyperhomocysteinemia [170] – MTHFR gene polymorphism can contribute to progression, as well as complications such as nephropathy and retinopathy, particularly in individuals with poorly managed blood glucose levels [171]
JAZF1	The JAZF1 gene harbors an intron variant linked to psoriasis, operating through an undisclosed mechanism. Additionally, this gene functions as a transcriptional repressor, exerting a negative impact on glucose metabolism and contributing to beta-cell impairment, probably by growth retardation, hypoglycemia, and reduced gluconeogenesis [172]
ST6GAL1	– ST6GAL1 is a glycosyltransferase involved in modifying glycoproteins, influencing cell-surface carbohydrate determinants and antigens differentiation – The glycosyltransferase activity of ST6GAL1 is crucial for lymphocyte function. ST6GAL1 is highly expressed during T-lymphocyte activation, suggesting a potential role in immune response
CDKAL1	– CDKAL1 gene to psoriasis, which is also implicated in Crohn's disease and T2DM [173] – CDKAL1 transcripts are absent from skin keratinocytes, while are expressed in immune cells, particularly in CD4+ and CD19+ lymphocytes, with downregulation during immune cell activation [174]

Table 21.8 Role of miR-21 in psoriasis and diabetes

Role of miR-21	Functions
Psoriasis	– Upregulated miR-21 in psoriasis skin lesions, correlated with disease activity [175] – Inhibits apoptosis in activated T cells – Induces Th17 polarization [176] – TNF-α shedding is needed for TNF-α signaling activation, miR-21 reduces TIMP-3 expression, activating the TNF-α sheddase TACE/ADAM17, leading to TNF-α overexpression [177] – Elevated miR-21 may result from impaired Jun/AP-1 transcriptional activity, activating IL-6/Stat3 pathway [178] – Overexpression of miR-21 contributes to T cell-mediated inflammation in psoriatic skin
Diabetes and obesity	– miR-21 plays a central role in differentiation and function of white and brown adipose tissue [179] – miR-21 correlates positively with BMI in subcutaneous adipose tissue – In human adipose tissue-derived mesenchymal stem cells, miR-21 modulates TGF-β signaling in adipogenic differentiation [180]
Diabetes and kidney	– Renal miR-21 expression is upregulated in type 2 diabetes mellitus – Overexpression of miR-21 magnifies high glucose-induced abundance of fibrotic markers in mesangial and tubular epithelial cells – Correlates with the development of microalbuminuria, renal fibrosis, and inflammation [181]
Pancreatic β cells	– Protective role in pancreatic β cells through the transcription factors c-Rel and p65 activate miR-21 gene promoter – miR-21 reduces levels of PDCD4, protecting against apoptosis mediated by the Bax family of proteins [182]

metabolic parameters in psoriasis patients, including blood lipid and glucose levels and blood pressure [187]. TNF-α plays a direct role in insulin resistance by initiating the activation of stress kinases, including IκB kinase, c-Jun N-terminal kinase, and p38 mitogen-activated protein kinase in both muscle and fat cells. This activation subsequently impedes insulin signal transduction pathways. Furthermore, TNF-α inhibits cell uptake of oxidized LDL, contributing to metabolic dysregulation [188]. Inhibition of TNF-α with adalimumab improves insulin sensitivity in patients with moderate-to-severe plaque psoriasis [189]. Serum IL-1β, IL-6, and IL-22 levels are elevated in patients with T2DM and obese individuals, cytokines which play an important part in the psoriasis pathogenesis. Moreover, experimental IFN-γ deletion improves insulin resistance and metabolic parameters in diet-induced obesity models [190].

IL-18, a pivotal cytokine in the Th1 response, exhibits pleiotropic effects crucial for immune defense against pathogens, primarily through the induction of IFNγ. It is a pro-inflammatory cytokine that triggers the expression of adhesion molecules; IL-18 demonstrates the capacity to enhance the synthesis of granulocyte macrophage colony-stimulating factor, TNF-α, and inducible nitric oxide synthase in both mononuclear and mesenchymal cells [190]. Besides that, IL-18 is produced in human adipose tissue, and its levels are associated with body weight and abdominal fat deposition. Increased IL-18 secretion from adipocytes in obese individuals correlates with higher BMI, adiposity, T2DM, insulin resistance, hypertriglyceridemia, and MetS [191]. IL-18 is implicated in the pathogenesis and progression of T1DM. Increased IL-18 expression in pancreatic β cells contributes to insulitis, inflammation, and cell death, and its presence is observed in the pancreatic islets of patients with fulminant T1DM. In psoriasis, IL-18 is constitutively expressed by keratinocytes, with higher levels in active lesions than stable ones. Furthermore, psoriatic patients exhibit increased serum IL-18 levels. Epidermal dendritic cells express the IL-18 receptor and, when stimulated by IL-18, demonstrate increased migratory tendency, suggesting a role in psoriasis pathophysiology [192]. The shared involvement of IL-18 in the pathogenesis of both psoriasis and T1DM is evident, contributing to insulitis and inflammation in pancreatic β cells, and influencing the inflammatory state in active psoriatic lesions, suggesting a potential link between these immune-mediated conditions.

21.2.3.4 Cellular Metabolism

Insulin resistance plays a crucial role in the pathophysiology of both diabetes and psoriasis, with a significant link with inflammation. In patients with psoriasis, dysregulation of inflammatory mediators, such as cytokines and adipokines, contributes to the development of insulin resistance [193]. This connection is noteworthy as insulin resistance has been identified in psoriasis patients, showing a substantial correlation with the extent and severity of the condition, even in the absence of concurrent MetS. Furthermore, in situations of hyperinsulinemia characteristic of T2DM, insulin can bind to IGF receptors, leading to increased proliferation of keratinocytes and fibroblasts. Additionally, diminished levels of adiponectin, a promoter of insulin sensitivity and inducer of anti-inflammatory cytokines, are observed in both psoriasis and T2DM [155].

The phosphoinositide 3-kinase (PI3K)/Akt/mTOR cascade acts as a key mediator of inflammation and a master sensor of intracellular metabolic status. mTOR, a central player in nutrient and growth factor sensing, regulates cellular processes based on metabolic needs. Activated mTOR signaling is implicated in psoriasis pathogenesis, influencing cell proliferation, differentiation, and inflammatory mediator secretion [194]. The Akt/mTOR pathway is also linked to metabolic complications associated with psoriasis, such as insulin resistance and obesity. In particular, the activation of mTOR is indispensable for the differentiation of T-helper effector cell lineages, facilitating the development toward Th1, Th2, and Th17. Enhanced mTOR signaling has been identified in the proliferating γδ T cells that secrete IL-17, responding to innate stimuli such as IL-23 and IL-1β. Typically, mTORC1 activation occurs in the basal layer cells of healthy skin, promoting differentiation while reducing proliferative capacity. In contrast, in the upper epidermal keratinocytes, mTORC1 is usually deactivated [195]. Persistent mTORC1 activation in keratinocytes has been proposed as a pivotal mechanism in the development of psoriasis. Exposure of keratinocytes to inflammatory cytokines such as IL-1β, IL-17A, IL-22, and TNF-α activates mTORC1 and its downstream targets, resulting in increased proliferation and stalled differentiation [196]. Furthermore, the Akt/mTOR pathway increased secretion of IL-6, CXCL8, or VEGF from keratinocytes exposed to TNF-α, augmenting the immune response [195].

21.2.3.5 Endothelial Dysfunction

Atherosclerosis, a key component of cardiovascular disease, is recognized as a process fueled by inflammation. Additionally, the underlying pathophysiology of psoriasis is deeply rooted in inflammatory cytokines that induce insulin resistance, eventually leading to downstream endothelial dysfunction and hyperproliferation [197]. Markers of endothelial dysfunction and plaque alteration, such as soluble intercellular adhesion molecule-1 (sICAM-1), soluble vascular cell adhesion molecule-1 (sVCAM-1), soluble E-selectin (sE-selectin), and metalloproteinases MMP-2 and MMP-9, are elevated in both diabetes and psoriasis [1]. Fibrinolytic and vascular markers such as plasminogen activator inhibitor-1 (PAI-1) and homocysteine (Hct) are increased in diabetes and psoriasis as well. High levels of plasminogen activator inhibitor-1 (PAI-1), a powerful inhibitor of fibrinolysis, were observed in individuals with psoriasis compared to healthy subjects. However, during treatment with ranitidine, there was a subsequent decrease in PAI-1 levels, and this reduction was found to be correlated with improvements in the PASI [198]. Moreover, earlier findings of endothelial dysfunction associated with subclinical atherosclerosis have been identified in patients with psoriasis compared to individuals without the condition, measured by high-resolution Doppler ultrasound. There is as yet no established mechanism to linking anti-IL-17A directly to flow-mediated dilation (FMD) improvement in psoriasis patients, and it is speculated that such an effect may be mediated, either directly or indirectly, through the influence of IL-17A on the reduction of systemic inflammation and oxidative stress, ultimately enhancing endothelial vasodilatory capacity [199].

21.2.3.6 Adipocyte

White adipose tissue has been recognized as an active endocrine organ, releasing soluble mediators termed adipokines, cytokines that play a pivotal role in various physiological processes, including immunity and inflammation [200]. Therefore, adipokines contribute to a low-grade inflammatory state observed in individuals with obesity [201]. Importantly, the intricate interplay between adipokines and inflammation has broader implications for psoriasis and diabetes. A list of adipokines and their implication in inflammation are listed in Table 21.9 [190].

Table 21.9 List of adipokines implicated in psoriasis and diabetes

Adipokine	Functions	Regulation in obesity	Implications in inflammation
Leptin	Regulates satiety and energy expenditure	Elevated expression in adipose tissue and circulation in obese individuals	Promotes pro-inflammatory cytokines release (TNF-α, IL-12, IL-6) in response to inflammatory mediators (TNF-α, IL-1β, insulin). Contributes to reduction in Treg cells, exacerbating local inflammation
Adiponectin	Involved in metabolic regulation, with insulin-sensitizing properties	Decreased serum levels in overweight individuals, increased with calorie restriction. Pro-inflammatory cytokines (TNF-α, IL-6) inhibit adiponectin secretion	Reduces secretion and activity of TNF-α and IL-6. Promotes anti-inflammatory mediators (IRAK-1) in macrophages, monocytes, and dendritic cells. Enhances Treg cell abundance
Resistin	Resists insulin action and impairs glucose homeostasis	Expression increased in human peripheral blood mononuclear cells with obesity Stimulated by pro-inflammatory cytokines (TNF-α, IL-1β, IL-6)	Implicated in inflammatory processes rather than glucose homeostasis modulation
Visfatin	Enhances production of inflammatory cytokines by leukocytes	Upregulated by inflammatory cytokines IL-6, TNF-α, and IL-1β	Plays a crucial role in T-cell activation, influences B- and T-lymphocyte development Acts as a chemotactic factor for lymphocytes and monocytes

21.2.4 Management

Lifestyle modifications, such as diet, weight reduction, smoking cessation, and increased physical activity, have shown benefits in both diabetes and psoriasis patients. Pharmacologic treatments such as glucagon-like peptide-1 receptor agonists (GLP-1R), thiazolidinediones, and metformin may have positive effects on both conditions. The reported positive effects of various drugs highlight a potential correlation between these diseases. Thiazolidinediones demonstrated antiproliferative and anti-inflammatory effects in human cells, with the expression of PPAR-γ observed in human keratinocytes. Activation of PPAR-γ was found to inhibit proliferation of keratinocytes in psoriasis as well as reduction of PASI [202]. Beyond its role as an antidiabetic medication, metformin exhibits a direct anti-inflammatory effect and proliferation inhibition in keratinocytes attributed to the activation of AMP-activated protein kinase and inhibition of mTOR pathways. Metformin reduces the risk of psoriasis development in diabetic patients. Significant success has been noted in effectively treating patients with both psoriasis and MetS using metformin [203]. Osteopontin, linked to vessel formation and inflammation through

Table 21.10 Effects of psoriasis management on metabolic syndrome

Medication	Effects on metabolic syndrome
Methotrexate	Associated with hepatotoxicity; reduces metabolic syndrome (MetS); decreases risk of type 2 diabetes (T2DM). No significant impact on glycemic index in psoriatic arthritis (PsA) patients
Cyclosporine	Worsens serum lipid and glucose levels Diabetogenic effect by inhibiting insulin secretion from pancreatic β cells
Acitretin	Results in hypertriglyceridemia, especially as part of hyperlipidemia
Anti-TNF-α	Mixed results. Insulin resistance improvement with infliximab in RA patients; etanercept augments insulin sensitivity in psoriasis patients; adalimumab improves β-cell function. However, increase in body weight and BMI with TNF-α inhibitors, potentially impacting on insulin resistance. No consistent effect on dyslipidemia; potential decrease in blood pressure with infliximab
Ustekinumab	No significant changes in fasting glucose levels; potential correlation with severe cardiovascular events in high-risk patients
Anti-IL-17 agents	Secukinumab leads to decreased body weight Ixekizumab shows no significant changes in glucose, lipid parameters, or blood pressure
Anti-IL-23 agents	Tildrakizumab is associated with weight increase; guselkumab impact not specified
Apremilast	Associated with weight loss; reduces total cholesterol, LDL, and HDL. No significant impact on Hb1Ac or endothelial function
JAK inhibitors	JAK inhibitors may induce hypoglycemia by increasing insulin sensitivity and consequently may reduce the need for antidiabetic medication

IL-1, is implicated in conditions such as psoriasis, insulin resistance, obesity, and T2DM. Metformin mitigates its upregulation, suggesting a potential dual regulatory role in both diseases [204]. Liraglutide, a GLP-1R agonist, is effective in treating plaque psoriasis coexisting with T2DM. GLP-1R treatment significantly reduced PASI scores, along with lower fasting plasma glucose levels. The effect of liraglutide may be related to the inhibition of inflammatory factors such as IL-23, IL-17, and TNF-α [205]. Current psoriasis therapies may have the potential to address MetS and diabetes. Notably, TNF-α inhibitors, such as adalimumab, demonstrate potential in improving insulin sensitivity [206]. Ustekinumab inhibits both IFN-γ and IL-17 signaling pathways that play critical roles in the pathogenesis of both psoriasis and the loss of β cells in T1DM [207]. Nevertheless, traditional systemic therapies may exacerbate MetS, as detailed in Table 21.10, outlining the impact of psoriasis management on MetS [79, 208].

Acknowledgements We extend our gratitude to Dr. Tatiana Sezin for her invaluable assistance in capturing the histological pictures.

Competing Interests The authors declare no competing financial or nonfinancial interests associated with the content of the book.

References

1. Brazzelli V, Maffioli P, Bolcato V, et al. Psoriasis and diabetes, a dangerous association: evaluation of insulin resistance, lipid abnormalities, and cardiovascular risk biomarkers. Front Med (Lausanne). 2021;8:605691. https://doi.org/10.3389/fmed.2021.605691.
2. Parisi R, Iskandar IYK, Kontopantelis E, et al. National, regional, and worldwide epidemiology of psoriasis: systematic analysis and modelling study. BMJ. 2020;369:m1590. https://doi.org/10.1136/bmj.m1590.
3. Damiani G, Bragazzi NL, Karimkhani Aksut C, et al. The global, regional, and national burden of psoriasis: results and insights from the Global Burden of disease 2019 study. Front Med (Lausanne). 2021;8:743180. https://doi.org/10.3389/fmed.2021.743180.
4. Armstrong AW, Mehta MD, Schupp CW, et al. Psoriasis prevalence in adults in the United States. JAMA Dermatol. 2021;157(8):940–6. https://doi.org/10.1001/jamadermatol.2021.2007.
5. Icen M, Crowson CS, McEvoy MT, et al. Trends in incidence of adult-onset psoriasis over three decades: a population-based study. J Am Acad Dermatol. 2009;60(3):394–401. https://doi.org/10.1016/j.jaad.2008.10.062.
6. Khalid JM, Globe G, Fox KM, et al. Treatment and referral patterns for psoriasis in United Kingdom primary care: a retrospective cohort study. BMC Dermatol. 2013;13:9. https://doi.org/10.1186/1471-5945-13-9.
7. Tollefson MM, Crowson CS, McEvoy MT, et al. Incidence of psoriasis in children: a population-based study. J Am Acad Dermatol. 2010;62(6):979–87. https://doi.org/10.1016/j.jaad.2009.07.029.
8. Liang Y, Sarkar MK, Tsoi LC, et al. Psoriasis: a mixed autoimmune and autoinflammatory disease. Curr Opin Immunol. 2017;49:1–8. https://doi.org/10.1016/j.coi.2017.07.007.
9. Rendon A, Schäkel K. Psoriasis pathogenesis and treatment. Int J Mol Sci. 2019;20(6):1475. https://doi.org/10.3390/ijms20061475.
10. Zhou X, Chen Y, Cui L, et al. Advances in the pathogenesis of psoriasis: from keratinocyte perspective. Cell Death Dis. 2022;13(1):81. https://doi.org/10.1038/s41419-022-04523-3.
11. Di Meglio P, Villanova F, Nestle FO. Psoriasis. Cold Spring Harb Perspect Med. 2014;4(8):a015354. https://doi.org/10.1101/cshperspect.a015354.
12. Morizane S, Yamasaki K, Mühleisen B, et al. Cathelicidin antimicrobial peptide LL-37 in psoriasis enables keratinocyte reactivity against TLR9 ligands. J Invest Dermatol. 2012;132(1):135–43. https://doi.org/10.1038/jid.2011.259.
13. Kim TG, Kim DS, Kim HP, et al. The pathophysiological role of dendritic cell subsets in psoriasis. BMB Rep. 2014;47(2):60–8. https://doi.org/10.5483/bmbrep.2014.47.2.014.
14. Chan TC, Hawkes JE, Krueger JG. Interleukin 23 in the skin: role in psoriasis pathogenesis and selective interleukin 23 blockade as treatment. Ther Adv Chronic Dis. 2018;9(5):111–9. https://doi.org/10.1177/2040622318759282.
15. Lowes MA, Kikuchi T, Fuentes-Duculan J, et al. Psoriasis vulgaris lesions contain discrete populations of Th1 and Th17 T cells. J Invest Dermatol. 2008;128(5):1207–11. https://doi.org/10.1038/sj.jid.5701213.
16. Witte E, Kokolakis G, Witte K, et al. IL-19 is a component of the pathogenetic IL-23/IL-17 cascade in psoriasis. J Invest Dermatol. 2014;134(11):2757–67. https://doi.org/10.1038/jid.2014.308.
17. Sachen KL, Arnold Greving CN, et al. Role of IL-36 cytokines in psoriasis and other inflammatory skin conditions. Cytokine. 2022;156(155897):155897. https://doi.org/10.1016/j.cyto.2022.155897.
18. Macleod T, Ainscough JS, Hesse C, et al. The proinflammatory cytokine IL-36γ is a global discriminator of harmless microbes and invasive pathogens within epithelial tissues. Cell Rep. 2020;33(11):108515. https://doi.org/10.1016/j.celrep.2020.108515.
19. Taheri Sarvtin M, Shokohi T, Hajheydari Z, et al. Evaluation of candidal colonization and specific humoral responses against Candida albicans in patients with psoriasis. Int J Dermatol. 2014;53(12):e555–60. https://doi.org/10.1111/ijd.12562.

20. Ran D, Cai M, Zhang X. Genetics of psoriasis: a basis for precision medicine. Precis Clin Med. 2019;2(2):120–30. https://doi.org/10.1093/pcmedi/pbz011.
21. Tsoi LC, Spain SL, Knight J, et al. Identification of 15 new psoriasis susceptibility loci highlights the role of innate immunity. Nat Genet. 2012;44(12):1341–8. https://doi.org/10.1038/ng.2467.
22. Jordan CT, Cao L, Roberson EDO, et al. Rare and common variants in CARD14, encoding an epidermal regulator of NF-kappaB, in psoriasis. Am J Hum Genet. 2012;90(5):796–808. https://doi.org/10.1016/j.ajhg.2012.03.013.
23. Nestle FO, Conrad C, Tun-Kyi A, et al. Plasmacytoid predendritic cells initiate psoriasis through interferon-alpha production. J Exp Med. 2005;202(1):135–43. https://doi.org/10.1084/jem.20050500.
24. Di Cesare A, Di Meglio P, Nestle FO. The IL-23/Th17 axis in the immunopathogenesis of psoriasis. J Invest Dermatol. 2009;129(6):1339–50. https://doi.org/10.1038/jid.2009.59.
25. Mateu-Arrom L, Puig L. Genetic and epigenetic mechanisms of psoriasis. Genes (Basel). 2023;14(8):1619. https://doi.org/10.3390/genes14081619.
26. Xiang Z, Yang Y, Chang C, et al. The epigenetic mechanism for discordance of autoimmunity in monozygotic twins. J Autoimmun. 2017;83:43–50. https://doi.org/10.1016/j.jaut.2017.04.003.
27. Gao L, Lu Q. The critical importance of epigenetics in autoimmune-related skin diseases. Front Med. 2023;17(1):43–57. https://doi.org/10.1007/s11684-022-0980-8.
28. Zhang P, Su Y, Chen H, et al. Abnormal DNA methylation in skin lesions and PBMCs of patients with psoriasis vulgaris. J Dermatol Sci. 2010;60(1):40–2. https://doi.org/10.1016/j.jdermsci.2010.07.011.
29. Li H, Yao Q, Mariscal AG, et al. Epigenetic control of IL-23 expression in keratinocytes is important for chronic skin inflammation. Nat Commun. 2018;9(1):1420. https://doi.org/10.1038/s41467-018-03704-z.
30. Ovejero-Benito MC, Reolid A, Sánchez-Jiménez P, et al. Histone modifications associated with biological drug response in moderate-to-severe psoriasis. Exp Dermatol. 2018;27(12):1361–71. https://doi.org/10.1111/exd.13790.
31. Wei T, Folkersen L, Biskup E, et al. Ubiquitin-specific peptidase 2 as a potential link between microRNA-125b and psoriasis. Br J Dermatol. 2017;176(3):723–31. https://doi.org/10.1111/bjd.14916.
32. Duan Q, Wang G, Wang M, et al. LncRNA RP6-65G23.1 accelerates proliferation and inhibits apoptosis via p-ERK1/2/p-AKT signaling pathway on keratinocytes. J Cell Biochem. 2020;121(11):4580–9. https://doi.org/10.1002/jcb.29685.
33. Ghosh D, Ganguly T, Chatterjee R. Emerging roles of non-coding RNAs in psoriasis pathogenesis. Funct Integr Genomics. 2023;23(2):129. https://doi.org/10.1007/s10142-023-01057-5.
34. Hampton PJ, Jans R, Flockhart RJ, et al. Lithium regulates keratinocyte proliferation via glycogen synthase kinase 3 and NFAT2 (nuclear factor of activated T cells 2). J Cell Physiol. 2012;227(4):1529–37. https://doi.org/10.1002/jcp.22872.
35. Brown G, Wang E, Leon A, et al. Tumor necrosis factor-α inhibitor-induced psoriasis: systematic review of clinical features, histopathological findings, and management experience. J Am Acad Dermatol. 2017;76(2):334–41. https://doi.org/10.1016/j.jaad.2016.08.012.
36. Weisenseel P, Laumbacher B, Besgen P, et al. Streptococcal infection distinguishes different types of psoriasis. J Med Genet. 2002;39(10):767–8. https://doi.org/10.1136/jmg.39.10.767.
37. Fife DJ, Waller JM, Jeffes EW, et al. Unraveling the paradoxes of HIV-associated psoriasis: a review of T-cell subsets and cytokine profiles. Dermatol Online J. 2007;13(2):4. https://doi.org/10.5070/d34sf63339.
38. Lee EB, Wu KK, Lee MP, et al. Psoriasis risk factors and triggers. Cutis. 2018;102(5S):18–20.
39. Zhou H, Wu R, Kong Y, et al. Impact of smoking on psoriasis risk and treatment efficacy: a meta-analysis. J Int Med Res. 2020;48(10):300060520964024. https://doi.org/10.1177/0300060520964024.

40. Wei J, Zhu J, Xu H, et al. Alcohol consumption and smoking in relation to psoriasis: a Mendelian randomization study. Br J Dermatol. 2022;187(5):684–91. https://doi.org/10.1111/bjd.21718.
41. Gerdes S, Zahl VA, Weichenthal M, et al. Smoking and alcohol intake in severely affected patients with psoriasis in Germany. Dermatology. 2010;220(1):38–43. https://doi.org/10.1159/000265557.
42. Poikolainen K, Reunala T, Karvonen J, et al. Alcohol intake: a risk factor for psoriasis in young and middle aged men? BMJ (Clin Res Ed). 1990;300(6727):780–3. https://doi.org/10.1136/bmj.300.6727.780.
43. Cassano N, Vestita M, Apruzzi D, et al. Alcohol, psoriasis, liver disease, and anti-psoriasis drugs. Int J Dermatol. 2011;50(11):1323–31. https://doi.org/10.1111/j.1365-4632.2011.05100.x.
44. Kirby B, Richards HL, Mason DL, et al. Alcohol consumption and psychological distress in patients with psoriasis. Br J Dermatol. 2008;158(1):138–40. https://doi.org/10.1111/j.1365-2133.2007.08299.x.
45. Tobin AM, Higgins EM, Norris S, et al. Prevalence of psoriasis in patients with alcoholic liver disease. Clin Exp Dermatol. 2009;34(6):698–701. https://doi.org/10.1111/j.1365-2230.2008.03140.x.
46. Kelly-Sell MK, Gudjonsson JE, Wu JJ, Feldman SR, Lebwohl MG. Chapter 1: Overview of psoriasis. In: Wu JJ, Feldman SR, Lebwohl MG, editors. Therapy for severe psoriasis. 1st ed. Amsterdam: Elsevier; 2016. p. 1–15.
47. Yan BX, Chen XY, Ye LR, et al. Cutaneous and systemic psoriasis: classifications and classification for the distinction. Front Med (Lausanne). 2021;8:649408. https://doi.org/10.3389/fmed.2021.649408.
48. Saleh D, Tanner LS. Guttate psoriasis. In: StatPearls. Treasure Island (FL): StatPearls Publishing; 2023. https://www.ncbi.nlm.nih.gov/books/NBK482498/.
49. Galili E, Levy SR, Tzanani I, et al. New-onset guttate psoriasis: a long-term follow-up study. Dermatology. 2023;239(2):188–94. https://doi.org/10.1159/000527737.
50. Micali G, Verzì AE, Giuffrida G, et al. Inverse psoriasis: from diagnosis to current treatment options. Clin Cosmet Investig Dermatol. 2019;12:953–9. https://doi.org/10.2147/CCID.S189000.
51. Hong JJ, Mosca ML, Hadeler EK, et al. Genital and inverse/intertriginous psoriasis: an updated review of therapies and recommendations for practical management. Dermatol Ther (Heidelb). 2021;11(3):833–44. https://doi.org/10.1007/s13555-021-00536-6.
52. Dopytalska K, Sobolewski P, Błaszczak A, et al. Psoriasis in special localizations. Reumatologia. 2018;56(6):392–8. https://doi.org/10.5114/reum.2018.80718.
53. Choon SE, Navarini AA, Pinter A. Clinical course and characteristics of generalized pustular psoriasis. Am J Clin Dermatol. 2022;23(Suppl. 1):21–9. https://doi.org/10.1007/s40257-021-00654-z.
54. Rivera-Díaz R, Daudén E, Carrascosa JM, et al. Generalized pustular psoriasis: a review on clinical characteristics, diagnosis, and treatment. Dermatol Ther (Heidelb). 2023;13(3):673–88. https://doi.org/10.1007/s13555-022-00881-0.
55. Romiti R, Hirayama ALDS, Arnone M, et al. Generalized pustular psoriasis (von Zumbusch). An Bras Dermatol. 2022;97(1):63–74. https://doi.org/10.1016/j.abd.2021.05.011.
56. Ruggiero A, Lauro W, Fabbrocini G, et al. A case of recalcitrant circinate generalized (Lapière) psoriasis successfully treated with risankizumab. Case Rep Dermatol. 2022;14(2):138–43. https://doi.org/10.1159/000523756.
57. Zheng M, Jullien D, Eyerich K. The prevalence and disease characteristics of generalized pustular psoriasis. Am J Clin Dermatol. 2022;23(Suppl. 1):5–12. https://doi.org/10.1007/s40257-021-00664-x.
58. Kondo RN, Araújo FM, Pereira AM, et al. Pustular psoriasis of pregnancy (impetigo herpetiformis)—case report. An Bras Dermatol. 2013;88(6 Suppl. 1):186–9. https://doi.org/10.1590/abd1806-4841.20132134.

59. Brunasso AMG, Puntoni M, Aberer W, et al. Clinical and epidemiological comparison of patients affected by palmoplantar plaque psoriasis and palmoplantar pustulosis: a case series study. Br J Dermatol. 2013;168(6):1243–51. https://doi.org/10.1111/bjd.12223.
60. Marsland AM, Chalmers RJG, Hollis S, et al. Interventions for chronic palmoplantar pustulosis. Cochrane Database Syst Rev. 2006;2016(1):CD001433. https://doi.org/10.1002/14651858.CD001433.pub2.
61. Sevrain M, Richard MA, Barnetche T, et al. Treatment for palmoplantar pustular psoriasis: systematic literature review, evidence-based recommendations and expert opinion. J Eur Acad Dermatol Venereol. 2014;28(s5):13–6. https://doi.org/10.1111/jdv.12561.
62. Kromer C, Loewe E, Schaarschmidt ML, et al. Treatment of acrodermatitis continua of Hallopeau: a case series of 39 patients. J Dermatol. 2020;47(9):989–97. https://doi.org/10.1111/1346-8138.15466.
63. Piraccini BM, Fanti PA, Morelli R, et al. Hallopeau's acrodermatitis continua of the nail apparatus: a clinical and pathological study of 20 patients. Acta Derm Venereol. 1994;74(1):65–7. https://doi.org/10.2340/00015555746567.
64. Assan F, Husson B, Hegazy S, et al. Palmoplantar pustulosis and acrodermatitis continua of Hallopeau: demographic and clinical comparative study in a large multicentre cohort. J Eur Acad Dermatol Venereol. 2022;36(9):1578–83. https://doi.org/10.1111/jdv.18127.
65. Chularojanamontri L, Rattanakorn K, Julanon N, et al. Acrodermatitis continua of Hallopeau and generalised pustular psoriasis: Should they be the same or different entities? Exp Dermatol. 2023;32(8):1235–45. https://doi.org/10.1111/exd.14805.
66. Jiaravuthisan MM, Sasseville D, Vender RB, et al. Psoriasis of the nail: anatomy, pathology, clinical presentation, and a review of the literature on therapy. J Am Acad Dermatol. 2007;57(1):1–27. https://doi.org/10.1016/j.jaad.2005.07.073.
67. Thomas L, Azad J, Takwale A. Management of nail psoriasis. Clin Exp Dermatol. 2021;46(1):3–8. https://doi.org/10.1111/ced.14314.
68. Edwards F, de Berker D. Nail psoriasis: clinical presentation and best practice recommendations. Drugs. 2009;69(17):2351–61. https://doi.org/10.2165/11318180-000000000-00000.
69. Bardazzi F, Starace M, Bruni F, et al. Nail psoriasis: an updated review and expert opinion on available treatments, including biologics. Acta Derm Venereol. 2019;99(6):516–23. https://doi.org/10.2340/00015555-3098.
70. Kishimoto M, Deshpande GA, Fukuoka K, et al. Clinical features of psoriatic arthritis. Best Pract Res Clin Rheumatol. 2021;35(2):101670. https://doi.org/10.1016/j.berh.2021.101670.
71. Kehl AS, Corr M, Weisman MH. Review: enthesitis: new insights into pathogenesis, diagnostic modalities, and treatment. Arthritis Rheumatol. 2016;68(2):312–22. https://doi.org/10.1002/art.39458.
72. Brockbank JE, Stein M, Schentag CT, et al. Dactylitis in psoriatic arthritis: a marker for disease severity? Ann Rheum Dis. 2005;64(2):188–90. https://doi.org/10.1136/ard.2003.018184.
73. Gottlieb AB, Merola JF. Axial psoriatic arthritis: an update for dermatologists. J Am Acad Dermatol. 2021;84(1):92–101. https://doi.org/10.1016/j.jaad.2020.05.089.
74. Gladman DD. Clinical features and diagnostic considerations in psoriatic arthritis. Rheum Dis Clin N Am. 2015;41(4):569–79. https://doi.org/10.1016/j.rdc.2015.07.003.
75. Sticherling M. Psoriasis and autoimmunity. Autoimmun Rev. 2016;15(12):1167–70. https://doi.org/10.1016/j.autrev.2016.09.004.
76. Ju HJ, Kim KJ, Kim DS, et al. Increased risks of autoimmune rheumatic diseases in patients with psoriasis: a nationwide population-based study. J Am Acad Dermatol. 2018;79(4):778–81. https://doi.org/10.1016/j.jaad.2018.06.026.
77. Katz U, Zandman-Goddard G. Drug-induced lupus: an update. Autoimmun Rev. 2010;10(1):46–50. https://doi.org/10.1016/j.autrev.2010.07.005.
78. Wilczek A, Sticherling M. Concomitant psoriasis and bullous pemphigoid: coincidence or pathogenic relationship? Int J Dermatol. 2006;45(11):1353–7. https://doi.org/10.1111/j.1365-4632.2006.02861.x.

79. Gisondi P, Fostini AC, Fossà I, et al. Psoriasis and the metabolic syndrome. Clin Dermatol. 2018;36(1):21–8. https://doi.org/10.1016/j.clindermatol.2017.09.005.
80. Snekvik I, Smith CH, Nilsen TIL, et al. Obesity, waist circumference, weight change, and risk of incident psoriasis: Prospective data from the HUNT study. J Invest Dermatol. 2017;137(12):2484–90. https://doi.org/10.1016/j.jid.2017.07.822.
81. Takeshita J, Grewal S, Langan SM, et al. Psoriasis and comorbid diseases: Epidemiology. J Am Acad Dermatol. 2017;76(3):377–90. https://doi.org/10.1016/j.jaad.2016.07.064.
82. Kimball AB, Szapary P, Mrowietz U, et al. Underdiagnosis and undertreatment of cardiovascular risk factors in patients with moderate to severe psoriasis. J Am Acad Dermatol. 2012;67(1):76–85. https://doi.org/10.1016/j.jaad.2011.06.035.
83. Marsche G, Saemann MD, Heinemann A, et al. Inflammation alters HDL composition and function: implications for HDL-raising therapies. Pharmacol Ther. 2013;137(3):341–51. https://doi.org/10.1016/j.pharmthera.2012.12.001.
84. Shih CM, Chen CC, Chu CK, et al. The roles of lipoprotein in psoriasis. Int J Mol Sci. 2020;21(3):859. https://doi.org/10.3390/ijms21030859.
85. Barros G, Duran P, Vera I, et al. Exploring the links between obesity and psoriasis: a comprehensive review. Int J Mol Sci. 2022;23(14):7499. https://doi.org/10.3390/ijms23147499.
86. Ko SH, Chi CC, Yeh ML, et al. Lifestyle changes for treating psoriasis. Cochrane Database Syst Rev. 2019;7(7):CD011972. https://doi.org/10.1002/14651858.CD011972.pub2.
87. Zhou BR, Zhang JA, Zhang Q, et al. Palmitic acid induces production of proinflammatory cytokines interleukin-6, interleukin-1β, and tumor necrosis factor-α via a NF-κB-dependent mechanism in HaCaT keratinocytes. Mediat Inflamm. 2013;2013:530429. https://doi.org/10.1155/2013/530429.
88. Kanemaru K, Matsuyuki A, Nakamura Y, et al. Obesity exacerbates imiquimod-induced psoriasis-like epidermal hyperplasia and interleukin-17 and interleukin-22 production in mice. Exp Dermatol. 2015;24(6):436–42. https://doi.org/10.1111/exd.12691.
89. Chen L, Li J, Zhu W, et al. Skin and gut microbiome in psoriasis: Gaining insight into the pathophysiology of it and finding novel therapeutic strategies. Front Microbiol. 2020;11:589726. https://doi.org/10.3389/fmicb.2020.589726.
90. Chávez-Castillo M, Ortega Á, Cudris-Torres L, et al. Specialized pro-resolving lipid mediators: the future of chronic pain therapy? Int J Mol Sci. 2021;22(19):10370. https://doi.org/10.3390/ijms221910370.
91. Gelfand JM, Neimann AL, Shin DB, et al. Risk of myocardial infarction in patients with psoriasis. JAMA. 2006;296(14):1735–41. https://doi.org/10.1001/jama.296.14.1735.
92. Boehncke WH, Boehncke S, Tobin AM, et al. The 'psoriatic march': a concept of how severe psoriasis may drive cardiovascular comorbidity. Exp Dermatol. 2011;20(4):303–7. https://doi.org/10.1111/j.1600-0625.2011.01261.x.
93. Armstrong AW, Voyles SV, Armstrong EJ, et al. A tale of two plaques: convergent mechanisms of T-cell-mediated inflammation in psoriasis and atherosclerosis. Exp Dermatol. 2011;20(7):544–9. https://doi.org/10.1111/j.1600-0625.2011.01308.x.
94. Cerman AA, Bozkurt S, Sav A, et al. Serum leptin levels, skin leptin and leptin receptor expression in psoriasis. Br J Dermatol. 2008;159(4):820–6. https://doi.org/10.1111/j.1365-2133.2008.08742.x.
95. Ruan Z, Lu T, Chen Y, et al. Association between psoriasis and nonalcoholic fatty liver disease among outpatient US adults. JAMA Dermatol. 2022;158(7):745–53. https://doi.org/10.1001/jamadermatol.2022.1609.
96. Lonardo A, Ballestri S, Marchesini G, et al. Nonalcoholic fatty liver disease: a precursor of the metabolic syndrome. Dig Liver Dis. 2015;47(3):181–90. https://doi.org/10.1016/j.dld.2014.09.020.
97. Tang Y, Bian Z, Zhao L, et al. Interleukin-17 exacerbates hepatic steatosis and inflammation in non-alcoholic fatty liver disease. Clin Exp Immunol. 2011;166(2):281–90. https://doi.org/10.1111/j.1365-2249.2011.04471.x.

98. Zheng Y, Danilenko DM, Valdez P, et al. Interleukin-22, a T(H)17 cytokine, mediates IL-23-induced dermal inflammation and acanthosis. Nature. 2007;445(7128):648–51. https://doi.org/10.1038/nature05505.
99. Alinaghi F, Tekin HG, Burisch J, et al. Global prevalence and bidirectional association between psoriasis and inflammatory bowel disease—a systematic review and meta-analysis. J Crohns Colitis. 2020;14(3):351–60. https://doi.org/10.1093/ecco-jcc/jjz152.
100. Hedin CRH, Sonkoly E, Eberhardson M, et al. Inflammatory bowel disease and psoriasis: modernizing the multidisciplinary approach. J Intern Med. 2021;290(2):257–78. https://doi.org/10.1111/joim.13282.
101. Cai Q, Teeple A, Wu B, et al. Prevalence and economic burden of comorbid anxiety and depression among patients with moderate-to-severe psoriasis. J Med Econ. 2019;22(12):1290–7. https://doi.org/10.1080/13696998.2019.1638788.
102. Singh S, Taylor C, Kornmehl H, et al. Psoriasis and suicidality: a systematic review and meta-analysis. J Am Acad Dermatol. 2017;77(3):425–440.e2. https://doi.org/10.1016/j.jaad.2017.05.019.
103. Bu J, Ding R, Zhou L, et al. Epidemiology of psoriasis and comorbid diseases: a narrative review. Front Immunol. 2022;13:880201. https://doi.org/10.3389/fimmu.2022.880201.
104. Tsai SY, Chen HJ, Chen C, et al. Increased risk of chronic fatigue syndrome following psoriasis: a nationwide population-based cohort study. J Transl Med. 2019;17(1):154. https://doi.org/10.1186/s12967-019-1888-1.
105. Köse B, Uzlu D, Erdöl H, et al. Psoriasis and uveitis. Int Ophthalmol. 2022;42(7):2303–10. https://doi.org/10.1007/s10792-022-02225-5.
106. Demerdjieva Z, Mazhdrakova I, Tsankov N, et al. Ocular changes in patients with psoriasis. Clin Dermatol. 2019;37(6):663–7. https://doi.org/10.1016/j.clindermatol.2019.07.029.
107. Fotiadou C, Lazaridou E. Psoriasis and uveitis: links and risks. Psoriasis (Auckl). 2019;9:91–6. https://doi.org/10.2147/PTT.S179182.
108. Weinstein JE, Pepple KL. Cytokines in uveitis. Curr Opin Ophthalmol. 2018;29(3):267–74. https://doi.org/10.1097/ICU.0000000000000466.
109. Paiva ES, Macaluso DC, Edwards A, et al. Characterisation of uveitis in patients with psoriatic arthritis. Ann Rheum Dis. 2000;59(1):67–70. https://doi.org/10.1136/ard.59.1.67.
110. Margolis D, Bilker W, Hennessy S, et al. The risk of malignancy associated with psoriasis. Arch Dermatol. 2001;137(6):778–83.
111. Watanabe T, Watanabe Y, Asai C, et al. Risks of malignancies among patients with psoriasis: a cohort study of 360 patients. J Dermatol. 2023;50(5):615–21. https://doi.org/10.1111/1346-8138.16644.
112. Chiesa Fuxench ZC, Shin DB, Ogdie Beatty A, et al. The risk of cancer in patients with psoriasis: a population-based cohort study in the Health Improvement Network. JAMA Dermatol. 2016;152(3):282–90. https://doi.org/10.1001/jamadermatol.2015.4847.
113. Geller S, Xu H, Lebwohl M, et al. Malignancy risk and recurrence with psoriasis and its treatments: a concise update. Am J Clin Dermatol. 2018;19(3):363–75. https://doi.org/10.1007/s40257-017-0337-2.
114. Stern RS, Laird N. The carcinogenic risk of treatments for severe psoriasis. Photochemotherapy follow-up study. Cancer. 1994;73(11):2759–64. https://doi.org/10.1002/1097-0142(19940601)73:11<2759::aid-cncr2820731118>3.0.co;2-c.
115. Paul CF, Ho VC, McGeown C, et al. Risk of malignancies in psoriasis patients treated with cyclosporine: a 5 y cohort study. J Invest Dermatol. 2003;120(2):211–6. https://doi.org/10.1046/j.1523-1747.2003.12040.x.
116. Burmester GR, Panaccione R, Gordon KB, et al. Adalimumab: long-term safety in 23 458 patients from global clinical trials in rheumatoid arthritis, juvenile idiopathic arthritis, ankylosing spondylitis, psoriatic arthritis, psoriasis and Crohn's disease. Ann Rheum Dis. 2013;72(4):517–24. https://doi.org/10.1136/annrheumdis-2011-201244.
117. Raychaudhuri SK, Maverakis E, Raychaudhuri SP. Diagnosis and classification of psoriasis. Autoimmun Rev. 2014;13(4–5):490–5. https://doi.org/10.1016/j.autrev.2014.01.008.

118. Nicolescu AC, Ionescu MA, Constantin MM, et al. Psoriasis management challenges regarding difficult-to-treat areas: therapeutic decision and effectiveness. Life (Basel). 2022;12(12):2050. https://doi.org/10.3390/life12122050.
119. Kimmel GW, Lebwohl M. Psoriasis: overview and diagnosis. In: Bhutani T, Liao W, Nakamura M, editors. Evidence-based psoriasis. Updates in clinical dermatology. New York: Springer; 2018. p. 1–16. https://doi.org/10.1007/978-3-319-90107-7_1.
120. Murphy M, Kerr P, Grant-Kels JM. The histopathologic spectrum of psoriasis. Clin Dermatol. 2007;25(6):524–8. https://doi.org/10.1016/j.clindermatol.2007.08.005.
121. Aydin O, Engin B, Oğuz O, et al. Non-pustular palmoplantar psoriasis: is histologic differentiation from eczematous dermatitis possible? J Cutan Pathol. 2008;35(2):169–73.
122. Elmets CA, Korman NJ, Prater EF, et al. Joint AAD-NPF Guidelines of care for the management and treatment of psoriasis with topical therapy and alternative medicine modalities for psoriasis severity measures. J Am Acad Dermatol. 2021;84(2):432–70. https://doi.org/10.1016/j.jaad.2020.07.087.
123. Zhang P, Wu MX. A clinical review of phototherapy for psoriasis. Lasers Med Sci. 2018;33(1):173–80. https://doi.org/10.1007/s10103-017-2360-1.
124. Elmets CA, Lim HW, Stoff B, et al. Joint American Academy of Dermatology-National Psoriasis Foundation guidelines of care for the management and treatment of psoriasis with phototherapy. J Am Acad Dermatol. 2019;81(3):775–804. https://doi.org/10.1016/j.jaad.2019.04.042.
125. Chowdhari S, Saini N. hsa-miR-4516 mediated downregulation of STAT3/CDK6/UBE2N plays a role in PUVA induced apoptosis in keratinocytes. J Cell Physiol. 2014;229(11):1630–8. https://doi.org/10.1002/jcp.24608.
126. Gui J, Gober M, Yang X, et al. Therapeutic elimination of the type 1 interferon receptor for treating psoriatic skin inflammation. J Invest Dermatol. 2016;136(10):1990–2002. https://doi.org/10.1016/j.jid.2016.06.608.
127. Weatherhead SC, Farr PM, Reynolds NJ. Spectral effects of UV on psoriasis. Photochem Photobiol Sci. 2013;12(1):47–53. https://doi.org/10.1039/c2pp25116g.
128. Marsili F, Travaglini M, Stinco G, et al. Effectiveness of cyclosporine A in patients with moderate to severe plaque psoriasis in a real-life clinical setting in Italy: the TRANSITION study. J Dermatolog Treat. 2022;33(1):401–7. https://doi.org/10.1080/09546634.2020.1757017.
129. Nast A, Amelunxen L, Augustin M, et al. S3-Leitlinie zur Therapie der psoriasis vulgaris update—Kurzfassung Teil 1—systemische therapie. J Dtsch Dermatol Ges. 2018;16(5):645–70. https://doi.org/10.1111/ddg.13516_g.
130. Jindal RM, Sidner RA, Milgrom ML. Post-transplant diabetes mellitus. The role of immunosuppression. Drug Saf. 1997;16(4):242–57. https://doi.org/10.2165/00002018-199716040-00002.
131. Haustein UF, Rytter M. Methotrexate in psoriasis: 26 years' experience with low-dose long-term treatment. J Eur Acad Dermatol Venereol. 2000;14(5):382–8. https://doi.org/10.1046/j.1468-3083.2000.00058.x.
132. Sbidian E, Maza A, Montaudié H, et al. Efficacy and safety of oral retinoids in different psoriasis subtypes: a systematic literature review. J Eur Acad Dermatol Venereol. 2011;25(s2):28–33. https://doi.org/10.1111/j.1468-3083.2011.03993.x.
133. Balak DM. Fumaric acid esters in the management of psoriasis. Psoriasis (Auckl). 2015;5:9–23. https://doi.org/10.2147/PTT.S51490.
134. De Luca DA. Dimethyl fumarate. A therapeutic alternative in psoriasis. Dermatol Argent. 2020;26(3):114–20. https://doi.org/10.47196/da.v26i3.2100.
135. Mrowietz U, Barker J, Boehncke WH, et al. Clinical use of dimethyl fumarate in moderate-to-severe plaque-type psoriasis: a European expert consensus. J Eur Acad Dermatol Venereol. 2018;32(Suppl. 3):3–14. https://doi.org/10.1111/jdv.15218.
136. Schafer P. Apremilast mechanism of action and application to psoriasis and psoriatic arthritis. Biochem Pharmacol. 2012;83(12):1583–90. https://doi.org/10.1016/j.bcp.2012.01.001.

137. Gao JC, Wu AG, Contento MN, et al. Apremilast in the treatment of plaque psoriasis: differential use in psoriasis. Clin Cosmet Investig Dermatol. 2022;15:395–402. https://doi.org/10.2147/CCID.S266036.
138. Berekmeri A, Mahmood F, Wittmann M, et al. Tofacitinib for the treatment of psoriasis and psoriatic arthritis. Expert Rev Clin Immunol. 2018;14(9):719–30. https://doi.org/10.1080/1744666X.2018.1512404.
139. Jo CE, Gooderham M, Beecker J. TYK 2 inhibitors for the treatment of dermatologic conditions: the evolution of JAK inhibitors. Int J Dermatol. 2022;61(2):139–47. https://doi.org/10.1111/ijd.15605.
140. Estevinho T, Lé AM, Torres T. Deucravacitinib in the treatment of psoriasis. J Dermatolog Treat. 2023;34(1):2154122. https://doi.org/10.1080/09546634.2022.2154122.
141. Al-Janabi A, Yiu ZZN. Biologics in psoriasis: updated perspectives on long-term safety and risk management. Psoriasis (Auckl). 2022;12:1–14. https://doi.org/10.2147/PTT.S328575.
142. Thatiparthi A, Martin A, Liu J, et al. Biologic treatment algorithms for moderate-to-severe psoriasis with comorbid conditions and special populations: a review. Am J Clin Dermatol. 2021;22(4):425–42. https://doi.org/10.1007/s40257-021-00603-w.
143. Piaserico S, Messina F, Russo FP. Managing psoriasis in patients with HBV or HCV infection: practical considerations. Am J Clin Dermatol. 2019;20(6):829–45. https://doi.org/10.1007/s40257-019-00457-3.
144. Nidegger A, Jenelten R, Conrad C. Anti-IL17 induced eczema and the yin-yang of Th2 and Th17. Rev Med Suisse. 2022;18(775):574–7. https://doi.org/10.53738/REVMED.2022.18.775.574.
145. Silfvast-Kaiser AS, Homan KB, Mansouri B. A narrative review of psoriasis and multiple sclerosis: links and risks. Psoriasis (Auckl). 2019;9:81–90. https://doi.org/10.2147/PTT.S186637.
146. Vashist S, Mahajan VK, Mehta KS, et al. Association of psoriasis with autoimmune disorders: results of a pilot study. Indian Dermatol Online J. 2020;11(5):753–9. https://doi.org/10.4103/idoj.IDOJ_648_19.
147. Jaberi-Douraki M, Schnell S, Pietropaolo M, et al. Unraveling the contribution of pancreatic β-cell suicide in autoimmune type 1 diabetes. J Theor Biol. 2015;375:77–87. https://doi.org/10.1016/j.jtbi.2014.05.003.
148. Emamaullee JA, Davis J, Merani S, et al. Inhibition of Th17 cells regulates autoimmune diabetes in NOD mice. Diabetes. 2009;58:1302–11. https://doi.org/10.2337/db08-1113.
149. Bartlett HS, Million RP. Targeting the IL-17-TH17 pathway. Nat Rev Drug Discov. 2015;14:11–2. https://doi.org/10.1038/nrd4518.
150. Bovenschen HJ, van de Kerkhof PC, van Erp PE, et al. Foxp3+ regulatory T cells of psoriasis patients easily differentiate into IL-17A-producing cells and are found in lesional skin. J Invest Dermatol. 2011;131:1853–60. https://doi.org/10.1038/jid.2011.139.
151. Wang C, Guan Y, Yang J. Cytokines in the progression of pancreatic β-cell dysfunction. Int J Endocrinol. 2010;2010:515136. https://doi.org/10.1155/2010/515136.
152. Holm JG, Thomsen SF. Type 2 diabetes and psoriasis: links and risks. Psoriasis (Auckl). 2019;9:1–6. https://doi.org/10.2147/PTT.S159163.
153. Henseler T, Christophers E. Disease concomitance in psoriasis. J Am Acad Dermatol. 1995;32(6):982–6. https://doi.org/10.1016/0190-9622(95)91336-x.
154. Nas K, Karkucak M, Durmus B, et al. Comorbidities in patients with psoriatic arthritis: a comparison with rheumatoid arthritis and psoriasis. Int J Rheum Dis. 2015;18(8):873–9. https://doi.org/10.1111/1756-185X.12580.
155. Abramczyk R, Queller JN, Rachfal AW, Schwartz SS. Diabetes and psoriasis: different sides of the same prism. Diabetes Metab Syndr Obes. 2020;13:3571–7. https://doi.org/10.2147/DMSO.S273147.
156. Wang H, Wang Z, Rani PL. Identification of PTPN22, ST6GAL1 and JAZF1 as psoriasis risk genes demonstrates shared pathogenesis between psoriasis and diabetes. Exp Dermatol. 2017;26(11):1112–7. https://doi.org/10.1111/exd.13393.

157. Gyldenløve M, Storgaard H, Holst JJ, et al. Patients with psoriasis are insulin resistant. J Am Acad Dermatol. 2015;72(4):599–605. https://doi.org/10.1016/j.jaad.2015.01.004.
158. Karadag AS, Ertugrul DT, Kalkan G, et al. The effect of acitretin treatment on insulin resistance, retinol-binding protein-4, leptin, and adiponectin in psoriasis vulgaris: a noncontrolled study. Dermatology. 2013;227(2):103–8. https://doi.org/10.1159/000351769.
159. Rajappa M, Rathika S, Munisamy M, et al. Effect of treatment with methotrexate and coal tar on adipokine levels and indices of insulin resistance and sensitivity in patients with psoriasis vulgaris. J Eur Acad Dermatol Venereol. 2015;29(1):69–76. https://doi.org/10.1111/jdv.12451.
160. Bottini N, Musumeci L, Alonso A, et al. A functional variant of lymphoid tyrosine phosphatase is associated with type I diabetes. Nat Genet. 2004;36(4):337–8. https://doi.org/10.1038/ng1323.
161. Tizaoui K, Shin JI, Jeong GH, et al. Genetic polymorphism of PTPN22 in autoimmune diseases: a comprehensive review. Medicina (Kaunas). 2022;58(8):1034. https://doi.org/10.3390/medicina58081034.
162. Menard L, Saadoun D, Isnardi I, et al. The PTPN22 allele encoding an R620W variant interferes with the removal of developing autoreactive B cells in humans. J Clin Invest. 2011;121(9):3635–44. https://doi.org/10.1172/JCI45790.
163. Habib T, Funk A, Rieck M, et al. Altered B cell homeostasis is associated with type I diabetes and carriers of the PTPN22 allelic variant. J Immunol. 2012;188(1):487–96. https://doi.org/10.4049/jimmunol.1102176.
164. Perri V, Pellegrino M, Ceccacci F, et al. Use of short interfering RNA delivered by cationic liposomes to enable efficient down-regulation of PTPN22 gene in human T lymphocytes. PLoS One. 2017;12(4):e0175784. https://doi.org/10.1371/journal.pone.0175784.
165. Garg G, Tyler JR, Yang JHM, et al. Type 1 diabetes-associated IL2RA variation lowers IL-2 signaling and contributes to diminished CD4+CD25+ regulatory T cell function. J Immunol. 2012;188(9):4644–53. https://doi.org/10.4049/jimmunol.1100272.
166. Bowes J, Loehr S, Budu-Aggrey A, et al. PTPN22 is associated with susceptibility to psoriatic arthritis but not psoriasis: evidence for a further PsA-specific risk locus. Ann Rheum Dis. 2015;74(10):1882–5. https://doi.org/10.1136/annrheumdis-2014-207187.
167. Benham H, Norris P, Goodall J, et al. Th17 and Th22 cells in psoriatic arthritis and psoriasis. Arthritis Res Ther. 2013;15(5):R136. https://doi.org/10.1186/ar4317.
168. Liew SC, Gupta ED. Methylenetetrahydrofolate reductase (MTHFR) C677T polymorphism: epidemiology, metabolism and the associated diseases. Eur J Med Genet. 2015;58(1):1–10. https://doi.org/10.1016/j.ejmg.2014.10.004.
169. Ruchusatsawat K, Wongpiyabovorn J, Shuangshoti S, et al. SHP-1 promoter 2 methylation in normal epithelial tissues and demethylation in psoriasis. J Mol Med. 2006;84(2):175–82. https://doi.org/10.1007/s00109-005-0020-6.
170. Chen AR, Zhang HG, Wang ZP, et al. C-reactive protein, vitamin B12 and C677T polymorphism of N-5,10-methylenetetrahydrofolate reductase gene are related to insulin resistance and risk factors for metabolic syndrome in Chinese population. Clin Invest Med. 2010;33(5):E290–7. https://doi.org/10.25011/cim.v33i5.14354.
171. Meng Y, Liu X, Ma K, et al. Association of MTHFR C677T polymorphism and type 2 diabetes mellitus (T2DM) susceptibility. Mol Genet Genomic Med. 2019;7(12):e1020. https://doi.org/10.1002/mgg3.1020.
172. Grarup N, Andersen G, Krarup NT, et al. Association testing of novel type 2 diabetes risk alleles in the JAZF1, CDC123/CAMK1D, TSPAN8, THADA, ADAMTS9, and NOTCH2 loci with insulin release, insulin sensitivity, and obesity in a population-based sample of 4,516 glucose-tolerant middle-aged Danes. Diabetes. 2008;57(9):2534–40. https://doi.org/10.2337/db08-0436.
173. Pascoe L, Tura A, Patel SK, et al. Common variants of the novel type 2 diabetes genes CDKAL1 and HHEX/IDE are associated with decreased pancreatic beta-cell function. Diabetes. 2007;56(12):3101–4. https://doi.org/10.2337/db07-0634.

174. Quaranta M, Burden AD, Griffiths CEM, et al. Differential contribution of CDKAL1 variants to psoriasis, Crohn's disease and type II diabetes. Genes Immun. 2009;10(7):654–8. https://doi.org/10.1038/gene.2009.51.
175. Meisgen F, Xu N, Wei T, et al. MiR-21 is up-regulated in psoriasis and suppresses T cell apoptosis. Exp Dermatol. 2012;21(4):312–4. https://doi.org/10.1111/j.1600-0625.2012.01462.x.
176. Murugaiyan G, da Cunha AP, Ajay AK, et al. MicroRNA-21 promotes Th17 differentiation and mediates experimental autoimmune encephalomyelitis. J Clin Invest. 2015;125(3):1069–80. https://doi.org/10.1172/JCI74347.
177. Guinea-Viniegra J, Zenz R, Scheuch H, et al. TNFalpha shedding and epidermal inflammation are controlled by Jun proteins. Genes Dev. 2009;23(22):2663–74. https://doi.org/10.1101/gad.543109.
178. Guinea-Viniegra J, Jiménez M, Schonthaler HB, et al. Targeting miR-21 to treat psoriasis. Sci Transl Med. 2014;6(225):225re1. https://doi.org/10.1126/scitranslmed.3008089.
179. Kurylowicz A. MicroRNAs in human adipose tissue physiology and dysfunction. Cells. 2021;10(12):3342. https://doi.org/10.3390/cells10123342.
180. Kim YJ, Hwang SJ, Bae YC, et al. MiR-21 regulates adipogenic differentiation through the modulation of TGF-beta signaling in mesenchymal stem cells derived from human adipose tissue. Stem Cells. 2009;27(12):3093–102. https://doi.org/10.1002/stem.235.
181. Zhong X, Chung ACK, Chen HY, et al. miR-21 is a key therapeutic target for renal injury in a mouse model of type 2 diabetes. Diabetologia. 2013;56(3):663–74. https://doi.org/10.1007/s00125-012-2804-x.
182. Ruan Q, Wang T, Kameswaran V, et al. The microRNA-21-PDCD4 axis prevents type 1 diabetes by blocking pancreatic beta cell death. Proc Natl Acad Sci U S A. 2011;108(29):12030–5. https://doi.org/10.1073/pnas.1101450108.
183. Boehncke WH, Schön MP. Psoriasis. Lancet. 2015;386(9997):983–94. https://doi.org/10.1016/S0140-6736(14)61909-7.
184. Tilg H, Moschen AR. Inflammatory mechanisms in the regulation of insulin resistance. Mol Med. 2008;14(3–4):222–31. https://doi.org/10.2119/2007-00119.Tilg.
185. Abdel-Moneim A, Bakery HH, Allam G. The potential pathogenic role of IL-17/Th17 cells in both type 1 and type 2 diabetes mellitus. Biomed Pharmacother. 2018;101:287–92. https://doi.org/10.1016/j.biopha.2018.02.103.
186. Ikumi K, Odanaka M, Shime H, et al. Hyperglycemia is associated with psoriatic inflammation in both humans and mice. J Invest Dermatol. 2019;139(6):1329–1338.e7. https://doi.org/10.1016/j.jid.2019.01.029.
187. Botelho KP, Pontes MA, Rodrigues CE, Freitas MV. Prevalence of metabolic syndrome among patients with psoriasis treated with TNF inhibitors and the effects of anti-TNF therapy on their lipid profile: a prospective cohort study. Metab Syndr Relat Disord. 2020;18(3):154–60. https://doi.org/10.1089/met.2019.0092.
188. Arjuman A, Chandra NC. Differential pro-inflammatory responses of TNF-α receptors (TNFR1 and TNFR2) on LOX-1 signalling. Mol Biol Rep. 2015;42(6):1039–47. https://doi.org/10.1007/s11033-014-3841-y.
189. Pina T, Armesto S, Lopez-Mejias R, et al. Anti-TNF-α therapy improves insulin sensitivity in non-diabetic patients with psoriasis: a 6-month prospective study. J Eur Acad Dermatol Venereol. 2015;29(7):1325–30. https://doi.org/10.1111/jdv.12814.
190. Granata M, Skarmoutsou E, Trovato C, et al. Obesity, type 1 diabetes, and psoriasis: an autoimmune triple flip. Pathobiology. 2017;84(2):71–9. https://doi.org/10.1159/000447777.
191. Olusi SO, Al-Awadhi A, Abraham M. Relations of serum interleukin 18 levels to serum lipid and glucose concentrations in an apparently healthy adult population. Horm Res. 2003;60(1):29–33. https://doi.org/10.1159/000070824.
192. Companjen A, van der Wel L, van der Fits L, et al. Elevated interleukin-18 protein expression in early active and progressive plaque-type psoriatic lesions. Eur Cytokine Netw. 2004;15(3):210–6. https://www.ncbi.nlm.nih.gov/pubmed/15542445

193. Sarandi E, Krueger-Krasagakis S, Tsoukalas D, et al. Psoriasis immunometabolism: progress on metabolic biomarkers and targeted therapy. Front Mol Biosci. 2023;10:1201912. https://doi.org/10.3389/fmolb.2023.1201912.
194. Cibrian D, de la Fuente H, Sánchez-Madrid F. Metabolic pathways that control skin homeostasis and inflammation. Trends Mol Med. 2020;26(11):975–86. https://doi.org/10.1016/j.molmed.2020.04.004.
195. Patel AB, Tsilioni I, Weng Z, et al. TNF stimulates IL-6, CXCL8 and VEGF secretion from human keratinocytes via activation of mTOR, inhibited by tetramethoxyluteolin. Exp Dermatol. 2018;27(2):135–43. https://doi.org/10.1111/exd.13461.
196. Buerger C, Shirsath N, Lang V, et al. Inflammation dependent mTORC1 signaling interferes with the switch from keratinocyte proliferation to differentiation. PLoS One. 2017;12(7):e0180853. https://doi.org/10.1371/journal.pone.0180853.
197. Boehncke WH. Systemic inflammation and cardiovascular comorbidity in psoriasis patients: causes and consequences. Front Immunol. 2018;9:579. https://doi.org/10.3389/fimmu.2018.00579.
198. Nielsen HJ, Christensen IJ, Svendsen MN, et al. Elevated plasma levels of vascular endothelial growth factor and plasminogen activator inhibitor-1 decrease during improvement of psoriasis. Inflamm Res. 2002;51(11):563–7. https://doi.org/10.1007/pl00012428.
199. von Stebut E, Reich K, Thaçi D, et al. Impact of secukinumab on endothelial dysfunction and other cardiovascular disease parameters in psoriasis patients over 52 weeks. J Invest Dermatol. 2019;139(5):1054–62. https://doi.org/10.1016/j.jid.2018.10.042.
200. Booth A, Magnuson A, Fouts J, et al. Adipose tissue: an endocrine organ playing a role in metabolic regulation. Horm Mol Biol Clin Investig. 2016;26:25–42. https://doi.org/10.1515/hmbci-2015-0073.
201. Versini M, Jeandel PY, Rosenthal E, et al. Obesity in autoimmune diseases: not a passive bystander. Autoimmun Rev. 2014;13:981–1000. https://doi.org/10.1016/j.autrev.2014.07.001.
202. Malhotra A, Shafiq N, Rajagopalan S, et al. Thiazolidinediones for plaque psoriasis: a systematic review and meta-analysis. Evid Based Med. 2012;17(6):171–6. https://doi.org/10.1136/ebmed-2011-100388.
203. Huang Z, Li J, Chen H, et al. The efficacy of metformin for the treatment of psoriasis: a meta-analysis study. Postepy Dermatol Alergol. 2023;40(5):606–10. https://doi.org/10.5114/ada.2023.130524.
204. Stanescu AMA, Simionescu AA, Florea M, et al. Is metformin a possible beneficial treatment for psoriasis? A scoping review. J Pers Med. 2021;11(4):251. https://doi.org/10.3390/jpm11040251.
205. Lin L, Xu X, Yu Y, et al. Glucagon-like peptide-1 receptor agonist liraglutide therapy for psoriasis patients with type 2 diabetes: a randomized-controlled trial. J Dermatolog Treat. 2022;33(3):1428–34. https://doi.org/10.1080/09546634.2020.1826392.
206. Barra L, Pope JE, Payne M. Real-world anti-tumor necrosis factor treatment in rheumatoid arthritis, psoriatic arthritis, and ankylosing spondylitis: cost-effectiveness based on number needed to treat to improve health assessment questionnaire. J Rheumatol. 2009;36(7):1421–8. https://doi.org/10.3899/jrheum.081122.
207. Marwaha AK, Tan S, Dutz JP. Targeting the IL-17/IFN-γ axis as a potential new clinical therapy for type 1 diabetes. Clin Immunol. 2014;154(1):84–9. https://doi.org/10.1016/j.clim.2014.06.006.
208. van Lint JA, van Hunsel FPAM, Tas SW, et al. Hypoglycaemia following JAK inhibitor treatment in patients with diabetes. Ann Rheum Dis. 2022;81(4):597–9. https://doi.org/10.1136/annrheumdis-2021-221840.

Chapter 22
Atopic Dermatitis and Diabetes

Adelina-Maria Sendrea and Carmen Maria Salavastru

Abstract Atopic dermatitis and diabetes represent chronic, inflammatory, and immune-mediated diseases, both with significant quality of life impact for the patient and patient's family but also considerable socio-economic burden. Although more and more studied in the past decades, the potential association and connection between these two medical entities is still debatable, as literature data is limited and, in some cases, even conflicting. However, their potential association relies on some commonly identified pathophysiological factors—such as perpetual inflammation, immunological responses, environmental factors, genetic background, and shared comorbidities. Therefore, some studies identified a positive association between atopic dermatitis and diabetes mellitus (either type 1 or type 2), while data from other studies revealed no connection between these diseases or, even more, showed that atopic dermatitis might reduce the risk of developing diabetes mellitus in some patients. Furthermore, these two chronic illnesses also share some clinical characteristics, which highlights a potential association. Up to this date, there is no conclusive scientific evidence in favor of a strong positive association between atopic dermatitis and diabetes mellitus, mainly due to a lack of studies on large and diversified populations. However, it is important for physicians to be aware of this potential association in both adult and pediatric populations and the importance of a multidisciplinary approach for atopic dermatitis. Future research on adequate population groups is needed in order to establish any potential association between atopic dermatitis and diabetes mellitus.

A.-M. Sendrea
Carol Davila University of Medicine and Pharmacy, Bucharest, Romania

Pediatric Dermatology Department, Colentina Clinical Hospital, Bucharest, Romania

Dermatology Research Unit, Colentina Clinical Hospital, Bucharest, Romania

C. M. Salavastru (✉)
Carol Davila University of Medicine and Pharmacy, București, Romania

Pediatric Dermatology Department, Colentina Clinical Hospital, Bucharest, Romania

K. Fritz, G.-S. Tiplica (eds.), *Cutaneous Manifestations in Diabetes*,
https://doi.org/10.1007/978-3-031-65300-1_22

22.1 Introduction

Atopic dermatitis and diabetes mellitus represent chronic diseases, both with complex and multifactorial pathogenesis, determined by an interplay between immune dysregulation and environmental factors in genetically predisposed individuals. Both disorders present with continuously increasing prevalence rates worldwide and are associated with significant socio-economic burdens.

Although initially thought to be a skin-limited condition, emerging data support the theory that atopic dermatitis is actually a systemic disease, in which patients (regardless of the age group) associate extra-cutaneous afflictions, including diabetes mellitus. Still, the connection between these two entities is currently under debate, with some data presented in the literature being conflicting.

22.2 Atopic Dermatitis: General Data

Atopic dermatitis is an inflammatory, immune-mediated skin condition, characterized by relapsing episodes of highly pruritic eczema lesions with different morphology and distribution according to patient's age, associated with skin xerosis. It affects mainly pediatric patients, with a prevalence up to 20% in children, while in adults it is present in a lesser percentage, up to 10% [1, 2].

The development of this condition relies on a complex interplay between a variety of factors, such as skin barrier dysfunction, genetic background, chronic inflammation, skin microbiome alterations, environmental factors, and Th2-driven immunological impairment, its pathogenesis being incompletely elucidated so far [3].

Patients with atopic dermatitis associate various comorbidities, the most well-known and universally recognized being the ones that comprise "the atopic march" (the gradual development of certain allergic conditions—from food allergies in infancy to allergic rhinitis and asthma in childhood) [4].

Besides the atopic march, recent data support the idea that atopic dermatitis is a systemic disorder, associating multiple comorbidities that affect different systems. Therefore, various conditions ranging from neuropsychiatric [5] and ocular diseases [6] to gastrointestinal, renal, and autoimmune afflictions [7] and, moreover, cardiovascular disorders and components of metabolic syndrome (including insulin resistance or diabetes mellitus) have been found in patients with atopic dermatitis [8, 9].

22.3 Diabetes Mellitus: General Data

Diabetes mellitus represents a complex and chronic metabolic disorder, with an increasing worldwide prevalence, determined by an impairment in glucose metabolism, which results in elevated blood glucose levels (hyperglycemia). Hyperglycemia, the main clinical characteristic, is determined by certain insulin-related disturbances (either an impairment in its secretion—relative or absolute—or a peripheral resistance to its actions in variable degrees, or both) [10].

The pathophysiology of diabetes mellitus is complex and multifactorial, with various factors (such as genetic background, environmental and life-style vectors, autoimmunity, chronic inflammation) being important pathogenic key factors in the development of this disease. There are four types of diabetes mellitus—type 1, type 2, gestational, and maturity-onset diabetes of the young (MODY).

Type 1 diabetes is characterized by an autoimmune T cell-driven destruction of the pancreatic ß cells, resulting in an absolute insulin deficiency. It comprises about 10% of diabetes mellitus cases, and it can affect both pediatric patients—juvenile onset (with rapid development) and adult population (with slower, gradual development) [10]. Patients with type 1 diabetes mellitus present with a ten times higher risk of cardiovascular events compared to non-diabetic ones [11].

Type 2 diabetes represents the most common diabetes mellitus type encountered in adult population (up to 95%), and it's caused by both insulin resistance and a relative insulin deficiency, being mainly determined by a complex interplay between genetic and environmental factors. This particular subtype of diabetes develops gradually and slowly, being asymptomatic for many years [10, 12]. Patients with type 2 diabetes mellitus associate a variety of other metabolic disturbances (such as dyslipidemia and atherosclerosis) and also present with a high risk of cardiovascular events [11].

Still, the distinction between type 1 and type 2 diabetes is currently faint as an increasing number of cases of type 1 are being encountered in adult population and type 2 is becoming more prevalent among younger patients [13].

Gestational diabetes represents, according to the American Diabetes Association, the diagnosis of diabetes mellitus during the first or third trimester of pregnancy. Most pregnant females return to normal blood glucose levels after giving birth; still they should be closely monitored due to a potential risk of developing type 2 diabetes mellitus [14].

MODY (maturity-onset diabetes of the young) represents an autosomal dominant genetic variant of type 2 diabetes mellitus that develops at a young age (usually before 25 years old) determined by some insulin secretion disturbances, but with normal insulin action [15].

22.4 Atopic Dermatitis-Diabetes Mellitus: The Pathophysiological Interplay

The potential interplay between atopic dermatitis and diabetes mellitus relies for the most part on some shared pathophysiological factors, starting with the perpetual pro-inflammatory status and the immunological crosstalk and going further to genetic background, some shared risk factors, and common comorbidities.

22.4.1 Shared Inflammatory Pathways and the Common Immunological Cross talk: The Revised "Th1/Th2 Paradigm"

Chronic inflammation and certain immunological disturbances represent hallmark pathophysiological features for both atopic dermatitis and diabetes mellitus.

According to the classic T-helper (Th) 1/Th2 paradigm, certain inflammatory diseases are conventionally driven by either a Th1- or a Th2-induced response [16]. The type 1 inflammatory responses are guided through Th1 CD4+ T cells and characterized by production of IFN-γ, while, on the other spectrum ending, the type 2 inflammatory responses, helmed by Th2 CD4+ T cells, are recognizable by specific interleukin production, such as interleukin (IL)-4, IL-5, and IL-13 [17].

Although atopic dermatitis is mainly a Th2-driven inflammatory disease, while diabetes mellitus type 1 is a predominantly Th1-induced one [18], some pro-inflammatory cytokines involved in atopic dermatitis may contribute to the inflammatory milieu encountered also in diabetes mellitus.

As new lymphocytic subgroups have been identified (such as Th17, T regulatory cells, or Th3), a new approach to immunologically driven disorders (including a potential association in between) was explored [17, 19]. Moreover, some experimental animal models showed that both subtypes of T-helper cytokines can be co-expressed within the same T-helper cell concurrently [20].

Therefore, the conventional Th1/Th2 paradigm, in which these two diseases tend to be mutually exclusive, is now considered to be oversimplified, with new data indicating that Th1- and Th2-driven diseases can coexist, suggesting that other factors, such as genetic background and environmental factors, might contribute as well, leading to a new, revised Th1/Th2 paradigm, serving as part of the reasoning for explanation for a potential association between atopic disease and diabetes mellitus. Moreover, the simultaneous presence of both diseases can be attributed to abnormalities in the immune system's response, influenced by specific genetic and environmental factors.

22.4.2 The Shared Impact of the "Hygiene Hypothesis"

The "hygiene hypothesis"—first postulated by Strachan in 1989 in connection to hay fever [21]—highlights the fact that the declining occurrence of various infections in developed and, more recently also in developing countries, due to modern lifestyles, can be attributed to an uprising prevalence of autoimmune and atopic diseases [22, 23].

While in relation to atopic dermatitis, this hypothesis has been more and more studied, recent data suggest that it also has a significant role in diabetes mellitus type 1 development. A study conducted in Northern Ireland identified an inversely proportional relationship between hygiene status and diabetes mellitus type 1 development, identifying the fact that areas with the least satisfactory hygiene conditions (e.g., overcrowded households or scarce sanitary facilities) present with the lowest occurrence of insulin-dependent diabetes mellitus [24].

Over time, several new discoveries have contributed to the revision of this hypothesis, leading to certain extensions of the initial hypothesis, known as "the old friends" and "microflora" hypotheses." *The old friends hypothesis* takes into consideration a certain coevolution of micro- and macroorganisms (such as helminths) with the human immune system improvement, implying that such organisms are necessary for normal development of the immune system, more exactly that a suitable level of early-life exposure to such organisms might exhibit protective features against immune dysregulation and atopic diseases development [25, 26]. *The microflora hypothesis* represents also a more modern expansion of the hygiene hypothesis, proposing that some disturbances in the early life of the intestinal microbiota, caused by various factors (such as antibiotic usage, infections, or nutrition), might disrupt the usual mechanism by which the microbiota supports the normal immunological tolerance; this can further lead to an immune system shift towards hypersensitivity diseases [26].

Therefore, according to some data present in the literature, similar to atopic disease, in the development of type 1 diabetes mellitus, certain characteristics more prevalent in industrialized countries (such as food, antibiotic exposure, and less exposure to various pathogens) might have a role.

22.4.3 The Epithelial Barrier Hypothesis

This represents another potential physiopathological common feature between atopic dermatitis and diabetes mellitus.

This theory postulates that chronic, perpetual peri-epithelial inflammation, triggered by exposure to various factors, determines various disruptions in the epithelial linings that serve as main barriers (physical, chemical, and immunological). This disruption in the normal epithelial linings contributes to development and aggravation of certain immunological conditions. Initially, this theory was demonstrated in diseases such as atopic dermatitis, followed by asthma, chronic rhinosinusitis, and inflammatory bowel diseases and, more recently, diabetes mellitus [23, 27].

While in atopic dermatitis, the disrupted epithelial barrier refers to the skin barrier (determined by a complex interplay between immune disturbances, filaggrin mutation, antimicrobial peptides deficiency, and cutaneous dysbiosis) [28], in diabetes it has been proven that the intestinal epithelial barrier dysfunction has a role—in type 1 diabetes mellitus, intestinal permeability determined by zonulin and insulin resistance precedes the development of disease, while in type 2 diabetes mellitus, the gut microbial dysbiosis along with thigh junctions and intestinal barrier rupture has implications in disease development [29].

22.4.4 *Genetic Background in Atopic Dermatitis and Diabetes Mellitus*

Although not completely understood, some data suggests there's a potential genetic linkage between atopic dermatitis and diabetes mellitus, with evidence that certain genetic factors may contribute to an increased risk in both conditions. Family and twin studies have provided evidence for the hereditary component in both atopic dermatitis and diabetes mellitus with the occurrence of these conditions among members of the same families suggesting a potential genetic predisposition—heritability rates estimated to be between 70% and 80% in atopic dermatitis [30], while in diabetes mellitus they vary between 20% and 80% [15].

22.4.5 *Shared Risk Factors and Common Comorbidities in Atopic Dermatitis and Diabetes Mellitus*

Although environmental factors and genetic predisposition contribute to the development of atopic dermatitis and diabetes mellitus, some modifiable risk factors are encountered in both diseases, like obesity, improper physical activity levels, and other cardiovascular diseases.

Obesity is considered a potential catalyst for the development of type 2 diabetes mellitus, and, according to literature data, there is a correlation between childhood and adolescent obesity and an increased chance of developing type 2 diabetes mellitus in young adults [31]. Moreover, obesity seems to be involved in type 1 diabetes mellitus as well, with an inverse relationship between the BMI and patient's age at diagnosis, implying that elevated body weight in young patients increases the risk for type 1 diabetes mellitus development [32].

When it comes to atopic dermatitis, the relationship with obesity is hazier. It has been identified that obesity might have a role in certain key factors involved in atopic dermatitis pathophysiology—such as switching from a Th2-predominant disorder to a more severe disease course driven by Th17 inflammation or increasing of the transepidermal water loss [33]. Some comprehensive research consisting of a systematic review and meta-analysis revealed a significant association between the presence of atopic dermatitis and increased likelihood of overweight or obese status in both children and adults, comprising studies from North America and Asia, but not Europe [9]. Moreover, a systematic review of observational studies has identified a positive correlation between atopic dermatitis and obesity, regardless of patient's age (infants, children, adolescents, and adults) [34].

Sedentarism represents another factor, identified in both atopic dermatitis and diabetes mellitus. In diabetes mellitus type 2 is known that higher physical activity levels are associated with a decreased chance of developing diabetes; consequently, a sedentary lifestyle can increase the risk of developing the disease by contributing to obesity, glycemic uptake, and insulin resistance [35]; therefore patients with high rates of sedentary behavior present an increased risk of developing type 2 diabetes mellitus compared to general population.

When it comes to atopic dermatitis, adult patients were found to exhibit low rates of moderate to vigorous physical exercise, which can be explained by various factors: the presence of eczema lesions, increased body temperature along with perspiration known as atopic dermatitis triggers and sleep disturbances and depression identified in such patients [9, 36].

Cardiovascular diseases are known to be linked with the presence of diabetes mellitus as it follows: an increased risk of cardiovascular disease mortality has been identified in diabetes patients regardless of gender, with such death rates 1.7 times higher in adult patients with diabetes mellitus compared to those without, mainly due to an increased risk of myocardial infarction and stroke; moreover, some cardiovascular risk factors (such as obesity, arterial hypertension, and dyslipidemia) are commonly identified among patients with diabetes mellitus, especially in those with type 2 [37]. In atopic dermatitis, few observational studies proposed the association with an increased risk of cardiovascular diseases development, some stating that atopic dermatitis itself is a potential cardiovascular disease risk factor; in a meta-analysis it was identified that atopic dermatitis patients present a high risk of developing heart failure, stroke, and myocardial infarction, with the risk of cardiovascular diseases being correlated with the severity of atopic dermatitis [38, 39]. However, no definitive causal relationship was demonstrated between these entities; in a Mendelian randomization study, such causal relationship was identified only between atopic dermatitis and heart failure, but not coronary artery disease, myocardial infarction, stroke, or atrial fibrillation [40], making the association between atopic dermatitis and diabetes mellitus still debatable and controversial.

22.5 Atopic Dermatitis and Diabetes Mellitus: Facts

Given the potential, but not fully proven common features displayed between these two chronic, inflammatory, non-curable diseases, the literature data regarding their interplay is currently debatable and controversial, some providing arguments in favor of this association, while others counterarguments.

22.5.1 Pros

Data from a population-based retrospective cohort study from Taiwan revealed a notable increased chance of atopic dermatitis occurrence in children with type 1 diabetes mellitus compared to healthy controls, especially in those under the age of 8; additionally, the same study excluded the potential co-influence of various comorbidities in the development of atopic dermatitis in such children, as patients with type 1 diabetes mellitus with no comorbidities presented with higher chances of atopic dermatitis [41].

Moreover, a Mendelian randomization study identified that genetically predicted atopic dermatitis is positively correlated with an elevated risk of developing both type 1 and type 2 diabetes mellitus [11].

Additionally, data from a cross-sectional study on adult atopic dermatitis from the USA showed that such patients present with higher chances of self-reported various comorbidities, among diabetes was listed (along with obesity, arterial hypertension, and heart diseases), these associations being directly proportional with atopic dermatitis severity [42].

22.5.2 Cons

A case-control study performed on a pediatric population (children and adolescents) revealed no difference in insulin-dependent diabetic patients compared to controls in terms of atopy prevalence, either as clinical atopic dermatitis, total serum IgE levels, or airborne allergens sensitivity [43].

Moreover, data from another comprehensive study—a multicenter, population-based, case-control one (EURODIAB)—revealed a reduced occurrence of atopic illnesses in children already diagnosed with insulin-dependent diabetes mellitus; however, this negative association was observed only in West Europe centers [44].

In adult atopic dermatitis, according to AAD guidelines for comorbidities management in this particular population subgroup, a potential negative correlation between atopic dermatitis and diabetes was identified, indicating a reduced risk of both diabetes in general and type 2 diabetes mellitus in particular in adults with atopic dermatitis [45]. Furthermore, a systematic literature review showed an unlikely association between atopic dermatitis and hyperglycemia, postulating that a positive association between type 2 diabetes mellitus and atopic dermatitis is improbable, analyzing data provided by adult population studies [46].

Additionally, a study identified a reduced risk of developing type 1 diabetes mellitus among atopic dermatitis patients [47], while another even postulated that atopic dermatitis might display protective properties against type 2 diabetes mellitus development [48].

22.6 Atopic Dermatitis in Patients with Diabetes Mellitus: Common Clinical Features

In about 30% of diabetes mellitus cases, patients might present with various dermatological manifestations, some of them even as diabetes precursors [49]. Among these skin manifestations of diabetes patients, some of them are also found in atopic dermatitis cases—such as pruritus, xerosis, or keratosis pilaris.

Pruritus in diabetic patients is frequently encountered (in up to 49% of cases), has a chronic character, and is commonly associated with skin xerosis or prurigo nodularis [49]. Skin xerosis is also frequent among diabetes mellitus patients, in some cases acquiring even an ichthyosiform aspect or being accompanied by keratosis pilaris [50].

Therefore, patients who associate these two medical entities—atopic dermatitis and diabetes mellitus—may present increased severities of these common clinical features (pruritus, xerosis, keratosis pilaris), leading to an even higher quality of life impairment in such selected cases.

22.7 Future Directions and Conclusions

To date, there is no conclusive evidence that finds a strongly positive association between atopic dermatitis and diabetes mellitus. Literature data varies considerably among various population subgroups, depending on age groups, comorbidities presence, geographical area, and subject's ethnicity.

Additional research into vast and diversified population groups (in terms of ethnicity, age, or geographical areas) regarding the co-occurrence of atopic dermatitis and diabetes mellitus and also future investigational molecular studies examining the potential involvement of the Th1-mediated diabetes mellitus in the emergence and course of Th2-driven atopic dermatitis and vice versa are needed.

Such future research developments might present with prognostic and therapeutic implications (e.g., early diagnosis and treatment of atopic dermatitis might reduce the chance of developing type 1 and type 2 diabetes mellitus and vice versa or might determine a better therapeutic response in both diseases).

To conclude, up to this date, it is important for physicians (dermatologists, pediatricians, endocrinologists, and nutrition specialists) to be aware of the likelihood of the association between atopic dermatitis and diabetes mellitus in both adults and children and the importance of multidisciplinary teams for management of atopic dermatitis.

References

1. Wollenberg A, Christen-Zach S, Taieb A, Paul C, Thyssen JP, de Bruin-Weller M, et al. ETFAD/EADV Eczema task force 2020 position paper on diagnosis and treatment of atopic dermatitis in adults and children. J Eur Acad Dermatol Venereol. 2020;34(12):2717–44.
2. Sacotte R, Silverberg JI. Epidemiology of adult atopic dermatitis. Clin Dermatol. 2018;36(5):595–605.
3. Kim J, Kim BE, Leung DYM. Pathophysiology of atopic dermatitis: Clinical implications. Allergy Asthma Proc. 2019;40(2):84–92.
4. Yang L, Fu J, Zhou Y. Research progress in atopic March. Front Immunol. 2020;11:1907.
5. Kage P, Zarnowski J, Simon JC, Treudler R. Atopic dermatitis and psychosocial comorbidities—what's new? Allergol Select. 2020;4:86–96.
6. Beck KM, Seitzman GD, Yang EJ, Sanchez IM, Liao W. Ocular co-morbidities of atopic dermatitis. Part I: Associated ocular diseases. Am J Clin Dermatol. 2019;20(6):797–805.
7. Darlenski RKJ, Hristakieva E, Fluhr JW. Atopic dermatitis as a systemic disease. Clin Dermatol. 2014;32(3):409–13.
8. Brunner PM, Silverberg JI, Guttman-Yassky E, Paller AS, Kabashima K, Amagai M, et al. Increasing comorbidities suggest that atopic dermatitis is a systemic disorder. J Invest Dermatol. 2017;137(1):18–25.
9. Silverberg JI. Comorbidities and the impact of atopic dermatitis. Ann Allergy Asthma Immunol. 2019;123(2):144–51.
10. Banday MZSA, Nissar S. Pathophysiology of diabetes: an overview. Avicenna J Med. 2020;10(04):174–88.
11. Lu F, Wu B, Wang Y. Mendelian randomization indicates that atopic dermatitis contributes to the occurrence of diabetes. BMC Med Genomics. 2023;16(1):132.
12. American Diabetes A. Diagnosis and classification of diabetes mellitus. Diabetes Care. 2014;37(Suppl. 1):S81–90.
13. Mirghani HO, Alhazmi K, Alghamdi S, Alraddadi M. The cross-talk between atopic dermatitis and diabetes mellitus: a meta-analysis. Cureus. 2021;13(3):e13750.
14. Sert UY, Ozgu-Erdinc AS. Gestational diabetes mellitus screening and diagnosis. Adv Exp Med Biol. 2021;1307:231–55.
15. Goyal S, Rani J, Bhat MA, Vanita V. Genetics of diabetes. World J Diabetes. 2023;14(6):656–79.
16. Mackay CR. Follicular homing T helper (Th) cells and the Th1/Th2 paradigm. J Exp Med. 2000;192(11):F31–4.
17. Rabin RL, Levinson AI. The nexus between atopic disease and autoimmunity: a review of the epidemiological and mechanistic literature. Clin Exp Immunol. 2008;153(1):19–30.
18. Cardwell CR, Carson DJ, Yarnell J, Shields MD, Patterson CC. Atopy, home environment and the risk of childhood-onset type 1 diabetes: a population-based case–control study. Pediatr Diabetes. 2008;9(3pt 1):191–6.
19. Kero J, Gissler M, Hemminki E, Isolauri E. Could TH1 and TH2 diseases coexist? Evaluation of asthma incidence in children with coeliac disease, type 1 diabetes, or rheumatoid arthritis: a register study. J Allergy Clin Immunol. 2001;108(5):781–3.
20. Assenmacher M, Lohning M, Scheffold A, Richter A, Miltenyi S, Schmitz J, Radbruch A. Commitment of individual Th1-like lymphocytes to expression of IFN-gamma versus IL-4

and IL-10: selective induction of IL-10 by sequential stimulation of naive Th cells with IL-12 and IL-4. J Immunol. 1998;161(6):2825–32.
21. Strachan DP. Hay fever, hygiene, and household size. BMJ. 1989;299(6710):1259–60.
22. Okada H, Kuhn C, Feillet H, Bach JF. The 'hygiene hypothesis' for autoimmune and allergic diseases: an update. Clin Exp Immunol. 2010;160(1):1–9.
23. D'Auria EMM, Colombo A, Sartorio MU, Zunica F, Zuccotti G, Lougaris V. Allergy and autoimmunity in children: non-mutually exclusive diseases. A narrative review. Front Pediatr. 2023;11:1239365.
24. Bach JF, Chatenoud L. The hygiene hypothesis: an explanation for the increased frequency of insulin-dependent diabetes. Cold Spring Harb Perspect Med. 2012;2(2):a007799.
25. Pfefferle PI, Keber CU, Cohen RM, Garn H. The hygiene hypothesis—learning from but not living in the past. Front Immunol. 2021;12:635935.
26. Stiemsma LT, Reynolds LA, Turvey SE, Finlay BB. The hygiene hypothesis: current perspectives and future therapies. Immunotargets Ther. 2015;4:143–57.
27. Kucuksezer UC, Ozdemir C, Yazici D, Pat Y, Mitamura Y, Li M, et al. The epithelial barrier theory: development and exacerbation of allergic and other chronic inflammatory diseases. Asia Pac Allergy. 2023;13(1):28–39.
28. Kim BE, Leung DYM. Significance of skin barrier dysfunction in atopic dermatitis. Allergy Asthma Immunol Res. 2018;10(3):207–15.
29. Akdis CA. Does the epithelial barrier hypothesis explain the increase in allergy, autoimmunity and other chronic conditions? Nat Rev Immunol. 2021;21(11):739–51.
30. Brown SJ, Elias MS, Bradley M. Genetics in atopic dermatitis: historical perspective and future prospects. Acta Derm Venereol. 2020;100(12):adv00163.
31. Malone JI, Hansen BC. Does obesity cause type 2 diabetes mellitus (T2DM)? Or is it the opposite? Pediatr Diabetes. 2019;20(1):5–9.
32. Al-Goblan AS, Al-Alfi MA, Khan MZ. Mechanism linking diabetes mellitus and obesity. Diabetes Metab Syndr Obes. 2014;7:587–91.
33. Mesjasz A, Zawadzka M, Chałubiński M, Trzeciak M. Is atopic dermatitis only a skin disease? Int J Mol Sci. 2023;24(1):837.
34. Ali ZSUC, Agner T, Thomsen SF. Is atopic dermatitis associated with obesity? A systematic review of observational studies. J Eur Acad Dermatol Venereol. 2018;32(8):1246–55.
35. Yuan S, Li X, Liu Q, Wang Z, Jiang X, Burgess S, Larsson SC. Physical activity, sedentary behavior, and type 2 diabetes: mendelian randomization analysis. J Endocr Soc. 2023;7:1–8.
36. Silverberg JI, Song J, Pinto D, Yu SH, Gilbert AL, Dunlop DD, Chang RW. Atopic dermatitis is associated with less physical activity in US Adults. J Invest Dermatol. 2016;136(8):1714–6.
37. Leon BM, Maddox TM. Diabetes and cardiovascular disease: epidemiology, biological mechanisms, treatment recommendations and future research. World J Diabetes. 2015;6(13):1246–58.
38. Ascott A, Mulick A, Yu AM, Prieto-Merino D, Schmidt M, Abuabara K, et al. Atopic eczema and major cardiovascular outcomes: a systematic review and meta-analysis of population-based studies. J Allergy Clin Immunol. 2019;143(5):1821–9.
39. Jung HJ, Lee DH, Park MY, Ahn J. Cardiovascular comorbidities of atopic dermatitis: using National Health Insurance data in Korea. Allergy Asthma Clin Immunol. 2021;17(1):94.
40. Chen H, Zhuo C, Zheng L. Assessing causal associations of atopic dermatitis with heart failure and other cardiovascular outcomes: a Mendelian randomization study. Front Cardiovasc Med. 2022;9:868850.
41. Lin CH, Wei CC, Lin CL, Lin WC, Kao CH. Childhood type 1 diabetes may increase the risk of atopic dermatitis. Br J Dermatol. 2015;174(1):88–94.
42. Silverberg JI, Gelfand JM, Margolis DJ, Boguniewicz M, Fonacier L, Grayson MH, et al. Association of atopic dermatitis with allergic, autoimmune, and cardiovascular comorbidities in US adults. Ann Allergy Asthma Immunol. 2018;121(5):604–12 e3.
43. Gazit V, Tasher D, Hanukoglu A, Landau Z, Ben-Yehuda Y, Somekh E, Dalal I. Atopy in children and adolescents with insulin-dependent diabetes mellitus. Isr Med Assoc J. 2008;10(12):858–61.

44. The EURODIAB Substudy 2 Study Group. Decreased prevalence of atopic diseases in children with diabetes. J Pediatr. 2000;137(4):470–4.
45. Davis DMR, Drucker AM, Alikhan A, Bercovitch L, Cohen DE, Darr JM, et al. American Academy of Dermatology Guidelines: awareness of comorbidities associated with atopic dermatitis in adults. J Am Acad Dermatol. 2022;86(6):1335–6 e18.
46. Ali Z, Ulrik CS, Agner T, Thomsen SF. Association between atopic dermatitis and the metabolic syndrome: a systematic review. Dermatology. 2018;234(3–4):79–85.
47. Schmitt J, Schwarz K, Baurecht H, Hotze M, Fölster-Holst R, Rodríguez E, et al. Atopic dermatitis is associated with an increased risk for rheumatoid arthritis and inflammatory bowel disease, and a decreased risk for type 1 diabetes. J Allergy Clin Immunol. 2016;137(1):130–6.
48. Drucker AM, Qureshi AA, Dummer TJB, Parker L, Li WQ. Atopic dermatitis and risk of hypertension, type 2 diabetes, myocardial infarction and stroke in a cross-sectional analysis from the Canadian Partnership for Tomorrow Project. Br J Dermatol. 2017;177(4):1043–51.
49. Lima AL, Illing T, Schliemann S, Elsner P. Cutaneous manifestations of diabetes mellitus: a review. Am J Clin Dermatol. 2017;18(4):541–53.
50. Mendes AL, Miot HA, Haddad VJ. Diabetes mellitus and the skin. An Bras Dermatol. 2017;92(1):8–20.

Chapter 23
Vitiligo in Diabetic Patients

Markus Böhm

Abstract Vitiligo is a common skin disorder characterized by white patches due to loss of melanin. Its major clinical subtype, non-segmental vitiligo (NSV), represents an autoimmune disorder in which melanocytes are destroyed by an interferon-γ-mediated immune response. NSV has a polygenetic background with susceptibility genes that predispose to other autoimmune-inflammatory diseases including diabetes mellitus type 1. According to most recent systematic reviews and meta-analyses, there is a significant association between vitiligo and diabetes mellitus type 1 but also type 2. Moreover, recent data suggest that early-onset and widespread vitiligo are independent risk factors for the development of diabetes mellitus. Medical practitioners should be alert to the association between vitiligo and diabetes. Screening for diabetes mellitus should be performed in patients with vitiligo, especially in those with NSV, if clinical signs of any metabolic dysfunction are present.

Vitiligo is an acquired skin disease with an estimated worldwide pooled prevalence of up to 2.1% based on a recent meta-analysis [1]. The disease is characterized by loss of melanin pigment in the skin and hair leading to white patches that may appear at any site of the human body including some mucosal surfaces, i.e., the lips and the anogenital area [2]. Importantly, vitiligo may lead to significant impairment of life quality with subsequent psychosocial disturbances depending on various factors such as extent of disease, skin phototype, and ethnicity or involvement of visible sites [3, 4]. Therefore, early detection, proper classification, and assessment of the disease are crucial to initiate a holistic therapeutic approach including shared decision-making with the patient [5] and best standard care based on national treatment guidelines and international consensus recommendations [6–8].

The major subtype of vitiligo is non-segmental vitiligo (NSV) which is characterized by symmetrically distributed white patches. Depending on the extent of the disease, NSV can involve only a limited portion of the skin like in acrofacial vitiligo, but it may also lead to generalization ("vitiligo vulgaris") and even to complete depigmentation (universal vitiligo) [2]. In contrast to segmental vitiligo (SV), whose

M. Böhm (✉)
Department of Dermatology, University of Münster, Münster, Germany
e-mail: bohmm@uni-muenster.de

K. Fritz, G.-S. Tiplica (eds.), *Cutaneous Manifestations in Diabetes*,
https://doi.org/10.1007/978-3-031-65300-1_23

etiology is still incompletely understood and which usually runs a self-limited course, NSV is regarded as an autoimmune disease [2]. A polygenetic disposition and environmental triggers result in intrinsic and metabolic abnormalities of melanocytes which activate the innate immune system. This is followed by an interferon-gamma (IFN-γ)-driven immune response in which melanocyte-specific CD8+ T lymphocytes finally destroy pigment cells [9]. Genome-wide association studies have identified more than 50 susceptibility genes that are associated with an increased risk for NSV [10, 11]. The identified loci include genes that are associated with other autoimmune-inflammatory diseases including diabetes type 1 and/or which encode crucial regulators of the immune system, e.g., HLA-DRB1/DQA1, CPVL, FASL, FOXP3, CTLA4, or IL-2RA.

Based on the genetic predisposition of NSV with susceptibility genes involved in immune regulation, the frequency of diabetes type 1 associated with vitiligo may be expected to be higher than in the general population. In a non-systematic review of associated comorbidities in patients, the frequency of diabetes type 1 was reported to range from 0.10 to 1.2 in vitiligo [12]. However, a large quantitative study recently addressed the association between vitiligo and diabetes mellitus in more detail [13]. This meta-analysis included 9 case-control studies with 15,657 patients. Seven studies reported the prevalence of diabetes mellitus (five studies with mixed-type and two with type 1 diabetes mellitus) in patients with vitiligo and two studies the prevalence of vitiligo in patients with diabetes type 2. The pooled estimate of the nine studies revealed that vitiligo was associated with diabetes mellitus (OR: 2.515; 95% CI: 1.972–3.208; $P < 0.001$). Of note, vitiligo was significantly associated with both types of diabetes (OR: 2.899; 95% CI; 1.532–5.482; $P = 0.001$ for type 1 and OR: 2.371; 95% CI: 1.712–3.283; $P < 0.001$ for type 2). Notably, the included studies did not provide data on the subtype of vitiligo or other clinical parameters which would have been useful for additional subgroup analysis [13]. The results of above study are supported by a recent systematic review and meta-analysis on the potential association between vitiligo and components of the metabolic syndrome [14]. Based on 32 studies and a total of 28,235 patients, a significant association between vitiligo and diabetes mellitus was detected with a pooled OR of 3.30 (95% CI: 2.10–5.17) which was higher than the association between vitiligo and obesity (OR: 2.08; 95% CI: 1.40–3.11).

Coexistent diabetes mellitus in patients with vitiligo in presence of a third autoimmune such as thyroid disease should raise suspicion for autoimmune polyglandular syndrome (APS). The precise frequency of the four different forms of APS is unknown in patients with vitiligo, but the polygenic forms, especially APS-3/4, appear more common and have been occasionally reported in anecdotal reports [15].

Whether coexisting diabetes mellitus in patients with vitiligo is associated with a distinct clinical profile of the skin disease or linked to a different treatment response and outcome has not been systematically investigated. In the qualitatively best, most recent, and large randomized placebo-controlled trials leading to approval of topical ruxolitinib, no differences were noted in the treatment outcome of patients with vitiligo and those with coexisting comorbidities [16]. Indeed, in diabetic patients with acute or rapidly progressing vitiligo, the risk-benefit ratio of systemic treatment with the corticosteroid mini-pulse therapy must be carefully weighed in a shared decision with the patient.

Interestingly, a recent study addressing the influence of vitiligo on diabetes mellitus suggests that early onset of vitiligo and greater body surface involvement are independent risk factors for the development of this metabolic disorder [17].

In summary, the current data indicate that the frequency of type 1 and 2 diabetes mellitus is elevated in patients with vitiligo. Medical practitioners need to be aware of diabetes mellitus as an important comorbidity in patients with vitiligo. Therefore, patients with vitiligo, especially those suffering from the autoimmune type of vitiligo, NSV, should be screened for diabetes if clinical signs point to this metabolic disorder or if additional symptoms of metabolic syndrome are present. In addition, medical practitioners should be alerted that early onset and widespread vitiligo diabetes mellitus may be risk factors for the development of subsequent diabetes mellitus.Conflict of InterestNone.

References

1. Zhang Y, Cai Y, Shi M, Jiang S, Cui S, Wu Y, Gao XH, Chen HD. The prevalence of vitiligo: a meta-analysis. PLoS One. 2016;11:e0163806.
2. Bergqvist C, Ezzedine K. Vitiligo: a review. Dermatology. 2020;236:571–92.
3. Ezzedine K, Eleftheriadou V, Jones H, Bibeau K, Kuo FI, Sturm D, Pandya AG. Psychosocial effects of vitiligo: a systematic literature review. Am J Clin Dermatol. 2021;22:757–74.
4. Chernyshov PV, Tomas-Aragones L, Manolache L, Pustisek N, Salavastru CM, Marron SE, Bewley A, Svensson A, Poot F, Suru A, Salek SS, Augustin M, Szepietowski JC, Koumaki D, Katoulis AC, Sampogna F, Abeni D, Linder DM, Speeckaert R, van Geel N, Seneschal J, Ezzedine K, Finlay AY. Quality of life measurement in vitiligo. Position statement of the European academy of dermatology and venereology task force on quality of life and patient oriented outcomes with external experts. J Eur Acad Dermatol Venereol. 2023;37:21–31.
5. Shourick J, Ahmed M, Seneschal J, Passeron T, Andreux N, Qureshi A, Cho E, Natella PA, Harris J, Tran V-T, Ezzedine K. Development of a shared decision-making tool in vitiligo: an international study. Br J Dermatol. 2021;185:787–96.
6. Böhm M, Schunter JA, Fritz K, Salavastru C, Dargatz S, Augustin M, Tanew A. S1 guideline: diagnosis and therapy of vitiligo. J Dtsch Dermatol Ges. 2022;20:365–78.
7. van Geel N, Speeckaert R, Taïeb A, Ezzedine K, Lim HW, Pandya AG, Passeron T, Wolkerstorfer A, Abdallah M, Alomar A, Bae JM, Bekkenk M, Benzekri L, Böhm M, Eleftheriadou V, Esmat S, Ghia D, Goh BK, Grimes P, Gupta S, Hamzavi IH, Harris JE, Oh SH, Huggins R, Katayama I, Lan E, Lee AY, Leone G, Le Poole C, Lui H, Maquignon N, Meurant JM, Monteiro P, Oiso N, Parsad D, Pliszewski G, Raboobee N, Rodrigues M, Rosmarin D, Suzuki T, Tanemura A, Thng S, Xiang F, Zhou Y, Picardo M, Seneschal J. Worldwide expert recommendations for the diagnosis and management of vitiligo: position statement from the international vitiligo task force part 1: towards a new management algorithm. J Eur Acad Dermatol Venereol. 2023;37:2173–84.
8. Seneschal J, Speeckaert R, Taïeb A, Wolkerstorfer A, Passeron T, Pandya AG, Lim HW, Ezzedine K, Zhou Y, Xiang F, Thng S, Tanemura A, Suzuki T, Rosmarin D, Rodrigues M, Raboobee N, Pliszewski G, Parsad D, Oiso N, Monteiro P, Meurant JM, Maquignon N, Lui H, Le Poole C, Leone G, Lee AY, Lan E, Katayama I, Huggins R, Oh SH, Harris JE, Hamzavi IH, Gupta S, Grimes P, Goh BK, Ghia D, Esmat S, Eleftheriadou V, Böhm M, Benzekri L, Bekkenk M, Bae JM, Alomar A, Abdallah M, Picardo M, van Geel N. Worldwide expert recommendations for the diagnosis and management of vitiligo: position statement from the inter-

national vitiligo task force-part 2: specific treatment recommendations. J Eur Acad Dermatol Venereol. 2023;37:2185–95.
9. Frisoli ML, Essien K, Harris JE. Vitiligo: mechanisms of pathogenesis and treatment. Ann Rev Immunol. 2020;38:621–48.
10. Jin Y, Andersen G, Yorgov D, Ferrara TM, Ben S, Brownson KM, Holland PJ, Birlea SA, Siebert J, Hartmann A, Lienert A, van Geel N, Lambert J, Luiten RM, Wolkerstorfer A, Wietze van der Veen JP, Bennett DC, Taïeb A, Ezzedine K, Kemp EH, Gawkrodger DJ, Weetman AP, Kõks S, Prans E, Kingo K, Karelson M, Wallace MR, McCormack WT, Overbeck A, Moretti S, Colucci R, Picardo M, Silverberg NB, Olsson M, Valle Y, Korobko I, Böhm M, Lim HW, Hamzavi I, Zhou L, Mi QS, Fain PR, Santorico SA, Spritz RA. Genome-wide association studies of autoimmune vitiligo identify 23 new risk loci and highlight key pathways and regulatory variants. Nat Genet. 2016;48:1418–24.
11. Spritz RA, Anderson GHL. Genetics of vitiligo. Dermatol Clin. 2017;35(2):245–55.
12. Seneschal J, Morice-Picard F, Taieb A. Vitiligo, associated disorders and comorbidities (autoimmune-inflammatory disorders, immunodeficiencies, rare monogenic diseases). In: Picardo M, Taieb A, editors. Vitiligo. 2nd ed. Springer Nature Switzerland; 2019. p. 125–39.
13. Chang HC, Lin MH, Huang YC, Hou TY. The association between vitiligo and diabetes mellitus: a systematic review and meta-analysis. J Am Acad Dermatol. 2019;81:1442–144.
14. Kang P, Zhang W-G, Ji Z-H, Shao Z-J, Li C-Y. Association between vitiligo and relevant components of metabolic syndrome: a systematic review and meta-analysis. J Dtsch Dermatol Ges. 2022;20:629–41.
15. Amerio P, Tracanna M, De Remigis P, Betterle C, Vianale L, Marra ME, Di Rollo D, Capizzi R, Feliciani C, Tulli A. Vitiligo associated with other autoimmune diseases: polyglandular autoimmune syndrome types 3B+C and 4. Clin Exp Dermatol. 2006;31:746–9.
16. Homey B, Böhm M. Thieme drug report, Ruxolitinib-Crème—Behandlungsansatz bei nicht-segmentaler Vitiligo. Thieme; 2024. p. 1–20.
17. Li B, Zhu G, Kang P, Chen J, He K, Wang X, Gao T, Li C, Li S. Influences of vitiligo-associated characteristics on the occurrence of diabetes mellitus: interactive analysis of a cross-sectional study. Exp Dermatol. 2023;32:1805–14.

Chapter 24
Autoimmune Connective Tissue Disorders in Diabetic Patients

Simona Caraiola and Razvan Adrian Ionescu

Abstract Since, on one hand, at least one type of diabetes mellitus is autoimmune in origin and, on the other hand, sometimes autoimmune diseases tend to coexist in the same patient, the potential association of diabetes mellitus and autoimmune diseases is of interest. As diabetes mellitus type 1 is, in many instances, an autoimmune glandular disease, there are other endocrine, as well as non-endocrine, autoimmune diseases associated with it. Recent years have highlighted the possibility that low-grade inflammation (which may be autoimmune-driven) is implicated in the pathogenesis of type 2 diabetes mellitus. It is therefore not surprising that several other autoimmune diseases are also associated to type 2 diabetes mellitus. This chapter reviews these potential associations and their possible implications.

24.1 Introduction

The immune system is essential for the functioning of the human body. A normal immune system provides accurate recognition of an organism's own cells and protects it against disease.

However, sometimes the immune system malfunctions: it can mistakenly identify the body's own cells as non-self-cells and unleash an immune attack against the body's organs and systems. This is mediated by antibodies (proteins normally produced by the immune system, which protect our bodies against non-self-structures) directed against the body's own structures, the so-called autoantibodies.

Autoimmune diseases (AIDs) reflect an interplay between genetic factors (such as gender, ethnicity, Human Leucocyte Antigen (HLA) patterns, etc.) which convey a certain likelihood of developing such a disease and environmental factors (such as exposure to certain chemical or physical agents) [1]; as such, not every person with

S. Caraiola · R. A. Ionescu (✉)
"Carol Davila" University of Medicine and Pharmacy, Bucharest, Romania

Third Internal Medicine Department, Colentina Clinical Hospital, Bucharest, Romania

K. Fritz, G.-S. Tiplica (eds.), *Cutaneous Manifestations in Diabetes*,
https://doi.org/10.1007/978-3-031-65300-1_24

a certain genetic profile is bound to develop the specific autoimmune disease to which that profile is associated.

There are more than 100 autoimmune diseases, affecting over 24 million people, in the United States [2]; these diseases can affect any organ of the body, resulting in various degrees of system malfunction which may, occasionally, develop into life-threatening conditions.

The symptoms of autoimmune diseases are extremely variable, and, sometimes, patients may go undiagnosed for a long time, especially if the specific autoimmune disease is quite rare. Most autoimmune diseases have no cure but can be controlled throughout one's life [3].

An important part of the autoimmune disease spectrum is autoimmune connective tissue disorders (AICTDs). This term refers to the group of AID that affect the connective tissue, that is, the tissue that supports cells within organs and organs within the body. Although AICTDs involve predominantly the joints, muscles, and skin (because of a greater predominance of connective tissue in these organs), since connective tissue is ubiquitous, AICTDs can also involve other organ systems (such as the lungs, the heart, the kidneys, the gut, the blood vessels, the eyes) [4].

AICTDS include polymyositis (PM), dermatomyositis (DM), rheumatoid arthritis (RA), systemic lupus erythematosus (SLE), Sjogren's syndrome, vasculitis, scleroderma (SSc), and mixed connective tissue disease (MCTD). All these conditions can be associated to diabetes mellitus (DM) in the same patient.

There are two major types of DM: type 1 DM (T1DM) and type 2 DM (T2DM). T1DM is caused by an inflammatory destruction of the pancreatic islets producing insulin, determined by an autoimmune process: presence of various auto antibodies directed against pancreatic tissue [5]. Because of its autoimmune pathogenesis, it is quite intuitive to presume that T1DM may be associated with other autoimmune diseases, especially endocrine ones.

T2DM, on the other hand, is considered, historically, a metabolic disease in which the two main metabolic determinants are aging and obesity [6]. Recent research focuses on low-grade inflammation as a main feature of T2DM pathogenesis. This is a state of subclinical systemic chronic inflammation that, when prolonged (such as with obesity and aging), can lead to profound disturbances with clinical consequences. Obesity and aging are so well-established promoters of inflammation that their influence on it is called metaflammation and inflammaging, respectively [7, 8]. Since the clinical presentation of AIDs is often preceded by low-grade inflammation [9], there might be a connection between the presence of T2DM and other autoimmune disorders.

24.2 T1DM and AICTD

24.2.1 Pathogenic Considerations

As previously stated, T1DM is an autoimmune disease, in which pancreatic islets are "attacked" by autoantibodies. It usually occurs in childhood, but more than 80% of people living with T1DM are adults [10]. The serologic markers of autoimmunity against pancreatic β cells are islet cell autoantibody (ICA), insulin autoantibody (IAA), glutamic acid decarboxylase antibody (GADA), and protein tyrosine phosphatase antibody (IA-2A), underlying the autoimmune nature of this disease [5]. With respect to AIDs, T1DM is most frequently associated with thyroid autoimmune dysfunction, and this association has been frequently described, in around 15–30% of patients [11, 12].

As to autoimmune connective tissue diseases, T1DM may be associated to several diseases (vitiligo, rheumatoid arthritis, and systemic lupus erythematosus [5]) in various proportion, but the most studied association of T1DM with AICTDs is with rheumatoid arthritis.

In autoimmune diseases, before the full-blown disease, there is a preclinical phase, in which, even though the patient experiences no symptoms, the immune system is activated, with laboratory signs of that activation. This preclinical phase, which can last for various lengths of time, is followed by symptoms that are nonspecific, which also can extend over a long period of time [13].

Upon analyzing the preclinical phase of T1DM and of RA and SLE, that is, their determinants (be they genetic, environmental, behavioral), one can find noteworthy similarities between these diseases that may account for their "predisposition" to coexist in the same patient [13]. For instance, in any geographical location, there seems to be a decrease in prevalence in the north-south direction [13, 14], which may mean there are genetic differences between northern and southern populations, on one hand, but it may also point to climatic, dietary habits and/or environmental differences across the north-south axis, on the other. In fact, very interestingly, when moving from Nordic countries to more southern ones, children have the same prevalence of T1DM (and multiple sclerosis, for that matter) as in the country they moved to [15]. Moreover, the same is true for RA: a higher prevalence was observed in South African RA patients, when people moved from rural to urban areas [16, 17], illustrating the possible importance of the environment in these diseases. There may be shared pathogenesis in terms of influence of the environment on development of T1DM and RA in the same individual.

When it comes to genetic factors involved in the clustering of T1DM with RA (or SLE), things are even more "obvious": some of the genetic factors of T1DM, RA, and SLE are shared [13]. It is well established that around 33% of the risk of developing RA is attributable to the *HLA-DRB1* molecule [18] and, in particular, to the small peptide sequence known as the "shared epitope" [19, 20], while *HLA-DRB1* in Caucasian people conveys a two- to threefold increase in the risk of development of SLE, as well [21, 22]. Finally, *HLA-DRB1*04*, is also a risk factor for *both* RA *and* T1DM [23, 24]. Moreover, RA, SLE, and T1DM also share non-HLA genetic risk factors; in fact, recent research showed that there are 89 overlapping genes, with 4 significant correlation regions and 107 significant correlation loci, between RA and T1DM [25]. For instance, the cell surface receptor *FLT3*, also known as CD135 (cluster of differentiation 135), present among others on dendritic cells (a type of antigen-presenting cells), is associated with an increased risk of T1DM, SLE, and RA [13]; *PTPN22* gene (coding for a protein involved in T- and B-cell signaling) is one of the other non-HLA genes associated with the development of T1DM, as well as with the risk of development of RA in male seropositive people

[26, 27]. This allele may be responsible, at least, in part, for the risk of T1DM patients developing RA [25]. In fact, Liao et al. conducted a case-control study in RA patients and controls regarding the prevalence of T1DM and T2DM, while testing their sera for the presence of anti-cyclic citrullinated peptide (anti-CCP) antibodies, rheumatoid factor, and the *620WPTPN22* allele) [28]. The authors found that T1DM is associated specifically with anti-CCP-positive RA (odds ratio (OR) 7.3 with 95% confidence interval (CI) 2.7–20.0), with the risk for developing RA in T1DM patients being lowered when adjusting for the abovementioned allele, suggesting a possible common pathway for the pathogenesis of T1Dm and RA. No association was found between T2DM and RA, whether anti-CCP-positive or anti-CCP-negative [28].

Even though genetics plays an important role in the occurrence of T1DM and AICTD, in itself it cannot explain the risk of developing these diseases in all cases, leaving room for the involvement of environmental and lifestyle factors. For instance, smoking is an important risk factor for both RA and SLE [29, 30]. The lack of association of smoking and T1DM risk may be due to the fact that T1DM onset is usually in childhood, with no time for the patient to have started smoking [13].

Another lifestyle-related factor is body mass index. There are several studies indicating that being overweight or obese confers an increased risk of T1DM as well as RA or SLE [14, 31–34]. Also, chronic stress and, mainly, post-traumatic stress disorder (PTSD) have been suggested to be associated to AID, with an increase of the risk of T1DM [14] and almost a doubling of the risk of developing RA [35, 36].

Another common pathway in the development of T1DM and AICTD, as pointed out previously, is the presence of a preclinical phase in which autoantibodies are detectable in the sera of patients. Thus, the majority of RA patients are positive for rheumatoid factor as well as for anti-citrullinated protein antibodies (ACPA) well before the full-blown picture of RA [37, 38], while T1DM patients can develop, in their preclinical phase, different autoantibodies: young children usually develop IAA, while in teenagers the most commonly found antibodies are GADA [39, 40]. Completely asymptomatic first-degree relatives of patients with T1DM, RA, and SLE may have disease-specific antibodies in their serum [5, 41, 42]. Regarding the cellular immunity component, in preclinical RA, there is a drop in T regulatory cell levels with a shift toward the pro-inflammatory T helper 2 subset of cells [43]. In T1DM, autoreactive T cells are also targeted against islet cells autoantigens, in patients as well as in their relatives [13, 44]. Also, both in preclinical RA and in the pathogenesis of T1DM, there is a malfunction of B cells [45, 46]. On another level, there are some similarities in terms of malfunction of the complement system in the preclinical phase of both SLE (where there are low levels of fraction C1q) and T1DM (where the C4d component is increased) [47, 48].

All the elements highlighted here suggest that there might be a connection, even at the preclinical level, between the development of T1DM and AICTD, partly explaining why they sometimes cluster in the same patient.

24.2.2 Clinical Considerations

Using a large database (~75 million members), Rogers et al. [49] showed that 27.03% of patients having T1DM, were also having an AID, with thyroid disease, RA, and celiac disease being the most prevalent. RA diagnosis was found to be increasing with age, with a maximum of prevalence in the 60–64 years of age group, and was significantly more prevalent in women than in males [49]. In the same paper, the authors report an overall 1.43% prevalence of psoriasis in patients with T1DM, with a greater prevalence in middle-aged female patients; the same was found for SLE prevalence. For Sjogren's syndrome, data showed an almost sevenfold higher prevalence in women than in males with T1DM [49]. RA, SLE, and psoriasis associated to T1DM increased the risk for cardiovascular events (renal failure, ischemic stroke, and myocardial infarction), while Sjogren's syndrome had no influence on myocardial infarction risk, elevating the other two. SLE was the most burdensome of all four associated diseases, in terms of added cardiovascular risk [49].

To make things even more complicated, in another recent paper as well, the presence of AID in longstanding T1DM, even though frequent, was associated with lower odds of cardiovascular events [50].

In a large cross-sectional study comprising 158,865 patients, investigating the prevalence and risk factors for developing polyautoimmunity in patients with T1DM, Bao et al. [50] found that AICTDs are encountered in 3.4% of patients with the most common AICTD being RA—2.0% of patients. As this is a significantly higher RA prevalence than in US general population, it may show a possible common risk for developing T1DM and RA [51]. When looking at the gender distribution of AICTD occurrence in T1DM patients, the authors found a significant female predominance for RA (73% female; $p < 0.0001$), Sjogren's syndrome (87% female; $p < 0.0001$), and SLE (82% female; $p < 0.0001$); it is noteworthy that 52.5% of the whole T1DM population were females. Another interesting finding of this study is that Asians and Caucasians were at higher risk of AICTD than others (African Americans, Hispanics, or Native Americans) of developing an AICTD ($p < 0.0001$). The conclusion of the authors is that T1DM persons are at increased risk of developing AICTD (and non-endocrine autoimmune diseases for that matter) [51].

T1DM can also be associated with other AICTD. Michitsuji et al. [52] report the case of a woman in her 60 s with T1DM who developed mixed connective tissue disease with anti-U1-RNP antibodies as well as PR3-ANCA. It has been found that 12% of 94 patients with T1DM were positive for ANCA (either MPO-ANCA or PR2-ANCA) [52]. Interestingly, even though this high prevalence of ANCA positivity would possibly suggest a pathogenic role for it in T1DM, there is no difference between diabetic patients positive and negative for ANCA, with respect to control of diabetes and to T1DM complications [53].

24.3 T2DM and AICTD

24.3.1 Pathogenic Considerations

T2DM is, traditionally, a metabolic disease. It is, a very complex disease, characterized by alterations in glycemic control, most frequently, in overweight or obese patients. Hyperglycemia of T2DM is associated to insulin resistance and variable degrees of insulin deficiency [54]. There are now numerous data emphasizing that a status of hampered inflammation (the so-called low-grade inflammation) is not an "innocent bystander" but an "actor" in T2DM [7, 8, 55].

It is well-known that adiponectin is the most abundant protein with cytokine activity secreted by adipose tissue (adipokine), in human blood [56]. Adiponectin is found in blood in three isoforms; it is homologous to the C1q component of complement, being part of the soluble collagen superfamily [57].

Adiponectin has a dual effect on inflammation: it can have both anti-inflammatory and pro-inflammatory effects. Thus, it is known that adiponectin can activate anti-inflammatory cytokines as interleukin (IL)-10 and reduce pro-inflammatory ones (IL-6 and TNF-α, which are important players in RA pathogenesis, IFN-γ) [58], while inhibiting macrophage M1-type activation (which have pro-inflammatory actions) and promoting macrophage M2 type activation (which have anti-inflammatory actions) [59]. On the other hand, the low-molecular-weight isoform of adiponectin has been proven to significantly increase levels of the pro-inflammatory cytokines IL-8 and granulocyte macrophage colony-stimulating factor (GM-CSF) in colonic epithelial cells [57] and to have synergistic effects with TNF-α-mediated NOX-2 expression [60]. It is well-known that, when compared to healthy people, RA patients have high levels of adiponectin as well as other adipokines, such as leptin and visfatin [61]. Also, the high-molecular-weight isoform of adiponectin has higher levels in RA patients than in healthy controls [60]. This isoform of adiponectin has an active role in the inflammation of RA, as it upregulates the release of IL-6, IL-8, and MMP-3 in synovial fibroblasts, which have structural effects on bones in RA [62]. In another study [63], adiponectin increased the production of TGFβ, IL-1Ra, PGE2, VGEF, and, again, IL-8 and IL-6, showing once more the pro-inflammatory action of this isoform of adiponectin. Moreover, it can promote production of TNF-α [64], which has been proven to have a central role in RA pathogenesis.

In T2DM, adiponectin shows low serum levels which are associated with high production of pro-inflammatory cytokines, leading to the state of low-grade inflammation. Since in normal people, adiponectin acts like an insulin sensitizer [65], the abovementioned abnormalities eventually lead to the disruption of β-cell functioning [66].

Another cytokine that may promote the development of RA in T2DM patients is interleukin 1β (IL-1β). It is produced as an inactive precursor, pro-IL-1β, which is cleaved to the active form by caspase 1. This requires the assembly and functioning of the inflammasome (an intracellular proteic platform involved in pathogen recognition and neutralization, whose malfunction is at the base of autoinflammation) [67, 68]. In RA, IL-1β may play multiple roles: modulates leucocyte recruitment inside affected joints [69], stimulates osteoclast differentiation and activity [70], and stimulates production of matrix metalloproteinases [71], the ultimate effect of all these actions being joint destruction. There is also a role for IL-1β in T2DM. High glucose levels as well as free fatty acids can stimulate the overproduction of pro-inflammatory cytokines, with effects on the pancreatic islet cells. Hyperglycemia produces the dissociation of thioredoxin-interacting protein from thioredoxin, which interacts with a specific inflammasome, activating caspase 1, thus producing IL-1β from its inactive precursor [72]. As to the saturated free fatty acids, they seem to also stimulate the production of IL-1β, as well as of other cytokines, through various mechanisms (IL-6, TNF-α) [73]. Moreover, it has been observed that stimulation of β islet cells with IL-1β produces a "vicious" cycle that promotes even more secretion of IL-1β by these cells, self-perpetuating its production in a process of autoinflammation [74]. This process may be prevented by blocking IL-1R1 signaling [73]. In later stages of T2DM, there is also amyloid deposition in β islet cells (which then is a hallmark of T2DM), a process owed to the high production of IL-1β by β cells themselves and macrophages via the activation of the specific inflammasome [75]. Another interesting mechanism promoting inflammation in T2DM, representing thus a potential "bridge" to AICTD development in this otherwise metabolic disease, is related to type 2 macrophages (M2). This type of macrophage is directly involved into the embryonic development of the pancreas, becoming resident pancreatic macrophages, adapted to the pancreatic milieu similarly to other resident macrophages [76–78]. During T2DM, the phenotype of the β pancreatic islet macrophages changes to the pro-inflammatory M1 type, characterized by increased production of various pro-inflammatory cytokines (including IL-1β) and overexpression of the specific inflammasome [67, 79]. All the above data suggest that there is an important role of inflammation in T2D, especially low-grade, and that via the cells that are part of these processes, there might be some connections between T2DM and the occurrence of AICTD in the same patient.

Nevertheless, it is known that the presence of hyperglycemia exerts various effects on the capability of the immune system to function normally; host defense mechanisms do not function properly in a diabetic patient especially if poorly controlled. Thus, hyperglycemia reduces neutrophil functions (degranulation, chemotaxis, phagocytosis) [80, 81], inhibits Fc-γ receptor-mediated phagocytosis [82], and inhibits opsonization [83]. All these actions take place via various mechanisms: inhibition of glucose-6-phosphate dehydrogenase [84], activation of some kinases, direct binding of C3 complement component, etc. [82, 83]. Moreover, since T2DM is characterized also increased nonenzymatic glycation of amino groups, the formation of irreversible advanced glycation end products (AEGs) is one the contributors to malfunction of the immune response. AEGs can interfere with the proper function of immunoglobulins, cytokines, and/or their respective receptors; consequently, the immune system may be less responsive [85]. Considering these known facts, even though one would expect T2DM patients to have lower rates of AICTD (which are characterized by an aberrantly immune response in the context of loss of self-tolerance), the question whether preexisting T2DM can be more frequently associated with AICTD via modulation of the inflammatory response remains.

24.3.2 Clinical Considerations

Tentolouris et al., in 2018, prospectively compared the prevalence of RA in a T2DM patient population, matched with the same number of controls [85]. The prevalence of RA in already diagnosed patients with T2DM was 0.25%, which is threefold lower than in matched controls (0.80%). This difference was statistically significant ($p = 0.029$) [85]. Moreover, the odds ratio for T2DM patients to develop RA was 0.30 (95% CI: 0.10–0.64), significantly lower ($p = 0.038$) than that of matched controls without T2DM. Interestingly, RA occurred at a significantly older age in T2DM patients than in matched controls (64 ± 15 years versus 48 ± 18 years; $p = 0.004$) [85]. Even though this was a cross-sectional study, thus providing associations without explaining them, it found a significantly lower prevalence of RA in T2DM patients, probably due to a variety of factors, some of which are aforementioned.

Searching a large database in the United States (Healthcare Cost and Utilization Project) for the 2019 data, Abugharbyeh et al. examined some of the AICTD prevalence in type 1 and type 2 diabetes mellitus, comparing them to nondiabetic control group [86]. In more than 1.5 million patients with T2DM, there was a lower prevalence of SLE, SSc, and Sjogren's syndrome than in the nondiabetic population (0.0007 vs. 0.001, p-value <0.0001 for SSc, 0.0015 vs. 0.0018, p-value <0.001 for Sjogren's syndrome). Interestingly, organ involvement characteristic to the AICTD considered also had a significantly lower incidence in T2DM patients compared to nondiabetic population: lung involvement in SSc had a prevalence of 0.0005 in T2DM group vs. 0.0008 in controls, p-value <0.0001, while lupus nephritis prevalence was 0.0004 (T2DM) vs. 0.0009 (nondiabetics), p-value <0.001 [86]. These findings suggest that T2DM and/or T2DM treatment may have a favorable effect on the prevalence as well as on the specific organ involvement of some AICTD.

Bearing in mind that observational studies may be biased by confounding factors not always known and/or considered, Inamo et al. performed a Mendelian randomization analysis using genome-wide association studies (GWAS) datasets of T2DM and RA [87]. Mendelian randomization has an advantage on casual relation because it assumes that the causal effect from the genetic variant to the outcome (i.e., RA) is mediated completely via the exposure (i.e., T2DM) and not by any confounding factor [87, 88]. In their study, the authors found a protective effect of T2DM on the risk of developing RA, no matter the ancestry (European or Asian) of the analyzed patients.

Some of the drugs used to treat T2DM also have immunomodulatory properties that might mitigate the risk of developing RA. In a large database, Zemedikun et al. retrospectively investigated the risk of developing RA in T2DM patients as well as the importance of different treatments used for glycemic control [89]. They demonstrated statistically significant lower risk of RA development in T2DM patients compared to controls, irrespective of gender. The risk was higher with smoking, which is a well-known environmental factor implicated in RA pathogenesis. Noteworthy, when patients with a history of statin use were excluded from the analysis, the risk for RA increased. The authors concluded that statin use, unlike other medicines (e.g., dipeptidyl peptidase-4 inhibitors), appears to consistently reduce the risk of development of RA in T2DM patients, even having a protective effect [89]. These findings, that need to be further investigated, might change the way we treat T2DM in the future.

Metformin is one of the first-line therapies used for T2DM treatment, due to its hypoglycemic and increased insulin sensitivity effects [90]. In addition, metformin also has some immune-modulatory and anti-inflammatory actions [91]. Based on these assumptions, Wang et al. investigated the potential role of metformin use in reducing the risk of development of Sjogren's syndrome in T2DM patients [92]. They found that the incidence of Sjogren's syndrome in metformin users was almost threefold lower than in metformin nonusers (16.82 per 100,000 person-years vs. 40.83 per 100,000 person-years). That is to say that metformin use could reduce the risk of development of Sjogren's syndrome in T2DM patients. Interestingly, T2DM patients aged 60 years or more were at lower risk to develop Sjogren's syndrome than those under the age of 60 [92]. This effect might be due to the ability of metformin to act on multiple levels of the immune system: it reduces autoreactive marginal B-cell formation, stimulates regulatory T-cell production, and suppresses T helper 17 cells [93, 94].

24.4 Additional Considerations

Another way of looking at the relationship between AICTD and diabetes mellitus is to search for the influence that AICTD may have on the risk of developing DM. In this respect, Taiwanese physicians investigated in a nationwide cohort study whether SSc is a risk factor for DM (irrespective of the type of DM) [95]. The authors found that the incidence of DM was, overall, reduced in SSc patients compared to controls. This is probably due to the specific cytokine environment present in SSc (IL-13, IL-10, and tumor necrosis factor-related apoptosis-inducing ligand (TRAIL) being the most important ones), which prevents the occurrence of both type 1 and type 2 diabetes mellitus [95]. There are certainly other factors involved in the "protective" role of SSc against DM, as the physical activity limitation due to SSc, higher blood pressure level often found in SSc, or higher cholesterol levels in SSc, all of which can interfere with the development of DM [96–98]. Additionally, it has been demonstrated that long-standing SSc is associated to liver fibrosis, which impairs gluconeogenesis and hepatic glucose production [99, 100]. This may also add to the mechanisms of a lower risk of T2DM development in SSc [101].

Sometimes, the presence of an autoimmune constellation may trigger unexpected consequences. Petersen et al. [102] reported a case of a 55-year-old woman with mixed connective tissue disease, presenting progressive myopathy evolving parallel to recurrent episodes of severe hypoglycemia. Anti-insulin receptor antibodies were present, which is very interesting, because usually their presence produces hyperglycemia. Hypoglycemia in the context of the presence of anti-insulin receptor antibodies is thought to result from a partial agonist activity of the aforementioned antibodies, when in low titer [103]. It is noteworthy that, usually, insulin receptor antibody-mediated disease occurs in a patient already having a systemic autoimmune disease (as it was shown in a case series of SLE patients), which was not the case in this female patient [104, 105].

24.5 Therapeutic Considerations

In the context of AICTD associated to diabetes mellitus, it is interesting to study whether any of the commonly used medications in T2DM are useful or not in treating the concomitant AICTD. It is well-known that one of the cornerstones of treatment in T2DM is the use of metformin. Metformin is part of the class of biguanides. To this day, it has an incompletely elucidated mechanism of action. Several such mechanisms have been proposed [106]. The most interesting, from an autoimmune perspective, is the one involving adenosine monophosphate-activated protein kinase (AMPK), which activates hepatocytes leading to the downregulation of gluconeogenic gene transcription [107–109]. On the other hand, AMPK has multiple interventions on the immune system. Through the mammalian target of rapamycin signaling pathway (mTOR), it controls the differentiation of T cells into effector or regulatory T cells [110]. AMPK also inhibits signal transducer and activator of transcription 3 (STAT3) which is involved in T-cell, memory B-cell, and plasma cell differentiation [111–113]. Via these implications in DM and AICTD pathogenesis, AMPK activation could be an interesting target for therapy of the autoimmune inflammatory disorders (AICTD).

In RA, fibroblast-like synoviocytes (FLS) are a central component of the synovial pannus, thus being involved in joint destruction [114]. Metformin has inhibitory actions on migration and proliferation of FLS [115, 116] as well as on the secretion of inflammatory cytokines by FLS [116]. In RA animal models, metformin was shown to be protective against bone erosion by inhibition of osteoclast differentiation and activation [117, 118]. These potentially beneficial effects of using metformin in the armamentarium of RA treatment have been translated into clinical practice as well. Metformin use in RA patients was associated with lower admission rates over 10 years of follow-up, compared to cyclooxygenase-2 inhibitors use [119]. In RA patients on a background methotrexate treatment, the addition of metformin to treatment was associated with better disease activity scores and higher rates of remission [120]. Moreover, diabetic patients adhering to metformin treatment for 18 years had lower risk rates of developing RA, compared to placebo-treated patients [120]. All these data suggest that metformin treatment may be an adjunctive to RA treatment, even maybe a preventive method for RA development in diabetic patients.

In SLE, metformin use was associated with downregulation of mitochondrial DNA form neutrophil extracellular traps (NETs), thus lowering the interferon-α production form antigen-presenting dendritic cells [121]. This translated into reduction of required glucocorticoid dose and risk of SLE flares, in clinical trials [121, 122].

In a retrospective cohort study on 15,098 T2DM Taiwanese patients, treated with metformin and an equivalent number of matched controls, having as primary end point the incidence of Sjogren's syndrome, Wang et al. found that Sjogren's incidence rate was significantly lower in metformin users than in controls; the hazard ratio in T2DM patients using metformin for Sjogren's syndrome was 0.46 (95% CI 0.23–0.92) [92]. Men and T2DM patients aged 60 years or over taking metformin were at a lower risk of developing Sjogren's syndrome than matched controls. The authors concluded that in T2DM patients, metformin use is associated with a reduced risk of Sjogren's occurrence.

24.6 Final Considerations

The clinician treating diabetes mellitus should be aware of the potential concomitant occurrence of autoimmune connective tissue diseases in their patients, since this is a potential comorbidity that might complicate the course, evolution, and treatment of diabetes. The treating physician should, periodically, actively search for such coexisting diseases in their patients, to intercept it as soon as possible, with the aim of mitigating its potential consequences on the management of such a complex and diverse disease, as diabetes mellitus. Moreover, future research is needed to elucidate the common pathogenic mechanisms involved in the clustering of AICTD in DM patients, as well as the influence of treatments used in DM on AICTD. This latter research could change the therapeutical approach of rheumatologists as well, in that it might reveal the benefits of using some of the DM medication in AICTD.

References

1. Ramos PS, Shedlock AM, Langfeld CD. Genetics of autoimmune diseases: insights from population genetics. J Hum Genet. 2015;60(11):657–64.
2. Martins K. What is an autoimmune disease? 2023. https://www.webmed.com/a-to-z-guides/autoimmune-diseases. Accessed 13 January 2024.
3. National Institute for Environmental Health Sciences. Autoimmune diseases; 2022. https://www.niehs.nih.gov/health/topics/conditions/autoimmune-diseases. Accessed 13 January 2024.

4. Dunkin MA. Connective tissue disease. 2023. https://www.webmed.com/a-to-z-guides/connective-tissue-disease. Accessed 13 January 2024.
5. Frommer L, Kahaly GJ. Type 1 diabetes and associated autoimmune diseases. World J Diabetes. 2020;11(11):527–39. https://doi.org/10.4239/wjd.v11.i11.527.
6. de Candia P, Prattichizzo F, Garavelli S, et al. Type 2 diabates: how much of an autoimmune disease? Front Endocrinol. 2019;10:451. https://doi.org/10.3389/fendo.2019.00451.
7. Prattichizzo F, De Nigris V, Micheloni S, et al. Increases in circulating levels of ketone bodies and cardiovascular protection with SGLT2 inhibitors: is low-grade inflammation the neglected component? Diabetes Obes Metab. 2018;20:2515–22. https://doi.org/10.1111/dom.13488.
8. Prattichizzo F, De Nigris V, Spiga R, et al. Inflammaging and metaflammation: the yin and yang of type 2 diabetes. Ageing Res Rev. 2018;41:1–17. https://doi.org/10.1016/j.arr.2017.10.003.
9. Furman D, Campisi J, Verdin E, et al. Chronic inflammation in the etiology of disease across life span. Nat Med. 2019;25(12):1822–32. https://doi.org/10.1038/s41591-0190-0675-0.
10. Centers for Diseases Control and Prevention. National Diabetes Statistics Report: estimates of diabetes and its burden in the Unites States, 2014. Atlanta: US Department of Health and Human Services; 2014.
11. Triolo TJ, Armstrong TK, McFann K, et al. Additional autoimmune disease found in 33% of patients at type 1 diabetes onset. Diabetes Care. 2011;34:1211–3.
12. Biondi B, Kahaly GJ, Robertson RP. Thyroid dysfunction and diabetes mellitus: two closely associated disorders. Endocr Rev. 2019;40:789–824.
13. Frazeli G, van Vollenhoven RF, de Jong BA, et al. Preclinical autoimmune disease: a comparison of rheumatoid arthritis, systemic lupus erythematosus, multiple sclerosis and type 1 diabetes. Front Immunol. 2022;13:899372. https://doi.org/10.3389/fimmu.2022.899372.
14. Rewers M, Ludvigsson J. Environmental risk factors for type 1 diabetes. Lancet. 2016;387(10035):2340–8. https://doi.org/10.1016/S0140-6736(16)30507-4.
15. Tettey P, Simpson S, Taylor BV, et al. Co-occurrence of multiple sclerosis and type 1 diabetes: shared aetiologic features and clinical implication for MS aetiology. J Neurol Sci. 2015;348(1–2):126–31. https://doi.org/10.1016/j.jns.2014.11.019.
16. Viatte S, Plant D, Raychaudhuri S. Genetics and epigenetics of rheumatoid arthritis. Nat Rev Rheumatol. 2013;9(3):141–53. https://doi.org/10.1038/nrrheum.2012.237.
17. Solomon L, Robin G, Valkenburg HA. Rheumatoid arthritis in an urban south African negro population. Ann Rheum Dis. 1975;34(2):128–35. https://doi.org/10.1136/ard.34.2.128.
18. Cornelis F, Faure S, Martinez M, et al. New susceptibility locus for rheumatoid arthritis suggested by a Genime-wide linkage study. Proc Natl Acad Sci U S A. 1998;95(18):10746–50. https://doi.org/10.1073/pnas.95.18.10746.
19. Gregersen PK, Silver J, Winchester RJ. The shared epitope hypothesis. An approach to understanding the molecular genetics of susceptibility to rheumatoid arthritis. Arhtritis Rheum. 1987;30(11):1205–13. https://doi.org/10.1002/art1780301102.
20. Van der Woude D, Houwing-Duistermaat JJ, Toes REM, et al. Quantitative heritability of anti-citrullinated protein antibody-positive and anti-citrullinated protein antibody-negative rheumatoid arthritis. Arthritis Rheum. 2009;60(4):916–23. https://doi.org/10.1002/art24385.
21. Graham RR, Ortmann VA, Langefeld CD, et al. Visualizind human leucocyte antigen class II risk haplotypes in human systemic lupus erythematosus. Am J Hum Genet. 2002;71(3):543–53. https://doi.org/10.1086/432290.
22. Ramos PS, Brown EE, Kimberly RP, et al. Genetic factors predisposing to systemic lupus erythematosus and lupus nephritis. Semin Nephrol. 2010;30(2):164–76. https://doi.org/10.1016/j.semneprol.2010.01.007.
23. Handel AE, Handunnetthi L, Ebers GC, et al. Type 1 diabetes mellitus and multiple sclerosis: common etiological features. Nat Rev Endocrinol. 2009;5(12):655–64. https://doi.org/10.1038/nrendo.2009.216.

24. Van Der Helm-Van Mil AHM, Verpoort KN, Le CS, et al. The HLA-DRB1 epitope alleles differ in the interaction with smoking and predisposition to antibodies to cyclic citrullinated peptide. Arthritis Rheum. 2007;56(2):425–32. https://doi.org/10.1002/art22373.
25. Wen Y-P, Yu Z-G. Identifying shared genetic loci and common risk genes of rheumatoid arthritis associated with three autoimmune diseases based on large-scale cross-trait genome-wide association studies. Front Immunol. 2023;14:1160397. https://doi.org/10.3389/fimmu.2023.1160397.
26. Plenge RM, Padyukov L, Remmers EF, et al. Replication of putative candidate-gene associations with rheumatoid arthritis in >4000 samples from North America and Sweden: association of susceptibility with PTPN22, CTLA4 and PADI4. Am J Hum Genet. 2005;77(6):1044–60. https://doi.org/10.1086/498651.
27. Primavera M, Giannini C, Chiarelli F. Prediction and prevention of type 1 diabetes. Front Endocrinol. 2020;15:11. https://doi.org/10.3389/fendo2020.00248.
28. Liao KP, Gunnarsson M, Kallberg H, et al. A specific association exists between type 1 diabetes and anti-CCP positive rheumatoid arthritis. Arthritis Rheum. 2009;60(3):653–60. https://doi.org/10.1002/art24362.
29. Heliovaara M, Aho K, Aromaa A, et al. Smoking and risk of rheumatoid arthritis. J Rheumatol. 1993;33(4):652–8.
30. Barbhaiya M, Tedeschi SK, Lu B, et al. Cigarette smoking and the risk of systemic lupus erythematosus, overall and by anti-double stranded DNA antibody subtype, in the nurses' health study cohorts. Ann Rheum Dis. 2018;77(2):196–202. https://doi.org/10.1136/annrheumdis-2017-211675.
31. Choi MY, Hahn J, Malspeis S, et al. A combination of healthy lifestyle behaviors reduces risk of incident systemic lupus erythematosus. Arthritis Rheumatol. 2021;74(2):274–83.
32. De Hair MJH, Landewe RBM, Van De Sande MGH, et al. Smoking and overweight determine the likelihood of developing rheumatoid arthritis. Ann Rheum Dis. 2013;72(10):1654–8. https://doi.org/10.1136/annrheumdis-2012-202254.
33. Crowson CS, Matteson EL, Davis JM, et al. Contribution of obesity to the rise in incidence of rheumatoid arthritis. Arthritis Care Res. 2013;65(1):71–7. https://doi.org/10.1002/acr.21660.
34. Lu B, Hiraki LT, Sparks JA, et al. Overweight or obese and risk of developing rheumatoid arthritis among women: a prospective cohort study. Ann Rheum Dis. 2014;73(11):1914–32. https://doi.org/10.1136/annrheumdis-2014-205459.
35. O'Donovan A, Cohen BE, Seal KH, et al. Elevated risk for autoimmune disorders in Iraq and Afghanistan veterans with posttraumatic stress disorder. Biol Psychiatry. 2015;77(4):365–74. https://doi.org/10.1016/j.biopsych.2014.06.015.
36. Lee YC, Agnew-Blais J, Malspeis S, et al. Post-traumatic stress disorder and risk for incident rheumatoid arthritis. Arthritis Care Res. 2016;68(3):292–8. https://doi.org/10.1002/acr22683.
37. Van Steebergen HW, Magnus L, Reijnierse M, et al. Clinical factors, anticitrullinated peptide antibodies and MRI-detected subclinical inflammation in relation to progression from clinically suspect arthralgia to arthritis. Ann Rheum Dis. 2016;75(10):1824–30. https://doi.org/10.1136/annrheumdis-2015-208138.
38. Nielen MMJ, Van Schaardenburg D, Reesnik HW, et al. Specific autoantibodies precede the symptoms of rheumatoid arthritis: a study of serial measurments in blood donors. Arthritis Rheum. 2004;50(2):380–6. https://doi.org/10.1002/art.20018.
39. Bosi E, Boulware DC, Becker DJ, et al. Impact of age and antibody type on progression from single to multiple antibodies in type 1 diabetes relatives. J Clin Endocrinol Metab. 2017;102(8):2881–6. https://doi.org/10.1210/jc.2017-00569.
40. Ziegler AG, Rewers M, Simell O, et al. Seroconversion to multiple islet autoantibodies and risk of progression to diabetes in children. JAMA. 2013;309(23):2473–9. https://doi.org/10.1007/s00125-017-4296-1.
41. Arbuckle MR, McClain MT, Rubertone MV, et al. Development of autoantibodies before the clinical onset of systemic lupus erythematosus. N Engl J Med. 2003;349(16):1526–33. https://doi.org/10.1056/NEJMoa021933.

42. James JA, Chen H, Young KA, et al. Latent autoimmunity across disease-specific boundaries in at-risk first-degree relatives of SLE and RA patients. EBioMedicine. 2019;42:76–85. https://doi.org/10.1016/j.ebiom.2019.03.063.
43. Kokkonen H, Soderstrom I, Rocklov J, et al. Up-regulation of cytokines and chemokines predates the onset of rheumatoid arthritis. Arthritis Rheumatol. 2010;62(2):383–91. https://doi.org/10.1002/art27186.
44. Marrosu MG, Coco E, Lai M, et al. Patients with multiple sclerosis and risk of type 1 diabetes mellitus in Sardinia: a cohort study. Lancet. 2002;359(9316):1461–5. https://doi.org/10.1016/S0140-6736(02)08431-3.
45. Kinslow JD, Blum LK, Deane KD, et al. Elevated IgA plasmablast levels in subject at risk of developing rheumatoid arthritis. Arthritis Rheumatol. 2016;68(10):2372–83. https://doi.org/10.1002/art39771.
46. Pescovitz MD, Greenbaum CJ, Krause-Steinrauf H, et al. Rituximab, B-lymphocyte depletion and preservation of beta-cell function. N Engl J Med. 2009;361(22):2143–52. https://doi.org/10.1056/NEJMMoa0904452.
47. Bhattacharya J, Pappas K, Toz B, et al. Serologic features of cohorts with variable genetic risk for systemic lupus erythematosus. Mol Med. 2018;24(1):24. https://doi.org/10.1186/s10020-018-0019-4.
48. Rowe P, Wasserfall C, Crocker B, et al. Increased complement activation in human type 1diabetes pancreata. Diabetes Care. 2013;36(11):3815–7. https://doi.org/10.2337/dc13-0203.
49. Rogers MAM, Wei MY, Kim C, et al. Sex differences in autoimmune multimorbidity in type 1 diabetes mellitus and the risk of cardiovascular and renal disease: a longitudinal study in the United States, 2001–2017. J Women Health. 2020;29(4):465–602. https://doi.org/10.1089/jwh.2019.7935.
50. Cardinez NC, Lovblom LE, Orszag A, et al. The prevalence of autoimmune diseases in longstanding diabetes: results from the Canadian study of longevity in adults with type 1 diabetes. Can J Diabetes. 2021;45(6):512–8. https://doi.org/10.1016/j.jcjd.2020.10.010.
51. Bao YK, Weide LG, Ganesan VC, et al. High prevalence of comorbid autoimmune diseases in adults with type 1 diabetes from the HealthFacts database. J Diabetes. 2019;11(4):273–9. https://doi.org/10.1111/1753-0407.12856.
52. Michitsuji T, Horai Y, Sako A, et al. A case of mixed connective tissue disease positive for proteinase 2 antineutrophil cytoplasmic antibody in a patient with slowly progressive type1 diabetes mellitus and chronic thyroiditis. Jpn J Clin Immunol. 2017;40(6):467–70.
53. Schlaffke J, et al. Assessment of antineutrophil-cytoplasmic autoantibodies (ANCA) in type 1 diabetic patients (in polish). Pol Arch Med Wewn. 2005;113:552–6.
54. Sladek R. The many faces of diabetes: addressing heterogeneity of a complex disease. Lancet Diabetes Endocrinol. 2018;6:348–9. https://doi.org/10.1016/S2213-8587(18)30070-6.
55. Hotamisligil GS. Inflammation, metaflammation and immunometabolic disorders. Nature. 2017;543:177–85. https://doi.org/10.1038/nature21363.
56. Obata Y, Yamada Y, Takahi Y, et al. Realtionship between serum adiponectin levels and age in healthy subjects and patients with type 2 diabetes. Clin Endocrinol. 2013;79:204–10.
57. Choi HM, Doss HM, Kim KS. Multifaceted physiological roles of adiponectin in inflammation and diseases. Int J Mol Sci. 2020;21:1219. https://doi.org/10.3390/ijms21041219.
58. Wolf AM, Wolf D, Rumpold H, et al. Adiponectin induces the anti-inflammatory cytokines IL-10 and IL-1RA in human leucocytes. Biochem Biophys Res Commun. 2004;323:630–5.
59. Luo Y, Liu M. Adiponectin: a versatile player of innate immunity. J Mol Cell Biol. 2016;8:120–8.
60. Chedid P, Hurtado-Nedelec M, Marion-Gaber B, et al. Adiponectin and its globular fragment differentially modulate the oxidative burst of primary human phagocytes. Am J Pathol. 2012;180:682–92.
61. Otero M, Logo R, Gomez R, et al. Changes in plasma levels of fat-derived hormones adiponectin, leptin, resistin and visfatin in patients with rheumatoid arthritis. Ann Rheum Dis. 2006;65:1198–201.

62. Kontny E, Janicka I, Skalska U, et al. The effect of multicentric adiponectin isoforms and leptin on the function of rheumatoid fibroblast-like synoviocytes. Scand J Rheumatol. 2015;44:363–8.
63. Skalska U, Kontny E. Adiponectin isoforms and leptin impact on rheumatoid adipose mesenchymal stem cells function. Stem Cell Int. 2016;2016:6532860., 6 pages. https://doi.org/10.1155/2016/6532860.
64. Li BT, Zhang FZ, Xu TS, et al. Increasing production of matrix metalloproteinases, tumor necrosis factor-α, vascular endothelial growth factor and prostaglandin E2 in rheumatoid arthritis synovial fibroblasts by different adiponectin isoforms in a concentration-dependent manner. Cell Mol Biol. 2015;61:27–32.
65. Cao H. Adipocytokines in obesity and metabolic disease. J Endocrinol. 2014;220:T47–59.
66. van Greevenbroek MMJ, Schalkwijk CG, Stenhouwer CDA. Obesity-associated low-grade inflammation an type 2 diabetes mellitus: causes and consequences. Neth J Med. 2013;71:174–87.
67. Giacomelli R, Ruscitti P, Alvaro S, et al. IL-1β at the crossroad between rheumatoid arthritis and type 2 diabetes: may we kill two birds with one stone? Expert Rev Clin Immunol. 2016;12:849. https://doi.org/10.1586/1744666x.2016.1168293.
68. Martinon F, Mayor A, Tschopp J. The inflammasomes: guardians of the body. Annu Rev Immunol. 2009;27:229–65.
69. van den Berg WB, Bresnihan B. Pathogenesis of joint damage in rheumatoid arthritis: evidence of a dominant role for interleukin-1. Baillieres Best Prect Res Clin Rheumatol. 1999;13:577–97.
70. Gravallese EM. Bone destruction in arthritis. Ann Rheum Dis. 2002;61:ii84–6.
71. Johnson LL, Dyer R, Hupe DJ. Matrix metalloproteinases. Curr Opin Chem Biol. 1998;2:466–71.
72. Zhou R, Tardivel A, Thorens B, et al. Thioredoxin-interacting protein links oxidative stress to inflammasome activation. Nat Immunol. 2010;11(2):136–40. https://doi.org/10.1038/ni.1831.
73. Boni-Schnetzler M, Boller S, Debray S, et al. Free fatty acids induce a proinflammatory response in islets Vis the abundantly expressed interleukin-1 receptor I. Endocrinology. 2009;150:5218–29.
74. Boni-Schnetzler M, Thorne J, Parnaud G, et al. Increased interleukin (IL)-1beta messenger ribonucleic acid expression in beta-cells of individuals with type 2 diabetes and regulation of IL-1beta in human islets by glucose and autostimulation. J Clin Endocrinol Metab. 2008;93:4065–74.
75. Masters SL, Dunne A, Subramanian SL, et al. Activation of the NLRP3 inflammasome by islet amyloid polypeptide provides a mechanism for enhanced IL-1beta in type 2 diabetes. Nat Immunol. 2010;11:897–904.
76. Banaei-Bouchareb L, Peuchmaur M, Czernichow P, et al. A transient microenvironment loaded mainly with macrophages in the early developing human pancreas. J Endocrinol. 2006;188:467–80.
77. Eguchi K, Manabe I. Macrophages and islet inflammation in type 2 diabetes. Diabetes Obes Metab. 2013;15:152–8.
78. Akira S, Misawa T, Satoh T, et al. Macrophages control innate inflammation. Diabetes Obes Metab. 2013;15:10–8.
79. Lee HM, Kim JJ, Kim HJ, et al. Upregulated NLRP3 inflammasome activation in patients with type 2 diabetes. Diabetes. 2013;62(1):194–204.
80. Stegenga ME, van der Crabben SN, Blumer RM, et al. Hyperglycemia enhances coagulation and reduces neutrophil degranulation, whereas hyperinsulinemia inhibits fibrinolysis during human endotoxinemia. Blood. 2008;112:82–9.
81. Wierusz-Wysocka B, Wysocki H, Wykretowicz A, et al. The influence of increasing glucose concentration on selected functions of polymorphonuclear neutrophils. Acta Diabetol Lat. 1998;25:283–8.

82. Saiepour D, Sehlin J, Oldenborg PA. Hyperglycemia-induced protein kinase C activation inhibits phagocytosis of C3b- and immunoglobulin G-opsonised yeast particles in normal human neutrophils. Exp Diabesity Res. 2003;4:125–32.
83. Mauriello CT, Hair PS, Rohn RD, et al. Hyperglycemia inhibits complement-mediated immunological control of S. aureus in a rat model of peritonitis. J Diabetes Res. 2014;2014(1):762051.
84. Jafar N, Edriss H, Nugent K. The effect of short-term hyperglycemia on innate immune system. Am J Med Scu. 2016;351:201–11.
85. Tentolouris A, Thanopoulou A, Tentoluris N, et al. Low prevalence of rheumatoid arthritis among patients with pre-existing type 2 diabetes mellitus. Ann Transl Med. 2018;6(20):399.
86. Abugharbyeh A, Khuder S, Kahaleh B. Decreased prevalence of autoimmune connective tissue diseases in type 1 and type 2 diabetes. Arthritis Rheumatol. 2022;74(Suppl. 9) https://acrabstracts.org/abstract/decreased-prevalence-of-autoimmune-connective-tissue-diseases-in-type-1-and-type-2-diabetes/. Accessed January3, 2024
87. Inamo J, Kochi Y, Takeuchi T. Is type 2 diabetes mellitus an inverse risk factor dor the development of rheumatoid arthsitis? J Hum Genet. 2021;66(2):219–23. https://doi.org/10.1038/s10038-020-00837-2. Epub 2020 Sep 8. PMID:32901113
88. Burgess S, Smith GD, Davies NM, et al. Guidelines for performing Mendelian randomization investigations. Wellcome Open Res. 2019;4:186.
89. Zemedikun DT, Gokhale K, Chandan JS, et al. Type 2 diabetes mellitus, glycaemic control, associated therapies and risk of rheumatoid arthritis: a retrospective cohort study. Rheumatology. 2021;60:5567–75. https://doi.org/10.1093/rheumatology/keab148.
90. Yang X, Xu Z, Zhang C, et al. Metformin, beyond an insulin asnsitizer, targeting heart and pancreatic β cells. Biochem Biophys Acta: Mol Basis Dis. 2017;1863(8):1984–90.
91. Ursini F, Russo E, Pellino G, et al. Metformin and autoimmunity: a "new deal" of an old drug. Front Immunol. 2018;9:1236. https://doi.org/10.3389/fimmu.2018.01236.
92. Wang C-Y, Lai J-n, Liu C-H, et al. Metformin use was associated with reduced risk of incidental Sjogren's syndrome in patients with type 2 diabetes: a population-based cohort study. Front Med. 2021;8:796615. https://doi.org/10.3389/fmed.2021.796615.
93. Sun Y, Tian T, Gao J, et al. Metformin ameliorates the development of experimental autoimmune encephalomyelitis by regulating T helper 17 and regulatory T cells in mice. J Neuroimmunol. 2016;292:58–67. https://doi.org/10.1016/j.neuroim.2016.01.014.
94. Duan W, Ding Y, Yu X, et al. Metformin mitigates autoimmune insulitis by inhibiting Th1 and Th17 response while promoting Treg production. Am J Transl Res. 2019;11:2393–402.
95. Tseng C-C, Chang S-j, Tsa W-C, et al. Reduced incidence of type 1 diabetes and type 2 diabetes in systemic sclerosis: a nationwide cohort study. Joint Bone Spine. 2016;83:307–13.
96. Battaglia D, Bellia M, Serafino-Agrusa L, et al. Physical capacity in performing daily activities is reduced in scleroderma patients with early lung involvement. Clin Respir J. 2015;11:36–42. https://doi.org/10.1111/crj.12299.
97. Morelli S, Ferri C, Di Francesco L, et al. Plasma endothelin-1 levels in patients with systemic sclerosis: influence of pulmonary or systemic hypetension. Ann Rheum Dis. 1995;54:730–4.
98. Kotyla PJ, Gozdzik J, Lewicki M, et al. Serum lipid profile I patients with systemic sclerosis: relationship to the thyreometabolic state. Rheumatol Int. 2006;26:583–4.
99. Lee SW, Kim BK, Park JY, et al. Disease duration and Medsger's severity score are associated with significant liver fibrosis in patients with systemic sclerosis. Clin Exp Rheumatol. 2015;33(91):S68074.
100. Changani KK, Jalan R, Cox IJ, et al. Evidence for altered hepatic gluconeogenesis in patients with cirrhosis using in vivo 31-phosphorus magnetic resonance spectroscopy. Gut. 2021;49:557–64.
101. Ursini F, et al. Retrospective analysis of type 2 diabetes prevalence in a systemic sclerosis cohort from southern Italy: Commnet on "reduced incidence of type 1 diabetes and type 2 diabetes in systemic sclerosis: a nationwide cohort study" by Tseng et al. Joint Bone Spine. 2016;83:397–13.

102. Petersen MC, Graves JM, Yao T, et al. Insulin receptor antibody -mediated hypoglycemia in a woman with mixed connective tissue disease. J Endocr Soc. 2022;6(1):bvab182. https://doi.org/10.1210/jendso/bvab182.
103. Malek R, Chong AY, Lupsa BC, et al. Treatment of type B insulin resistance: a novel approach to reduce insulin receptor autoantibodies. J Clin Endocrinol Metab. 2010;95(8):3641–7.
104. Lupsa BC, Chong AY, Cochran EK, et al. Autoimmune forms of hypoglycemia. Medicine (Baltimore). 2009;88(3):141–53.
105. Arioglu E, Andewelt A, Diabo C, et al. Clincal course of the sybdrome of autoantibodies to the insulin receptor (type B insulin resistance): a 28-year perspective. Medicine (Baltimore). 2002;81(2):87–100.
106. Foretz M, Guigas B, Viollet B. Understanding the glucoregulatory mechanisms of metformin in type 2 diabetes mellitus. Nat Rev Endocrinol. 2019;15:569–89.
107. Kim J-W, Choe J-Y, Park S-H. Metformin and its therapeutic applications in autoimmune inflammatory rheumatic diseases. Korean J Intern Med. 2022;37:13–26. https://doi.org/10.3904/kjim.2021.363.
108. Zhou G, Myers R, Li Y, eta la. Role of AMP-activated protein kinas in mechanism of metformin action. J Clin Invest. 2001;108:1167–74.
109. Shaw RJ, Lamia KA, Vasquez D, et al. The kinase LKB1 mediates glucose homeostasis in liver and therapeutic effects of metformin. Science. 2005;310:1642–6.
110. Dlegoffe GM, Kole TP, Aheng Y, et al. The mTOR kinase differentially regulates effector and regulatory T cell lineage commitment. Immunity. 2009;30:832–44.
111. Ma CS, Avery DT, Chan A, et al. Functional STAT3 deficiency compromises the generator of human T follicular helper cells. Blood. 2012;119:3997–4008.
112. Avery DT, Deenick EK, Ma CS, et al. B-cell intrinsic signaling through IL-21 receptor and STAT3 is required for establishing long-lived antibody response in humans. J Exp Med. 2010;207:155–72.
113. Deenick EK, Avery DT, Chan A, et al. Naïve and memory human B cells have distinct requirements for STAT3 activation to differentiate into antibody-secreting plasma cells. J Exp Med. 2013;210(12):2739–53.
114. You S, Koh JH, Leng L, et al. The tumor-like phenotype of rheumatoid synovium: molecular profiling and prospects for precision medicine. Arthritis Rheumatol. 2018;70:637–52.
115. Chen K, Lin ZW, He SM, et al. Metformin inhibits the proliferation of rheumatoid arthritis fibroblast-like synoviocytes through IGF-IR/PI3K/AKT/m-TOR pathway. Biomed Pharmacother. 2019;115:108875.
116. Chen Y, Qiu F, Yu B, et al. Metformin, an AMPK activator, inhibits activation of FLSs but promotes HAPLN1 secretion. Mol Ther Methods Clin Dev. 2020;17:1202–14.
117. Jung SM, Kim KW, Yang CW, et al. Cytokine-mediated bone destruction in rheumatoid arthritis. J Immunol Res. 2014;2014(1):263625.
118. Kim HR, Kim KW, Kim BM, et al. N-acetyl-l-cysteine controls osteoclastogenesis through regulating Th17 differentiation and RANKL production in rheumatoid arthritis. Korean J Internal Med. 2019;34(1):210.
119. Lu CH, Chung CH, Lee CH, et al. Combination of COX-2 inhibitor and metformin attenuates rate of admission in patients with rheumatoid arthritis and diabetes in Taiwan. Medicine (Baltimore). 2019;98:e17371.
120. Abdallah MS, Alarfaj SJ, Saif DS, et al. The AMPK modulator metformin and the onset of rheumatoid arthritis: a population-based cohort study. Scand J Rheumatol. 2020;49:173–80.
121. Wang H, Li T, Chen S, et al. Neutrophil extracellular trap mitochondrial DNA and its autoantibody in systemic lupus erythematosus and a proof-of-concept trial of metformin. Arthritis Rheumatol. 2015;67:3190–200.
122. Sun F, Geng S, Wang H, et al. Effects of metformin on disease flares in patients with systemic lupus erythematosus: post hoc analyses from two randomized trials. Lupus Sci Med. 2020;7:e000429.

Chapter 25
Acne and Rosacea

Winston W. Liu, Choon Fong Liew, and Hazel H. Oon

Abstract Acne and rosacea are common inflammatory skin conditions that are associated with systemic inflammation and metabolic abnormalities. Here, we review the evidence for a connection between diabetes, acne, and rosacea. Acne has been linked to type 2 diabetes and insulin resistance. The pathophysiologic basis of this connection involves hyperandrogenism and activation of the mTORC1/FoxO1 pathway. However, rosacea has a less clear link to insulin resistance. While available evidence is insufficient to recommend routine screening of all acne and rosacea patients for diabetes, management of glucose intolerance shows promise in improving the severity of skin disease. Nevertheless, future studies involving larger cohorts and randomized controlled trials need to be conducted to clarify the role of diabetes in acne and rosacea.

25.1 Acne and Insulin Resistance

Acne vulgaris is a chronic inflammatory disease of the pilosebaceous unit that affects approximately 9.4% of people worldwide [1]. The disease is classically thought to be driven by four processes: (1) increased sebum production secondary to androgen stimulation, (2) comedonal formation due to changes in follicular

W. W. Liu
Duke University School of Medicine, Durham, NC, USA
e-mail: winston.w.liu@duke.edu

C. F. Liew
Specialist Care Group, Diabetes and Endocrinology Centre, Mount Elizabeth Medical Centre, Singapore, Singapore
e-mail: liew_stanley@specialistcaregroup.com

H. H. Oon (✉)
National Skin Centre and Skin Research Institute of Singapore, Singapore, Singapore

Yong Loo Lin School of Medicine, National University of Singapore, Singapore, Singapore
e-mail: derm@hazeloon.com

K. Fritz, G.-S. Tiplica (eds.), *Cutaneous Manifestations in Diabetes*,
https://doi.org/10.1007/978-3-031-65300-1_25

keratinization, (3) inflammatory signals in the pilosebaceous unit, and (4) follicular colonization by *Cutibacterium acnes* [2]. Patients present with comedones, papules, pustules, nodules, or cysts, often with postinflammatory erythema, hyperpigmentation, and scarring as sequelae. Lesions most commonly affect the face, neck, and trunk. Acne typically arises during the late teenage years, and mild cases often resolve before 25, though adult acne can present as new-onset acne at age 25 or beyond, persist from adolescent acne, or recur after a few years of recrudescence during adolescence (recidivant acne) [3, 4]. Though acne can cause pain and pruritus, a large toll of the disease is psychological, and it has been linked to numerous mood and anxiety disorders. Management is according to severity grading, with topical agents, systemic antibiotics, hormonal therapies, and vitamin A derivatives such as isotretinoin.

The relationship between diabetes and acne was first raised by the striking observation that though acne is quite common in westernized societies, its prevalence in civilizations with Paleolithic diets, lower in sugar and dairy, is negligible [5]. Subsequent epidemiologic studies have shown increased prevalence of insulin resistance in acne patients. A frequent marker of insulin resistance used in these studies is the Homeostatic Model Assessment for Insulin Resistance (HOMA-IR) score, which is the product of the fasting blood glucose and insulin level. HOMA-IR has been shown to be elevated in acne patients through case-control studies from the Americas, Europe, and Asia [6–10]. There have been some discrepancies with smaller studies showing no change in HOMA-IR or fasting blood glucose [11]. Moreover, a correlation between HOMA-IR and acne severity has also not been demonstrated [8, 12] though studies restricted to patients with severe acne have larger effect sizes when comparing HOMA-IR [7, 9]. The association between acne and insulin resistance as measured by hemoglobin A1c (HbA1c) has also been evaluated in one case-control study of 549 acne patients and 549 controls at one center in the USA. While mean HbA1c demonstrated a statistically significant increase, the effect size was modest (5.41% vs. 5.3%), though a regression did demonstrate a significant association after accounting for covariates including body mass index (BMI) [13]. Further studies using larger cohorts are needed to confirm these results and to help clarify the relationship between acne severity and insulin resistance.

Nevertheless, the insulin resistance that underlies type 2 diabetes is now recognized as a key contributor to the development of acne vulgaris [14]. Indeed, acne is recognized as a component of many systemic syndromes that involve insulin resistance such as seborrhea-acne-hirsutism-androgenetic alopecia (SAHA), hyperandrogenism-insulin resistance-acanthosis nigricans (HAIR-AN), and polycystic ovarian syndrome (PCOS) [15]. Nearly 70% of patients with PCOS are reported to have acne, and the prevalence of PCOS in patients with moderate to severe acne is estimated to be 37% [4, 16, 17]. In addition, a new subtype of acne termed "insulin resistance-associated acne" has also recently been proposed and is thought to be a part of the metabolic syndrome [18]. Specific differences in presentation or prognosis for acne patients with diabetes remain to be studied. While patients with severe acne may be screened for early signs of diabetes, current guidelines do not support routine endocrinologic testing [19]. However, patients who have other signs of metabolic dysfunction or hyperandrogenism should undergo further work-up.

25.2 Mechanisms Linking Diabetes and Acne

Patients with non-insulin-dependent diabetes classically develop hyperinsulinemia and insulin resistance. Increased insulin signaling can then lead to the development of acne through two mechanisms: (1) mechanistic target of rapamycin complex 1 (mTORC1)/forkhead box transcription factor O1 (FoxO1) signaling and (2) hyperandrogenism (Fig. 25.1).

mTOR is a highly conserved serine-threonine kinase that can associate with several other proteins in the cytoplasm to form mTORC1. It is reciprocally controlled by FoxO1, a transcription factor that is shuttled into and out of the nucleus in response to energy state. mTORC1 responds to increased energy availability (i.e., nutrients, insulin, IGF-1, and a high ATP/AMP ratio) by shifting cellular processes toward anabolism and the synthesis of proteins, lipids, and nucleotides [20]. In contrast, FoxO1 is active in the nucleus during low-energy states, where it attenuates androgen signaling, regulates sebaceous lipogenesis, and antagonizes mTORC1 [21]. Thus, in hyperinsulinemic states, FoxO1 is inactivated and mTORC1 is activated.

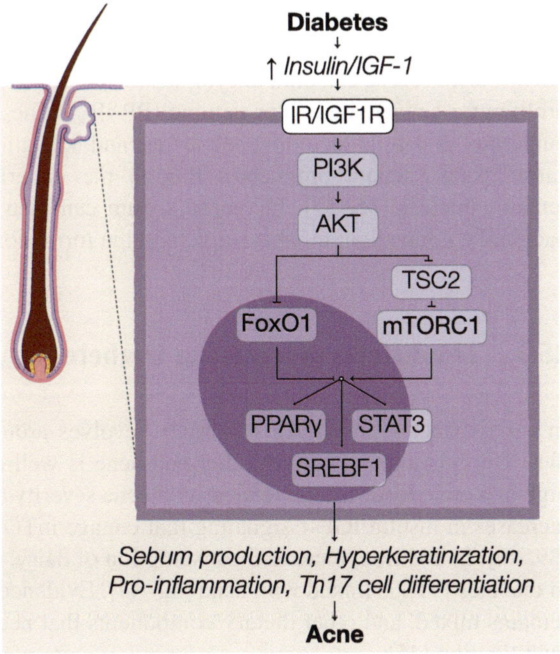

Fig. 25.1 Pathophysiological connection between diabetes and acne

In diabetes, mTORC1/FoxO1 signaling can be triggered via activation of both the insulin receptor (IR) and the IGF-1 receptor (IGF-1R), which are both expressed on keratinocytes and sebocytes [22]. Hyperinsulinemia is thought to lead to IGF-1R activation via reduction in IGF-1-binding globulins, which increases IGF-1 availability [23]. Increased insulin is also theorized to fully saturate epithelial IR, allowing excess insulin to cross-react with IGF-1R [24]. In either case, acne patients show elevated IR/IGF-1R signaling, inhibition of FoxO1, and activation of mTORC1 [25, 26]. Notably, patients with congenital IGF-1 absence have reduced rates of both diabetes and acne [27].

In vitro, IR/IGF-1R has been shown to activate the phosphoinositide 3-kinase (PI3K)/Akt pathway, which directly extrudes FoxO1 from the nucleus and disinhibits mTORC1 via TSC2. mTORC1 can increase expression of sterol response element-binding protein-1 (SREBP-1), a key transcription factor in lipogenesis, and acetyl CoA carboxylase, the rate-limiting step of fatty acid synthesis, both contributory to sebocyte overproduction [28, 29]. Interestingly, these lipid regulatory factors also can contribute to the Th17 cell inflammatory response seen in acne [30, 31]. Moreover, fatty acid overproduction by sebocytes allows for *C. acnes* biofilm formation [14]. FoxO1 inactivation promotes the transcription of inflammatory factors, peroxisome proliferator-activated receptor gamma (PPARɣ), and STAT3, which can contribute to inflammation, keratinocyte proliferation, and follicular hyperkeratinization [32, 33]. Given mTORC1's central role in metabolic syndrome, acne has been suggested to be a cutaneous manifestation of metabolic syndrome [14].

Hyperandrogenism has been classically associated with acne development [34]. In diabetes, insulin can act on ovarian and adrenal cells to secrete androgens as well as on hepatic cells to lower sex hormone-binding globulin production, which together increase androgen levels [35]. These elevated levels of testosterone and dihydrotestosterone can bind to cytoplasmic androgen receptors and the peroxisome proliferator-activated receptor gamma (PPARɣ). These receptors are expressed by numerous skin cells including sebocytes, and activation of sebocytes is thought to cause excess sebum production though the underlying intracellular signaling remains unclear [36, 37]. Increased sebum can then lead to hyperkeratinization, bacterial colonization, inflammation, and the formation of acne.

25.3 The Effects of Treating Diabetes on Acne

In early diabetes, management largely revolves around weight management and diet. The relationship between diet and acne is well-established [38]. Foods with high glycemic loads are correlated with acne severity and postulated to cause acute increases in insulin/IGF-1 signaling that engage mTORC1-dependent mechanisms [39, 40]. In addition, increased consumption of dairy, though potentially protective in diabetes [41], is linked with acne [42–44]. Evidence for the role of saturated fats remains mixed, and other dietary components that need to be monitored are under investigation [45].

Several small, randomized, controlled trials have been completed to assess the impact of a low glycemic load dietary intervention. When compared to high glycemic loads, patients demonstrated decreased numbers of lesions on the face after 10–12 weeks of diet [46–48], but not 2 weeks [49]. Patients in the trials also showed a significant reduction in weight and increases in IGF-1-binding protein. While variations in the specific foods and patient populations preclude specific recommendations, patients with diabetes and acne should be counseled to reduce dietary glycemic load.

Pharmacologic management of diabetes often begins with the biguanide metformin. Metformin activates the AMP-activated protein kinase (AMPK) pathway, which can inhibit mTORC1 [50]. In female PCOS patients, metformin is also known to reduce elevated IGF-1 and androgen levels, which also contribute to acne pathogenesis [51]. In PCOS, metformin has been shown to significantly reduce acne severity [52, 53]. Surprisingly, in a small study of PCOS patients with intractable acne, acne severity was more improved following metformin treatment as compared to isotretinoin [54].

In non-PCOS patients, small, randomized studies have shown improvement in acne severity with metformin when used as an adjunct to standard treatment [55–57]. When compared to doxycycline in a small randomized, controlled trial, metformin showed no significant difference [58]. A new topical metformin formulation has recently been shown to improve acne in a split-face, placebo-controlled trial [59]. Taken together, these results suggest that metformin may have a beneficial effect in treating acne. Further larger randomized controlled trials will be needed to substantiate these findings. A small randomized trial involving the thiazolidinedione pioglitazone demonstrated a qualitative reduction in the prevalence of acne in PCOS patients [60]. However, the effects of other antidiabetic medications such as GLP-1 analogues on acne remain to be studied. Moreover, whether improvement in diabetes management, independent of weight loss, improves acne remains an open question.

25.4 Rosacea and Diabetes

Rosacea is a chronic inflammatory disease that affects approximately 5.4% of people worldwide, with women more commonly affected starting in the third to fifth decade of life [61]. Patients typically present with persistent erythema, phymatous changes (i.e., skin thickening due to fibrosis or sebaceous hyperplasia), papules, pustules, and telangiectasias on the face. Patients will sometimes also report burning, stinging, edema, or a dry sensation [62]. Up to 75% of patients have involvement of the eyes, termed ocular rosacea. While the disease was once classified into subtypes, the recent ROSacea COnsensus (ROSCO) group has led the transition to a phenotypic approach [63]. The pathophysiologic basis of the disease remains unknown but is thought to involve genetic factors, dysregulated immune activation, neurovascular dysfunction, and microbes such as *Demodex folliculorum* [64].

Management involves general skin care as well as symptomatic management using alpha-adrenergic modulators, ivermectin cream, antibiotics, isotretinoin, as well as procedures including intense pulsed light, laser, and resections [63]. Flares are often triggered by sunlight, spicy foods, heat, stress, smoking, or alcohol, and patients are counseled to avoid triggers.

A link between rosacea and diabetes was raised in a case-control study of 53,927 patients, and controls from a UK-based database showed a significant reduction in rosacea risk with advanced diabetes and a negative correlation with HbA1c [65]. Subsequent studies have had mixed results, with the majority showing no relationship between diabetes and rosacea including several meta-analyses [66–69]. However, several studies using Korean cohorts have shown a positive association between taking diabetic medications and a diagnosis of diabetes mellitus with rosacea [70–72]. Interestingly, diabetic patients with rosacea from Taiwan have been shown to have increased risks of diabetic eye manifestations including glaucoma on medical treatment, cataract surgery, diabetic macular edema, and dry eyes, with subdistribution hazard ratio (SHR) of 1.11, 1.13, 1.31, and 1.55, respectively. This subset of patients also had an increased risk of other comorbidities including psoriasis, irritable bowel syndrome, anxiety, and depression [73]. Whether these findings represent a distinct subset of rosacea patients or rather reflect a subpopulation with poor underlying health status and sociocultural determinants remains to be carefully delineated.

Despite a lack of detected associations with diabetes, rosacea has been shown to be associated with several cardiometabolic risk factors including hyperlipidemia, hypercholesterolemia, and an elevated HOMA-IR [67, 69, 74–76]. However, an association with diagnosed metabolic syndrome has more mixed results [68, 69, 74, 77]. This is likely a function of heterogeneity in the criteria used to diagnose metabolic syndrome. At least four different criteria have been raised including the NCEP-ATP III, the International Diabetes Foundation, the World Health Organization, and the European Group for the Study of Insulin Resistance (Table 25.1). Indeed, such heterogeneity has led to unevenness when associating metabolic syndrome with other cutaneous diseases such as psoriasis [78]. Future meta-analyses will need to consider standardized criteria for diagnosis to properly assess the relationship between metabolic syndrome and rosacea.

Interestingly, in a case-control study involving 6759 rosacea patients and 33,795 matched controls from Denmark, an association between rosacea and autoimmune diseases was detected. Patients with rosacea were found to have a 2.59 odds ratio (OR) for type 1 diabetes [79]. Indeed, a genome-wide association study of European patients showed that rosacea patients were significantly more likely to have single-nucleotide polymorphisms that have been associated with type 1 diabetes [80]. Further studies in other cohorts and populations will be needed to confirm these observations.

In a retrospective, observational, single-center study at the Mount Sinai Health System network, 12,470 rosacea cases were propensity score-matched to controls based on 13 characteristics. Arterial (OR, 2.96), hypertensive (OR, 1.43), and cerebrovascular diseases (OR, 1.19) were significantly higher compared to controls

Table 25.1 Criteria for metabolic syndrome

	IDF	AHA	NCEP ATP III	WHO
	Number 1 + ≥2 other criteria	≥3 criteria	≥3 criteria	Number 2 + ≥2 other criteria
1.	Waist circumference: ≥94 cm (M); ≥80 cm (F)	Waist circumference: ≥102 cm (M); ≥89 cm (F)		Waist/hip ratio: >0.90 (M), >0.85 (F); or BMI > 30 kg/m^2
2.	Fasting glucose ≥100 mg/dL or Rx		Fasting glucose ≥110 mg/dL or Rx	Glucose intolerance, IGT, diabetes, and/or other evidence of IR
3.	TG ≥ 150 mg/dL or Rx			TG ≥ 150 mg/dL or HDL-C: <35 mg/dL (M); <39 mg/dL (F)
4.	HDL-C: <40 mg/dL (M), <50 mg/dL (F) or Rx			
5.	≥130/85 mmHg or Rx			≥140/90 mmHg

AHA American Heart Association, *WHO* World Health Organization, *NCEP ATP III* National Cholesterol Education Program, *IDF* International Diabetes Foundation

[81]. Systemic inflammatory markers of raised ESR ≥10 mm/h and CRP levels ≥10 mg/L were more prevalent in the rosacea participants (OR 1.90 and 1.32, respectively), suggesting inflammation beyond the skin as part of a systemic inflammatory process.

The antidiabetic medication metformin has also been proposed as a treatment for rosacea, though no trials have been performed to assess its efficacy [82]. Metformin is theorized to have antiangiogenic, anti-fibrotic, and anti-inflammatory effects that may benefit patients with rosacea [83]. Metformin has also been reported to cause a rosacea-like facial rash [84]. Randomized clinical trials assessing the efficacy of metformin for rosacea will be needed to understand its potential utility.

25.5 Conclusions

Acne and rosacea are common inflammatory skin conditions that have been associated with systemic inflammation and metabolic abnormalities. While diabetes and insulin resistance are linked to acne via activation of the mTORC1/FoxO1 pathway, a pathophysiologic and epidemiologic association with rosacea is less clear. However, rosacea has been associated with type 1 diabetes. Regardless, acne patients with PCOS will benefit for screening for diabetes and other metabolic comorbidities. Available evidence is insufficient to recommend routine screening of all acne and rosacea patients. Management of any glucose intolerance may also improve acne and rosacea. Interventions involving low glycemic diet improve acne severity, and pharmacologic intervention with metformin has been shown to improve acne and has been postulated to improve rosacea. The effect of newer, more potent agents for glycemic control such as dipeptidyl peptidase-4 inhibitors, sodium glucose cotransporter-2 inhibitors, and glucagon-like peptide-1 agonists and their impact on acne and rosacea subtypes remain to be explored.

References

1. Hay RJ, Johns NE, Williams HC, Bolliger IW, Dellavalle RP, Margolis DJ, Marks R, Naldi L, Weinstock MA, Wulf SK. The global burden of skin disease in 2010: an analysis of the prevalence and impact of skin conditions. J Invest Dermatol. 2014;134:1527–34.
2. Zaenglein AL. Acne vulgaris. N Engl J Med. 2018;379:1343–52.
3. Dréno B, Thiboutot D, Layton AM, Berson D, Perez M, Kang S, the Global Alliance to Improve Outcomes in Acne. Large-scale international study enhances understanding of an emerging acne population: adult females. Acad Dermatol Venereol. 2015;29:1096–106.
4. Carmina E, Dreno B, Lucky WA, Agak WG, Dokras A, Kim JJ, Lobo RA, Ramezani Tehrani F, Dumesic D. Female adult acne and androgen excess: a report from the multidisciplinary androgen excess and PCOS committee. J Endocr Soc. 2022;6:bvac003.
5. Cordain L, Lindeberg S, Hurtado M, Hill K, Eaton SB, Brand-Miller J. Acne vulgaris: a disease of Western civilization. Arch Dermatol. 2002;138:1584–90.

6. Del Prete M, Mauriello MC, Faggiano A, Di Somma C, Monfrecola G, Fabbrocini G, Colao A. Insulin resistance and acne: a new risk factor for men? Endocrine. 2012;42:555–60.
7. Emiroğlu N, Cengiz FP, Kemeriz F. Insulin resistance in severe acne vulgaris. Adv Dermatol Allergol/Postępy Dermatol Alergol. 2015;32:281–5.
8. Nagpal M, De D, Handa S, Pal A, Sachdeva N. Insulin resistance and metabolic syndrome in young men with acne. JAMA Dermatol. 2016;152:399–404.
9. Singh M, Shri D. Insulin resistance in moderate to severe acne vulgaris. Indian J Dermatol. 2022;67:205.
10. Carneiro ACA, De Carvalho JF, De Sá DC, Rodrigues CEM. Prevalence of metabolic syndrome and insulin resistance in adult patients with acne: association with traditional cardiovascular risk factors and acne severity. Metab Syndr Relat Disord. 2023;21:109–14.
11. Balta I, Ekiz O, Ozuguz P, Ustun I, Karaca S, Dogruk Kacar S, Eksioglu M. Insulin resistance in patients with post-adolescent acne. Int J Dermatol. 2015;54:662–6.
12. Sadowska-Przytocka A, Gruszczyńska M, Ostałowska A, Antosik P, Czarnecka-Operacz M, Adamski Z, Łącka K. Insulin resistance in the course of acne–literature review. Adv Dermatol Allergol/Postępy Dermatol Alergol. 2022;39:231–8.
13. Gu L, Ong M, Fan SX, Christos P, Lipner SR. Not just skin deep: association of acne with elevated hemoglobin A1c levels in a retrospective case-control study of 1098 patients at an academic center. J Cosmetic Dermatol. 2023;22:3520–1.
14. Melnik BC. Acne vulgaris: the metabolic syndrome of the pilosebaceous follicle. Clin Dermatol. 2018;36:29–40.
15. Chen W, Obermayer-Pietsch B, Hong J, et al. Acne-associated syndromes: models for better understanding of acne pathogenesis. Acad Dermatol Venereol. 2011;25:637–46.
16. Timpatanapong P, Rojanasakul A. Hormonal profiles and prevalence of polycystic ovary syndrome in women with acne. J Dermatol. 1997;24:223–9.
17. Borgia F, Cannavò S, Guarneri F, Cannavò SP, Vaccaro M, Guarneri B. Correlation between endocrinological parameters and acne severity in adult women. Acta Dermatovenereol Stockholm. 2004;84:201–4.
18. Kubba R. Insulin resistance associated acne. In: Suh DH, editor. Acne. Cham: Springer International Publishing; 2021. p. 95–110.
19. Reynolds RV, Yeung H, Cheng CE, Cook-Bolden F, Desai SR, Druby K, Freeman EE, Keri JE, Gold LFS, Tan JK. Guidelines of care for the management of acne vulgaris. J Am Acad Dermatol. 2024;90:1006.e1.
20. Ardestani A, Lupse B, Kido Y, Leibowitz G, Maedler K. mTORC1 signaling: a double-edged sword in diabetic β cells. Cell Metab. 2018;27:314–31.
21. Melnik BC, Zouboulis CC. Potential role of Fox O1 and m TORC 1 in the pathogenesis of Western diet-induced acne. Exp Dermatol. 2013;22:311–5.
22. Rudman SM, Philpott MP, Thomas GA, Kealey T. The role of IGF-I in human skin and its appendages: morphogen as well as mitogen? J Invest Dermatol. 1997;109:770–7.
23. Nam SY, Lee EJ, Kim KR, Cha BS, Song YD, Lim SK, Lee HC, Huh KB. Effect of obesity on total and free insulin-like growth factor (IGF)-1, and their relationship to IGF-binding protein (BP)-1, IGFBP-2, IGFBP-3, insulin, and growth hormone. Int J Obes (Lond). 1997;21:355–9.
24. Cruz PD Jr, Hud JA Jr. Excess insulin binding to insulin-like growth factor receptors: proposed mechanism for acanthosis nigricans. J Invest Dermatol. 1992;98:82S.
25. Monfrecola G, Lembo S, Caiazzo G, De Vita V, Di Caprio R, Balato A, Fabbrocini G. Mechanistic target of rapamycin (mTOR) expression is increased in acne patients' skin. Exp Dermatol. 2016;25:153–5.
26. Agamia NF, Abdallah DM, Sorour O, Mourad B, Younan DN. Skin expression of mammalian target of rapamycin and forkhead box transcription factor O1, and serum insulin-like growth factor-1 in patients with acne vulgaris and their relationship with diet. Br J Dermatol. 2016;174:1299–307.
27. Ben-Amitai D, Laron Z. Effect of insulin-like growth factor-1 deficiency or administration on the occurrence of acne. Acad Dermatol Venereol. 2011;25:950–4.

28. Smith TM, Cong Z, Gilliland KL, Clawson GA, Thiboutot DM. Insulin-like growth factor-1 induces lipid production in human SEB-1 sebocytes via sterol response element-binding protein-1. J Invest Dermatol. 2006;126:1226–32.
29. Smith TM, Gilliland K, Clawson GA, Thiboutot D. IGF-1 induces SREBP-1 expression and lipogenesis in SEB-1 sebocytes via activation of the phosphoinositide 3-kinase/Akt pathway. J Invest Dermatol. 2008;128:1286–93.
30. Kelhälä H-L, Palatsi R, Fyhrquist N, Lehtimäki S, Väyrynen JP, Kallioinen M, Kubin ME, Greco D, Tasanen K, Alenius H. IL-17/Th17 pathway is activated in acne lesions. PLoS One. 2014;9:e105238.
31. Angela M, Endo Y, Asou HK, Yamamoto T, Tumes DJ, Tokuyama H, Yokote K, Nakayama T. Fatty acid metabolic reprogramming via mTOR-mediated inductions of PPARγ directs early activation of T cells. Nat Commun. 2016;7:13683.
32. Kim H, Moon SY, Sohn MY, Lee WJ. Insulin-like growth factor-1 increases the expression of inflammatory biomarkers and sebum production in cultured sebocytes. Ann Dermatol. 2017;29:20–5.
33. Melnik BC. Acne transcriptomics: fundamentals of acne pathogenesis and isotretinoin treatment. Cells. 2023;12:2600.
34. Bloch B. Metabolism, endocrine glands and skindiseases, with special reference to acne vulgaris and xanthoma. Br J Dermatol. 1931;43:61–87.
35. Crave JC, Lejeune H, Brebant C, Baret C, Pugeat M. Differential effects of insulin and insulin-like growth factor I on the production of plasma steroid-binding globulins by human hepatoblastoma-derived (Hep G2) cells. J Clin Endocrinol Metabol. 1995;80:1283–9.
36. Arora MK, Yadav A, Saini V. Role of hormones in acne vulgaris. Clin Biochem. 2011;44:1035–40.
37. Del Rosso JQ, Kircik L. The cutaneous effects of androgens and androgen-mediated sebum production and their pathophysiologic and therapeutic importance in acne vulgaris. J Dermatol Treat. 2024;35:2298878.
38. Bowe WP, Joshi SS, Shalita AR. Diet and acne. J Am Acad Dermatol. 2010;63:124–41.
39. Melnik B. Dietary intervention in acne: attenuation of increased mTORC1 signaling promoted by Western diet. Dermatoendocrinol. 2012;4:20–32.
40. Burris J, Rietkerk W, Shikany JM, Woolf K. Differences in dietary glycemic load and hormones in New York city adults with no and moderate/severe acne. J Acad Nutr Diet. 2017;117:1375–83.
41. Gijsbers L, Ding EL, Malik VS, De Goede J, Geleijnse JM, Soedamah-Muthu SS. Consumption of dairy foods and diabetes incidence: a dose-response meta-analysis of observational studies. Am J Clin Nutr. 2016;103:1111–24.
42. Adebamowo CA, Spiegelman D, Berkey CS, Danby FW, Rockett HH, Colditz GA, Willett WC, Holmes MD. Milk consumption and acne in teenaged boys. J Am Acad Dermatol. 2008;58:787–93.
43. LaRosa CL, Quach KA, Koons K, Kunselman AR, Zhu J, Thiboutot DM, Zaenglein AL. Consumption of dairy in teenagers with and without acne. J Am Acad Dermatol. 2016;75:318–22.
44. Ulvestad M, Bjertness E, Dalgard F, Halvorsen JA. Acne and dairy products in adolescence: results from a Norwegian longitudinal study. Acad Dermatol Venereol. 2017;31:530–5.
45. Baldwin H, Tan J. Effects of diet on acne and its response to treatment. Am J Clin Dermatol. 2021;22:55–65.
46. Smith RN, Mann NJ, Braue A, Mäkeläinen H, Varigos GA. The effect of a high-protein, low glycemic–load diet versus a conventional, high glycemic–load diet on biochemical parameters associated with acne vulgaris: a randomized, investigator-masked, controlled trial. J Am Acad Dermatol. 2007;57:247–56.
47. Kwon HH, Yoon JY, Hong JS, Jung JY, Park MS, Suh DH. Clinical and histological effect of a low glycaemic load diet in treatment of acne vulgaris in Korean patients: a randomized, controlled trial. Acta Derm Venereol. 2012;92:241–6.

48. Morales-Sánchez MA, Camacho-Rosas LH, García-Becerril I, Peralta-Pedrero ML. Effect of adding a low glycemic load and index diet over 12 weeks in the treatment of moderate acne: a randomized controlled trial. Int J Dermatol. 2023;62:e39. https://doi.org/10.1111/ijd.16418.
49. Burris J, Shikany JM, Rietkerk W, Woolf K. A low glycemic index and glycemic load diet decreases insulin-like growth factor-1 among adults with moderate and severe acne: a short-duration, 2-week randomized controlled trial. J Acad Nutr Diet. 2018;118:1874–85.
50. Howell JJ, Hellberg K, Turner M, Talbott G, Kolar MJ, Ross DS, Hoxhaj G, Saghatelian A, Shaw RJ, Manning BD. Metformin inhibits hepatic mTORC1 signaling via dose-dependent mechanisms involving AMPK and the TSC complex. Cell Metab. 2017;25:463–71.
51. Mathur R, Alexander CJ, Yano J, Trivax B, Azziz R. Use of metformin in polycystic ovary syndrome. Am J Obstet Gynecol. 2008;199:596–609.
52. Sharma S, Mathur DK, Paliwal V, Bhargava P. Efficacy of metformin in the treatment of acne in women with polycystic ovarian syndrome: a newer approach to acne therapy. J Clin Aesthet Dermatol. 2019;12:34.
53. Yen H, Chang Y-T, Yee F-J, Huang Y-C. Metformin therapy for acne in patients with polycystic ovary syndrome: a systematic review and meta-analysis. Am J Clin Dermatol. 2021;22:11–23.
54. Elham B, Somayeh S, Afsaneh S-B, Azadeh G, Mohammadreza G, Saba S, Masoomeh R. The effect of metformin in the treatment of intractable and late onset acne: a comparison with oral isotretinoin. Iran J Dermatol. 2019;22:47–52.
55. Fabbrocini G, Izzo R, Faggiano A, Del Prete M, Donnarumma M, Marasca C, Marciello F, Savastano R, Monfrecola G, Colao A. Low glycaemic diet and metformin therapy: a new approach in male subjects with acne resistant to common treatments. Clin Exp Dermatol. 2016;41:38–42.
56. Robinson S, Kwan Z, Tang MM. Metformin as an adjunct therapy for the treatment of moderate to severe acne vulgaris: a randomized open-labeled study. Dermatol Ther. 2019;32(4):e12953.
57. Gabaton NA, Paliza AC, Letran EL. A double-blind randomized controlled trial on the efficacy and safety of metformin as an adjunct to lymecycline and topical adapalene plus benzoyl peroxide gel in the treatment of moderate to severe acne vulgaris. J Philippine Dermatol Soc. 2020;29:20–47.
58. Sadati MS, Yazdanpanah N, Shahriarirad R, Javaheri R, Parvizi MM. Efficacy of metformin vs. doxycycline in treating acne vulgaris: an assessor-blinded, add-on, randomized, controlled clinical trial. J Cosmetic Dermatol. 2023;22:2816–23.
59. EL-Komy MHM, Abdo NMK, Shamma RN, Bedair NI. Topical metformin 30% gel in the treatment of acne vulgaris in women, a split face, placebo-controlled study. Exp Dermatol. 2023;32:1663–73.
60. Shahebrahimi K, Jalilian N, Bazgir N, Rezaei M. Comparison clinical and metabolic effects of metformin and pioglitazone in polycystic ovary syndrome. Indian J Endocrinol Metab. 2016;20:805.
61. Gether L, Overgaard LK, Egeberg A, Thyssen JP. Incidence and prevalence of rosacea: a systematic review and meta-analysis. Br J Dermatol. 2018;179:282–9.
62. Van Zuuren EJ. Rosacea. N Engl J Med. 2017;377:1754–64.
63. Schaller M, Almeida LMC, Bewley A, Cribier B, Del Rosso J, Dlova NC, Gallo RL, Granstein RD, Kautz G, Mannis MJ. Recommendations for rosacea diagnosis, classification and management: update from the global ROSacea COnsensus 2019 panel. Br J Dermatol. 2020;182:1269–76.
64. Rainer BM, Kang S, Chien AL. Rosacea: epidemiology, pathogenesis, and treatment. Dermatoendocrinol. 2017;9:e1361574.
65. Spoendlin J, Voegel JJ, Jick SS, Meier CR. Risk of rosacea in patients with diabetes using insulin or oral antidiabetic drugs. J Invest Dermatol. 2013;133:2790–3.
66. Hua T-C, Chung P-I, Chen Y-J, Wu L-C, Chen Y-D, Hwang C-Y, Chu S-Y, Chen C-C, Lee D-D, Chang Y-T. Cardiovascular comorbidities in patients with rosacea: a nationwide case-control study from Taiwan. J Am Acad Dermatol. 2015;73:249–54.

67. Egeberg A, Hansen PR, Gislason GH, Thyssen JP. Assessment of the risk of cardiovascular disease in patients with rosacea. J Am Acad Dermatol. 2016;75:336–9.
68. Zhang J, Yan Y, Jiang P, Liu Z, Liu Y, Liu Y, Wang X, Li M, Xu Y. Association between rosacea and cardiovascular disease: a systematic review and meta-analysis. J Cosmetic Dermatol. 2021;20:2715–22.
69. Chen Q, Shi X, Tang Y, Wang B, Xie H, Shi W, Li J. Association between rosacea and cardiometabolic disease: a systematic review and meta-analysis. J Am Acad Dermatol. 2020;83:1331–40.
70. Son JH, Chung BY, Jung MJ, Choi YW, Kim HO, Park CW. The risk of rosacea according to chronic diseases and medications: a 5-year retrospective, multi-institutional case-control study. Ann Dermatol. 2018;30:676–87.
71. Woo YR, Kim HS, Lee SH, Ju HJ, Bae JM, Cho SH, Lee JD. Systemic comorbidities in Korean patients with rosacea: results from a multi-institutional case-control study. J Clin Med. 2020;9:3336.
72. Choi D, Choi S, Choi S, Park SM, Yoon H. Association of Rosacea with cardiovascular disease: a retrospective cohort study. JAHA. 2021;10:e020671.
73. Wang F-Y, Kang EY-C, Liu C-H, Ng CY, Shao S-C, Lai EC-C, Wu W-C, Huang Y-Y, Chen K-J, Lai C-C. Diabetic patients with rosacea increase the risks of diabetic macular edema, dry eye disease, glaucoma, and cataract. Asia-Pacific J Ophthalmol. 2022;11:505–13.
74. Akin Belli A, Ozbas Gok S, Akbaba G, Etgu F, Dogan G. The relationship between rosacea and insulin resistance and metabolic syndrome. Eur J Dermatol. 2016;26:260–4.
75. Ozbagcivan O, Ozturk T, Akarsu S, Ilknur T, Fetil E. Evaluation of metabolic syndrome and its components in patients with rosacea: a cross-sectional, case-control study. Hong Kong J Dermatol. 2020;28:55–62.
76. Tsung-Yu T, Chiang Y-Y, Huang Y-C. Cardiovascular risk and comorbidities in patients with rosacea: a systematic review and meta-analysis. Acta Derm Venereol. 2020;100(17):adv00300. https://doi.org/10.2340/00015555-3668.
77. Rainer BM, Fischer AH, Da Silva DLF, Kang S, Chien AL. Rosacea is associated with chronic systemic diseases in a skin severity–dependent manner: results of a case-control study. J Am Acad Dermatol. 2015;73:604–8.
78. Chan WMM, Yew YW, Theng TSC, Liew CF, Oon HH. Prevalence of metabolic syndrome in patients with psoriasis: a cross-sectional study in Singapore. Singapore Med J. 2020;61:194.
79. Egeberg A, Hansen PR, Gislason GH, Thyssen JP. Clustering of autoimmune diseases in patients with rosacea. J Am Acad Dermatol. 2016;74:667–72.
80. Chang ALS, Raber I, Xu J, Li R, Spitale R, Chen J, Kiefer AK, Tian C, Eriksson NK, Hinds DA. Assessment of the genetic basis of rosacea by genome-wide association study. J Invest Dermatol. 2015;135:1548–55.
81. Pagan AD, Jung S, Caldas S, Ungar J, Gulati N, Ungar B. Cross-sectional study of psoriasis, atopic dermatitis, rosacea, and alopecia areata suggests association with cardiovascular diseases. J Drugs Dermatol. 2023;22:576–81.
82. Li Y, Yang L, Wang Y, Deng Z, Xu S, Xie H, Zhang Y, Li J. Exploring metformin as a candidate drug for rosacea through network pharmacology and experimental validation. Pharmacol Res. 2021;174:105971.
83. Minah CHO, Woo YR, Cho SH, Lee JD, Kim HS. Metformin: a potential treatment for acne, hidradenitis suppurativa and rosacea. Acta Derm Venereol. 2023;103:adv18392.
84. Mumoli L, Gambardella A, Labate A, Succurro E, De Sarro G, Arturi F, Gallelli L. Rosacea-like facial rash related to metformin administration in a young woman. BMC Pharmacol Toxicol. 2014;15:3.

Chapter 26
Skin Disorders in Pregnancy

Valentina Broshtilova and Mary Gantcheva

Abstract Many endocrinopathies demonstrate dermatological manifestations that facilitate previously undiagnosed endocrine disorders with maternal and fetal ramifications. Maternal and fetal risks depend significantly on early diagnosis and management of these endocrinopathies in order to prevent perinatal mortality and increased overall morbidity. A plethora of systemic and dermatological inflammatory conditions may develop in the course of pregnancy complicated with diabetes. Maternal obesity and gestational insulin resistance also provoke low-grade inflammation, which downregulates placental leptin gene expression and diminishes tumor necrosis factor alpha and interleukin-6 in the fetus, causing placental morphometry changes and higher fetus weight. Markers of microangiopathy such as impaired endothelial permeability and increased intima thickness are detected in higher levels in pregnant diabetic patients. Hence, pregnancy acts as a "stress test" to identify women with diabetic predisposition and susceptibility to chronic persistent inflammation. Dermatological disorders that evolve during pregnancy are classified in two main categories: specific conditions that occur more commonly or exacerbate during pregnancy and diabetes-related skin diseases. Their prompt verification insured by a highly qualified multidisciplinary team of an obstetrician, a dermatologist, and an expert endocrinologist helps to optimize management and improve outcomes. Diabetes prevention requires lifestyle changes and exercise promotion to prevent a healthier mother and child's future. Insulin is the first choice of treatment in complicated cases. The role of other antihyperglycemic agents requires more sophisticated and larger randomized controlled studies to evaluate their efficacy and safety.

V. Broshtilova
Internal Diseases, Pharmacology and Clinical Pharmacology, Pediatrics, Epidemiology, Infectious Diseases, and Skin Diseases, Faculty of Medicine, Sofia University "St. Kliment Ohridski", Sofia, Bulgaria

M. Gantcheva (✉)
Acibadem City Clinic, Sofia, Bulgaria

Institute of Experimental Morphology, Pathology and Anthropology with Museum, Bulgarian Academy of Science, Sofia, Bulgaria

K. Fritz, G.-S. Tiplica (eds.), *Cutaneous Manifestations in Diabetes*,
https://doi.org/10.1007/978-3-031-65300-1_26

26.1 Introduction

Pregnancy is a specific physiological state, accompanied by a variety of skin-related problems that have to be diagnosed and addressed promptly in order to avoid potentially fatal maternal and fetal outcomes [1]. The upregulation of female sex hormones enhances higher cutaneous sensitivity, especially to external meteorological, bacterial, and viral triggers, thus increasing the susceptibility to systemic infections, metabolic diseases, and autoimmune dysregulation. Meanwhile, the decreased cell-mediated immunity accounts for exacerbation of dysbacteriosis and chronic persistent skin infections such as candidiasis [2]. Maternal obesity and gestational insulin resistance also provoke low-grade inflammation, which downregulates placental leptin gene expression and diminishes tumor necrosis factor alpha and interleukin-6 in the fetus, causing placental morphometry changes and higher fetus weight [3].

26.2 Epidemiology of Diabetes During Pregnancy

Diabetes mellitus is associated with a plethora of skin disorders, induced by increased blood glucose concentration. The impaired protein, fat, and carbohydrate metabolism that evolves as a consequence of insufficient insulin secretion or tissue insulin resistance causes macroangiopathic (cardiovascular) and/or microvascular (ocular, nephrotic, neuropathic, and skin) complications with lifelong morbidity. One third of diabetes patients experience dermatological disorders during the course of their disease [4].

Together with patients that have absolute insulin absence due to autoimmune beta-cell destruction (type 1 diabetes) and those with insulin resistance and relative insulin deficiency (type 2 diabetes), there is a unique group of women that express glucose intolerance for the first time during pregnancy—gestational diabetes (GD). Usually GD occurs at 24–28 weeks of gestation [5]. It is estimated that one of every ten pregnancies is complicated with elevation of blood glucose.

26.3 Pathogenetic Pathways

Minority of patients develop GD due to autoimmune destruction of insulin-producing pancreatic cells, analogous to type 1 diabetes monogenic mutations. Most of the GD cases, however, share the diabetes type 2 risk factors such as obesity, physical inactivity, positive family history, polycystic ovary syndrome, etc.

The high insulin requirements during late pregnancy provoke increased synthetic pressure over maternal pancreatic beta cells, impairing their ability to stimulate glucose disposal and its tissue utilization, giving rise to higher free blood circulation and elevating serum fatty acid levels. The insulin signaling pathway alterations, together with reduced PRAR gamma expression and insulin-mediated glucose transportation in skeletal muscles and fat cells, are the main GD pathogenetic mechanisms [6].

Interestingly, post-receptor defects in insulin signaling pathways are usually identified in the placenta, suggesting a major role of maternal metabolic dysfunction rather than fetus dysregulations. However, the increased antigenic load by the fetus, especially its human leukocyte antigen-G expression that protects from immune attacks inhibiting cytotoxic T-cell activity, interacts with nuclear factor-kappa B to trigger the diabetogenic process [7].

26.4 Diagnosis

Glycosuria, age over 30 years, obesity, family history of diabetes, past history of GD or glucose intolerance, and previous macrosomic child delivery as main GD risk factors constitute a patient cohort that obligatorily undergoes glucose challenge test screening [8]. However, it has been estimated that up to 40% of GD cases are left underdiagnosed since they have not been classified in this high-risk category. Therefore, the modern screening concept requires universal testing of all pregnant women except those considered of very low-risk. These include nulliparous women under 25 years with a body mass index under 25 kg/m^2 and multiparous women under 40 years with body mass index under 25 kg/m^2 that have no previous macrosomic child [9].

GD is diagnosed based on one or more abnormal values during glucose challenge test performed during 24th–28th week of pregnancy. Early testing between 12th or 16th week is recommended in cases of mothers with severe obesity (body mass index over 35 kg/m^2), previous history of GD, strong family history of diabetes, and glycosuria [10].

26.5 Obstetric and Perinatal Complications Due to Diabetes

Diabetes during pregnancy is associated with a high risk of macrosomia, shoulder dystocia, neonatal hypoglycemia, hyperbilirubinemia, and birth injuries [11]. The offspring's risk of obesity, metabolic syndrome, and diabetes is significantly increased. Children exposed to gestational diabetes show susceptibility to arterial hypertension and low high-density lipoprotein cholesterol. The placental hyperinsulinemia is an independent risk factor for glucose intolerance in children. Preeclampsia and other serious pregnancy disorders including perinatal death, prematurity, and intrauterine growth retardation are common GD complications [12]. Ten percent of GD women develop overt diabetes in a 10-year follow-up period, as the overall lifelong risk for developing diabetes increases with 40%. In the first 5 years after delivery, those women express higher levels of endothelial inflammatory markers and increased intima thickness of the carotid artery. They show elevated fat deposition in the liver and muscles, which increases and perpetuates obesity-related insulin resistance. GD prevention includes weight loss measures and dietary modifications, together with smoking cessation and intensification of physical activity. Antenatal exercise significantly reduces GD risk [13].

26.6 Skin Complications in Diabetic Pregnancies

26.6.1 Hormone-Driven Dermatoses

Traditionally, cutaneous disorders during pregnancy are classified as physiological (hormone-driven), exacerbated preexisting skin conditions, and pregnancy-specific dermatoses [14]. The physiological changes are referred to as pregnancy stigmas as they resolve postpartum and pose no harm to the mother and the fetus. They encompass the following conditions: (1) pigmentary (melasma, pseudoacanthotic changes, dermal melanocytosis, verrucous areola pigmentation, vulvar melanosis), (2) skin appendages changes (hirsutism, postpartum telogen hair loss, diffuse hair thinning, subungual hyperkeratosis, distal onycholysis, horizontal ridges, nail fragility and softening, hyperhidrosis, seborrhea and acne, diffuse xerosis), and (3) connective tissue disorders (stretch marks, soft prenatal fibrosis, spider angiomas, palm erythema, significant lip edema, microvascular instability, mucosal membranes hyperemia, varicose veins, and hemorrhoids).

26.6.2 Dermatoses That Exacerbate During Pregnancy

Any preexisting dermatosis can exacerbate during pregnancy. Atopic dermatitis, psoriasis, and hidradenitis suppurativa (HS) are the chronic skin inflammatory disorders that cause most severe morbidity and quality of life decline [15]. Pruritus occurs in 14–20% of all pregnancies and causes severe complications in up to 2% of them. Usually endocrinopathies and systemic hematologic dyscrasias underlie those most refractory cases. Up to 60% of psoriatic patients improve their skin condition during pregnancy, which is due to progesterone elevation, which downregulates T-cell proliferative response. It is now clear that 37% of HS patients experience spontaneous pregnancy loss, 25% give preterm birth, and 59% develop gestational diabetes and preeclampsia due to severe arterial hypertension.

26.6.3 *Pregnancy-Specific Dermatoses*

The pregnancy-specific dermatoses occur due to the interaction of hormonal, metabolic, immune, and microbiome dysregulation during pregnancy. Most of these skin pathologies are benign and resolve shortly after delivery; however, some increase the fetal risk and require antenatal surveillance [16]. The most prominent subjective symptom that is constantly associated with all pregnancy-related dermatoses is pruritus. Half of the patients usually have atopic predisposition, which exacerbates during pregnancy. Therefore, the most recent term used to classify this condition is "atopic eruption of pregnancy" (AEP). It includes three different inflammatory dermatoses with overlapping clinical features—eczema in pregnancy, early onset prurigo of pregnancy, and pruritic folliculitis.

26.6.3.1 AEP

AEP high prevalence during pregnancy is based on atopic background. The immune dysbalance toward increased Th2 cytokine production of interleukin-4 and interleukin-10 favors exacerbation of atopic dermatitis [17]. Moreover, 80% of all patients manifest their atopic dermatitis for the first time during pregnancy. The eruption is usually diffuse, affecting the face, trunk, and extremities, including palmoplantar areas. Prurigo of pregnancy affects 1 in 300 cases. The pruritic excoriated papules and nodules are often located on the extensor aspects of the upper arms and lower extremities. Despite taxonomy, pruritic folliculitis presents with non-itchy miliar follicular-centered papules and pustules, disseminated on the shoulders, upper trunk, and arms. It is often classified as an acneiform eruption, although no common pathophysiological background has been proven. It resolves spontaneously with no maternal-fetal morbidity.

26.6.3.2 Polymorphic Eruption of Pregnancy

Polymorphic eruption of pregnancy is synonymous to pruritic urticarial papules and plaques of pregnancy (PUPPP) and is the second most common dermatosis during pregnancy after atopic eczema [18]. It occurs once in 160 pregnancies and is associated with multiple gestation and maternal overweight. The pathogenesis remains elusive, although it is hypothesized that collagen fragmentation causes antigen formation, provoking skin eruption. Erythematous, non-follicular papules, plaques, and vesicles begin to appear in the third trimester in the areas of striae gravidarum, sparing the periumbilical site. The lesions are extremely pruritic and usually disappear postpartum, although there are a few cases that start after delivery. The condition does not increase mother or child morbidity.

26.6.3.3 Herpes Gestationis

Herpes gestationis, also known as pemphigoid gestationis (PG) is a subepidermal autoimmune bullous dermatosis that affects 1 in 50,000 pregnancies [16]. It starts in the second or third trimester. HLA-DR3 and HLA-DR4 are usually involved in its pathogenesis, which is suggestively triggered by a potential placental antigen, showing some cross-reactivity with skin antigens. Polymorphous urticarial, papulo-vesicular eruption spreads on the abdominal region. Histologically, it is verified by a subepidermal clefting. The immunofluorescent findings demonstrate linear IgG and C3 deposits on the dermal-epidermal junction. The disease may fade during late pregnancy to flare again after delivery. The IgG antibodies that cross the placenta cause transient vesiculobullous eruption in up to 10% of the newborns. Placentar failure is associated with premature delivery to small-for-gestation-age babies. Some patients suffer nongestational exacerbations under contraceptive triggers or menstrual cycles.

26.6.3.4 Intrahepatic Cholestasis of Pregnancy

Intrahepatic cholestasis of pregnancy (ICP) is characterized by pruritus with or without skin lesions that occur in the third trimester [19]. The pathognomonic diagnostic feature is the laboratory constellation of cholestasis (bile acid levels over 10 mcrmol/L and elevated alkaline phosphatase, with or without high bilirubin). The skin lesions appear secondary to itching and depend on its duration. Most often linear excoriations and prurigo papules are seen on the lateral aspects of the abdomen and lower legs. Genetic background of HLA-A31 and HLA-B8, family history of cholelithiasis, and higher risk of gallstones are commonly described. Premature delivery, intrauterine demise due to fetus anoxia, and meconium-stained amniotic fluid are the most common complications. Coagulopathies due to vitamin K insufficiency may often occur in prolonged cases.

26.6.3.5 Impetigo Herpetiformis

Impetigo herpetiformis (IP) is a form of generalized pustular psoriasis that may develop during pregnancy. A pathogenetic hypothesis suggests a dysbalance in calcium metabolism. Patients usually develop severe hypoproteinemia and electrolyte abnormalities. Intrauterine growth restriction, low birth weight, stillbirth, and neonatal death may develop [15].

26.6.4 Complications Specifically Related to Diabetes

Skin conditions are highly prevalent in diabetic patients. Nonspecific dermatological changes such as xerosis, itching, diffuse or palmar erythema, scarring, and edema are often accompanying cases of non-well-controlled diabetes [20].

26.6.4.1 Diabetic Dermopathy

Diabetic dermopathy affects about 30% of diabetic patients. It is characterized by asymptomatic erythematous or hyperpigmented macules and papules with fine pityriasiform scale, distributed on the shins, and less commonly on the anterior aspects of the thighs, forearm, dorsal feet, and scalp. Multiple lesions are pathognomonic for diabetes, and their presence should alert the clinician to perform blood testing to a previously non-diagnosed patient. The lesions are harmless and spontaneously resolve with optimization of blood control, which strengthens the pathogenetic hypothesis that they are a consequence of increased glycosylation of small vessels basal membrane [21].

26.6.4.2 Diabetic Blisters

Diabetic blisters, also referred to as bullosis diabeticorum, feature spontaneously evolving blisters on the dorsal aspects of feet and hands. They are considered a distinct sign of diabetes. The size of the lesions is the most striking clinical characteristic, since they may become very large—up to 17 centimeters in diameter. However, no discomfort or pain is present. Small nerve endings damage is suggestive to cause this condition. Neuropathy lessens skin sensation, increasing vulnerability and susceptibility to trauma or friction. Therefore, minor triggers such as repetitive impact by ill-fitting shoes provoke the disease. The blisters gradually reabsorb, dry out, and heal spontaneously. Their appearance is always suggestive of poor blood control, peripheral neuropathy, and microvascular dysfunction [22].

26.6.4.3 Digital Sclerosis

A lot of patients with a prolonged history of type 1 diabetes develop diabetic stiff skin (also known as digital cheiroarthropathy or digital sclerosis). It is characterized by thickening and induration of fingers and toes, which demonstrate waxy appearance and texture. The impaired microvasculature with an increase of glycation end products is believed to cause the condition. The skin becomes hard, losing its normal elasticity. As it progresses, the stiffness limits everyday range of motions and flexibility, even affecting balance and coordination. Patient's quality of life deteriorates, and the risk of associated mechanically prone erosions and ulcer formation increases.

26.6.4.4 Diabetic Foot Ulcers

Diabetic foot ulcers are common complications arising due to hyperglycemia, peripheral neuropathy, and poor blood circulation.

26.6.4.5 Diabetic Neuropathy

Peripheral nerves, exposed to hyperglycemia for a long time, lose their conductivity and sensitization, thus causing difficulty for the individuals to detect pain, discomfort, and injuries. Therefore, minor skin defects easily progress to severe ulcers and infections.

26.6.4.6 Skin Infections

High blood sugar levels weaken innate immunity and, together with chronic nerve damage, facilitate bacterial and fungal invasion through small and superficial skin defects. *Staphylococcus aureus* bacteria often invade eyelid oil glands, leading to chordeolum formation. Superficial and deep folliculitis, especially distributed to the scalp, arms, and legs, are commonly seen in diabetic patients. *Candida* and *Malassezia* species overgrowth can affect different body parts, especially inguinal folds, and oral and genital mucosa [23].

26.6.4.7 Acanthosis Nigricans

Acanthosis nigricans presents with hyperpigmented, velvety texture patches, localized to the body folds, such as the neck, armpits, groin, and elbows. The higher circulating levels of insulin and insulin-like growth factor in patients with diabetes stimulate keratinocytic proliferation, causing prominent acanthosis and hypermelanosis in the epidermis. Despite being harmless, acanthosis nigricans serves as an indicator for underlying metabolic dysfunction, polycystic ovary syndrome, certain medication intake (such as corticosteroids and oral contraceptives), insulin resistance, and obesity [24].

26.6.4.8 Other Dermatological Conditions Associated with Diabetes

Necrobiosis lipoidica, reactive perforating collagenosis, and Kyrle disease, especially in diabetic patients with chronic renal failure, scleredema (sclerodermiform changes with thickening of the neck and upper back), disseminated granuloma annulare, eruptive xanthoma on the hands, arms, feet, and buttocks, xanthelasma, skin tags, vitiligo, and cutaneous dysesthesia (due to small fiber neuropathy) can also occur more frequently in patients with diabetes [4].

26.7 Differential Diagnosis

The most common clinical symptom is itching. Sometimes the underlying course may not be related to pregnancy; however, a good understanding of the pathogenesis and clinical features of pregnancy-related specific dermatoses is extremely helpful [15]. The critical diagnostic issue is the discrimination of a dermatological lesion. If the pruritus is not objectivized by skin eruption, the diagnosis is limited to ICP or systemic conditions, incidentally occurring during pregnancy. Generalized pruritus occurs in liver, kidney, hematological, and endocrine diseases, as well as in any kind of malignancy, especially Hodgkin lymphoma [25]. Therefore, routine full blood count and biochemistry screening are recommended. Those cases that show dermatological substrate are discriminated according to the pregnancy duration. Atopic eczema usually exacerbates in the first trimester. AEP is still the most common pregnancy-specific dermatosis in the second trimester, albeit PG tends to have its onset in the same period. The differential diagnosis of pruritic skin changes in the third trimester is the most complicated. It consists of ICP, PG, PUPPP, and IP. Although rare, some morbilliform and urticarial drug eruptions may also occur. Beta-lactam antibiotics are commonly prescribed during pregnancy, and together with blood transfusion products and low-molecular-weight heparin are the most common triggers of macular-papular drug eruptions. Amoxicillin and propylthiouracil can also cause hypersensitivity vasculitis and even life-threatening conditions such as acute generalized exanthematous pustulosis and toxic epidermal necrolysis. Drug-induced bullous lesions may be mistaken with bullous pemphigoid; however, “thio” groups—containing medications such as penicillamine and captopril—are exceptionally used during pregnancy [26].

26.8 Therapeutic Management

Optimal serum glucose control is needed in order to ensure best management of skin complications in diabetes. The importance of regular skin assessments as part of routine diabetes care is essential [5]. Early detection usually prevents progression and ensures proper intervention in due time. Recommended fasting glycaemia goal is under 5.5 mmol/L. Insulin therapy is considered if the plasma glucose goals are not met in a 2-week period follow-up and particularly if clinical or ultrasonographic observations suggest macrosomia. Human insulin and insulin analogs such as insulin lispro, aspart insulin, and glargine are used due to their safety profile and optimal dosing. The risk of nocturnal hypoglycemia should be taken in consideration and strictly minimized. Oral hypoglycemic agents such as glyburide and metformin are possible alternatives to insulin treatment. Clinical trials showed no significant difference in maternal glycemic control and cesarean delivery rates between insulin- and glyburide-treated patients. No substantial fetal or maternal outcome differences were identified in cohorts treated with insulin compared to metformin. However, sufficient long-term data on metformin safety in respect to physical and psychological offspring health are still missing [27].

Dermatological therapeutic principles include proper patient education to adequate self-control. Patients should learn to cleanse, moisturize, and inspect their skin on a daily basis. Moisturizing provides sufficient skin integrity, enhancing skin barrier function to prevent dryness. Thus, the risk of inflammatory skin disorders, pruritus, and infections is minimized [28]. Regular emollient use reduces transepidermal water loss and protects from external irritants. The emollients' effectiveness in managing diabetic skin complications reveals their crucial role in skin health promotion and reduction of morbidity associated with this condition.

Most of the pregnancy-related conditions are benign and resolve spontaneously in the postpartum period [1]. Topical emollients should be considered as a first-line therapeutic option during pregnancy. Moderately potent corticosteroids in combination with oral antihistamines may be used in more generalized or prolonged cases. Topical benzyl peroxide gives a favorable outcome in pruritic folliculitis. Narrowband UV B therapy is a second-line therapeutic option in all cases of pruritus, refractory to topical agents. PG may require high doses of intravenous corticosteroids. Systemic steroids are used only in severe cases of PUPPP, ICP, BP, or IH. Induction of labor may be considered in near-term pregnancies. Epidural or spinal anesthesia should not be performed on sites of puncture occupied by skin lesions [29].

26.9 Conclusions

The diagnosis and proper management of skin-related problems during diabetic pregnancy is an extremely challenging task that requires a multidisciplinary comprehensive approach. Optimal control of underlying endocrinopathies minimizes maternal and fetus morbidity, associated with pregnancy-related specific dermatoses such as obstetric cholestasis, pemphigoid gestationis, and impetigo herpetiformis. Preconceptional counseling, close pregnancy monitoring, and optimal glucose control, provided by a highly qualified team of endocrinologist, dermatologist, and obstetric medicine physicians, are crucial in preventing maternal-fetus complications.

References

1. Sachdeva S. The dermatoses of pregnancy. Indian J Dermatol. 2008;53(3):103–5.
2. Kroumpouzos G, Cohen LM. Dermatoses of pregnancy. J Am Acad Dermatol. 2001;45:1–19.
3. Musa E, Salazar-Petres E, Arowolo A, Levitt N, Matjila M, Sferruzzi-Perri A. Obesity and gestational diabetes independently and collectively induce specific effects on placental structure, inflammation and endocrine function in a cohort of south African women. J Physiol. 2023;601(7):1287–306.
4. David P, Singh S, Ankar R. A comprehensive overview of skin complications in diabetes and their prevention. Cureus. 2023;15(5):e38961. https://doi.org/10.7759/cureus.38961.
5. Kaaja R, Ronnemaa T. Gestational diabetes: pathogenesis and consequences to mother and offspring. Rev Diabet Stud. 2008;5:194–202.
6. Buchanan TA, Xiang AH. Gestational diabetes mellitus. J Clin Invest. 2005;115(3):485–91.
7. Oztekin O. New insights into the pathophysiology of gestational diabetes mellitus: possible role of human leukocyte antigen-G. Med Hypotheses. 2007;69(3):526–30.
8. O'Sullivan JB, Mahan CM. Criteria for the oral glucose tolerance test in pregnancy. Diabetes. 1964;13:278–85.
9. Carpenter MW, Coustan DR. Criteria for screening tests for gestational diabetes. Am J Obstet Gynecol. 1982;144:768–73.
10. Ju H, Rumbold AR, Willson KJ, Crowther CA. Borderline gestational diabetes and pregnancy outcomes. BMC Pregnancy Childbirth. 2008;8:31.
11. Griffin ME, Coffey M, Johnson H, Scanlon P, Foley M, Stronge J, O'Meara NM, Firth RG. Universal vs risk factor-based screening for gestational diabetes mellitus: detection rates, gestation at diagnosis and outcomes. Diabet Med. 2000;17(1):26–32.
12. Boney CM, Verma A, Tucker R, Vorh BR. Metabolic syndrome in childhood: association with birth weight, maternal obesity and gestational diabetes. Pediatrics. 2008;115(3):E290–6.
13. Tam WH, Yang X, Ko GT, Tong PC, Cockram CS, Sahota DS, Rogers MS, Chn JC. Glucose intolerance and cardiometabolic risk in children exposed to maternal gestational diabetes mellitus in utero. Pediatrics. 2008;122:1229–34.
14. Snarskaya E, Olisova O, Makatsariya A, Kochergin N, Radetskaya L, Bitsadze V, Khizroeva J. Skin pathologies in pregnancy. J Perinat Med. 2019;47:371. https://doi.org/10.1515/jpm-2018-0338.
15. Mehta N, Chen K, Kroumpouz G. Skin disease in pregnancy: the approach of the obstetric medicine physician. Clin Dermatol. 2016;34:320–6.
16. Kroumpouzos G, Cohen LM. Specific dermatoses of pregnancy: an evidence-besed systematic review. Am J Obstet Gynecol. 2003;188:1083–92.
17. Koutroulis I, Papoutsis J, Kroumpouzos G. Atopic dermatitis in pregnancy: current status and challenges. Obstet Gyneol Surv. 2011;66:654–63.
18. Rudolph CM, Al-Fares S, Vaughan-Jones SA. Polymorphic eruption of pregnancy: clinicopathology and potential trigger factors in 181 patients. Br J Dermatol. 2006;154:54–60.
19. Ovadia C, Wilkinson C. Intrahepatic cholestasis of pregnancy. Clin Dermatol. 2016;34:327–34.
20. de Macedo GM, Nunes S, Barreto T. Skin disorders in diabetes: an epidemiology and physiopathology review. Diabetol Metab Syndr. 2016;8:63.
21. Forbes JM, Cooper ME. Mechanisms of diabetic complications. Physiol Rev. 2013;93:137–88.
22. Barrett E, Liu Z, Khamaisi M. Diabetic microvascular disease: an endocrine society scientific statement. J Clin Endocrinol Metab. 2017;102:4343–410.
23. Falcone M, Meier J, Marini MG, Caccialanza R, Aguado J, Del Plato S, Menichetti F. Diabetes and acute bacterial skin and skin structure infections. Diabetes Res Clin Pract. 2021;174:108732.
24. Wukich D. Diabetes and its negative impact on outcomes in orthopaedic surgery. World J Orthop. 2015;6:331–9.

25. Geenes V, Williamson C. Pruritus and obstetric cholestasis. In: Kroumpouzos G, editor. Text atlas of obstetric dermatology. Philadelphia, PA: Lippincott Williams & Wilkins; 2013. p. 164–75.
26. Valeyrie-Allanore L, Sassolas B, Roujeau JC. Drug-induced skin, nail, and hair disorders. Drug Saf. 2007;30:1011–30.
27. Rowan J, Hague W, Gao W, Battin M, Moore M, Mig Trial Investigators. Metformin versus insulin for the treatment of gestational diabetes. N Engl J Med. 2008;358(19):2003–15.
28. Kirsner R, Yosipovitch G, Hu S. Diabetic skin changes can benefit from moisturizers and cleanser use: a review. J Drugs Dermatol. 2019;18:1211–7.
29. Kaaja R, Greer I. Manifestations of chronic disease during pregnancy. JAMA. 2005;294:2751–7.

Chapter 27
Genetic Syndromes Associated with Diabetes Mellitus

Alexios Alexopoulos and Talia Kakourou

Abstract Genetic syndromes associated with diabetes mellitus (DM) have proven difficult to identify, given the clinical overlap, the genetic heterogeneity, and the exceptionally low prevalence these conditions demonstrate. Early neurologic deficits in the presence of diabetes mellitus especially in the neonatal-early childhood period should alert the clinicians to investigate for these conditions. The most common clinical manifestations of syndromic diabetes include sensorineural hearing loss, ataxia, seizures, vision loss, and other developmental abnormalities. The genetic etiologies of these syndromes contribute toward our understanding of the pathophysiology of more common forms of DM; moreover, they may lead to the development of more personalized medical treatments.

Diabetes mellitus (DM) is a disease of inadequate control of blood levels of glucose. It is a metabolic disease resulting from defects in insulin secretion, insulin action, or both. According to the genetic background, DM can be classified into three subtypes:

(a) polygenic diabetes with diabetes type 1 and diabetes type 2 as the main representatives,
(b) monogenic diabetes which is caused by single gene mutations including maturity-onset diabetes of the young and neonatal diabetes, and,
(c) syndromic diabetes which is defined as the presence of diabetes as part of a broader clinical syndrome [1, 2].

Syndromic diabetes is very diverse and presents exceptionally rare in the general population. Moreover, not all of these syndromes are genetically identified in the literature making their classification even more difficult. As syndromic DM demonstrates a very low prevalence, it can be frequently misdiagnosed as diabetes with complications. The diagnosis of syndromic DM is further complicated by clinical

A. Alexopoulos (✉)
Pediatric Dermatology Unit, First Department of Pediatrics, Athens University, Agia Sofia Children's Hospital, Athens, Greece

T. Kakourou
First Department of Pediatrics, Athens University, Agia Sofia Children's Hospital, IASO Children's Hospital, Athens, Greece

K. Fritz, G.-S. Tiplica (eds.), *Cutaneous Manifestations in Diabetes*,
https://doi.org/10.1007/978-3-031-65300-1_27

heterogeneity and the overlap of clinical features, which contribute to the difficulty of diagnosing specific syndromes. The most common clinical manifestations of syndromic diabetes are neurological deficits including sensorineural hearing loss, ataxia, seizures, vision loss, and developmental abnormalities. The onset and progression of these syndromes are sometimes similar; therefore a high clinical suspicion should be maintained in order to identify them.

Based on the age of onset and the mode of inheritance of the syndrome, the most frequently described DM syndromes are the following [3–5].

27.1 Diabetes Syndromes with Neonatal Onset

27.1.1 Insulin Resistance Syndromes

Insulin resistance syndromes differ from typical insulin resistance not only by their severity but also because patients demonstrate normal lipid profiles. Their etiology is directly linked to defects in insulin receptor signaling rather than obesity.

The most common type is type A insulin resistance syndrome, which is inherited by both autosomal dominant and autosomal recessive forms. It affects mainly non-obese females and presents with extreme insulin resistance, acanthosis nigricans, hirsutism, and polycystic ovarian disease [6].

Rabson-Mendenhall syndrome (RMS) is another form of insulin resistance with autosomal recessive inheritance. Patients with RMS have clinical features of extreme insulin resistance, acanthosis nigricans, hirsutism, dental precocity, thick nails, pineal hyperplasia, genital enlargement in both males and females, abdominal distension, and other distinctive dysmorphic features [7].

The most severe form is Donohue syndrome (DS), an autosomal recessive disorder in which patients rarely survive beyond infancy, and they present with failure to thrive, severe hyperinsulinemia, and fasting hypoglycemia [8].

27.1.2 Bone Abnormalities Syndromes

Wolcott-Rallison syndrome (WRS) is a rare autosomal recessive disease, characterized by insulin-requiring diabetes associated with skeletal dysplasia and growth retardation. Typically, diabetes occurs before 6 months of age, and skeletal dysplasia is diagnosed within the first 2 years of life. Other clinical manifestations include frequent episodes of acute liver failure, renal dysfunction, exocrine pancreas insufficiency, intellectual deficit, hypothyroidism, neutropenia, recurrent infections, and bone fractures. WRS is caused by mutations in the gene encoding eukaryotic translation initiation factor known as PKR-like endoplasmic reticulum kinase (PERK). WRS should be suspected in any infant who presents with permanent neonatal diabetes associated with skeletal dysplasia and/or episodes of acute liver failure. Early intervention is recommended, in order to avoid episodes of hepatic failure, which is a life-threatening complication. WRS should be differentiated from other forms of neonatal/early-onset insulin-dependent diabetes based on clinical presentation and genetic testing [9].

27.1.3 Intestinal Malformations Syndromes

Mitchell-Riley syndrome (MRS) is characterized by neonatal diabetes, pancreatic hypoplasia, gallbladder agenesis or hypoplasia, and duodenal atresia. It is caused by biallelic mutations in the regulatory factor X6 gene (RFX6) located on chromosome 6q22. Clinical management can be difficult, as neonatal diabetes in MRS is associated with severe complications from the intestine and the liver. Low birth weight, protracted diarrhea, and persisting feeding difficulties related to bowel surgery contribute to failure to thrive. Other abnormalities such as cholestasis, hepatic failure, anemia, thrombocytopenia, hemochromatosis, hypospadias, and metabolic disorders (acidosis) are described in MRS, but their physiopathology is not yet fully elucidated [10].

27.1.4 Syndromes Associated with Lipodystrophies

Monogenic lipodystrophy is a group of diseases featuring a complete or partial lack of adipose tissue and adipose tissue-derived hormones. These patients demonstrate insulin resistance, dyslipidemia, and other metabolic complications. Unlike insulin receptor defects, insulin resistance is caused by the formation of fat into ectopic areas, resulting in clinical features and consequences similar to obesity.

Based on the loss of adipose tissue, congenital lipodystrophies can be divided into congenital generalized lipodystrophy (CGL) which presents more frequently and familial partial lipodystrophy (FPLD). Body fat deficiency in FPLD is found mainly on the limbs, buttocks, and hips [11, 12].

27.1.5 Immune Dysregulation, Polyendocrinopathy, Enteropathy, and X-Linked Syndrome

Immune dysregulation, polyendocrinopathy, enteropathy, X-linked (IPEX) syndrome characterizes complex autoimmune reactions beginning in the perinatal period and caused by dysfunction of the transcription factor forkhead box P3 (FOXP3). This disorder is most common in the first year of life. IPEX syndrome is inherited in boys in an X-linked recessive manner. Mutations of FOXP3 gene cause malfunction of a protein localized in the DNA-binding domain (forkhead domain). The abnormal protein interferes with the normal development and function of T regulatory cells, with an observed loss of CD4 + CD25 + T regulatory cells and uncontrolled proliferation of activated CD4 + effector cells. The immune system attacks its own tissues and organs as a consequence of uncontrolled T-cell activation causing inflammation, autoimmunity, and metabolic disorders. IPEX syndrome is one of the autoimmune polyendocrine syndromes that lead to the dysfunction of multiple endocrine glands. The most common abnormalities are diabetes mellitus in the first month of life, severe atopic dermatitis (eczema), autoimmune thyroiditis, refractory diarrhea, hemolytic anemia, thrombocytopenia, neutropenia, and nephropathy [13, 14].

27.1.6 Developmental Delay, Epilepsy, and Neonatal Diabetes Syndrome

Developmental delay, epilepsy, and neonatal diabetes (DEND) syndrome is a form of permanent neonatal diabetes mellitus (PNDM) associated with developmental regression, epilepsy, and muscle weakness. It is a rare disorder with very few cases reported in the literature. DEND syndrome, which is a monogenic, autosomal recessive disorder, represents the most severe clinical form of PNDM. It is caused by activating mutations in the KATP channel subunit Kir 6.2 or SUR1 genes present on chromosome 11 (KCNJ11 and ABCC8).

Activating mutations lead to less KATP channel closure, causing membrane hyperpolarization, thus preventing Ca2+ influx and impairing insulin secretion causing neonatal DM. In the brain these mutations play a role by increasing spontaneous discharge rate of neurons in the ventromedial hypothalamus. It is postulated that epilepsy results from decreased activity of inhibitory interneurons in the hippocampus, as there is a greater density of KATP channels in the inhibitory neurons as compared to the excitatory neurons [15, 16].

27.2 Diabetes Syndromes with Childhood-Adult Onset

27.2.1 Alstrom Syndrome

Alstrom syndrome is a rare monogenic condition caused by mutations in the gene ALMS1. There are approximately 450 cases described in the literature. Its diagnosis may be challenging since there is considerable phenotypic variation within families.

The major phenotypes usually include retinal dystrophy beginning in infancy and leading to juvenile blindness, sensorineural hearing loss, insulin resistance, and obesity. In few cases infants also may present with congestive heart failure due to dilated cardiomyopathy (DCM). In adolescence, type 2 diabetes mellitus (T2DM), hypertriglyceridemia, and adolescent-onset DCM usually develop. In adulthood scoliosis, alopecia, male hypogonadism, and hyperandrogenism in female patients may be present. Fibrosis in multiple organs has also been reported as the disease progresses [17].

27.2.2 Wolfram Syndrome Type 1 and Type 2

Wolfram syndrome is a rare genetic form of syndromic diabetes caused by mutations in the genes WFS1 (Wolfram syndrome type 1) or CISD2 (Wolfram syndrome type 2), respectively [18].

Pathogenic WFS1 variants cause pathological endoplasmic reticulum (ER) stress in pancreatic β cells, neuron, retinal ganglion cells, and oligodendrocytes, resulting in the dysfunction and degeneration of affected tissues. Wolfram syndrome type 1 is thus a systemic disease caused by ER dysfunction. Cardinal manifestations in Wolfram syndrome type 1 are insulin-dependent diabetes mellitus, optic nerve atrophy, and neurodegeneration. Other symptoms often seen in these patients include diabetes insipidus, hearing loss, trigeminal neuralgia-like headaches, dysphagia, neurogenic bladder, anxiety, depression, and other neurologic conditions. Wolfram syndrome is also referred as *d*iabetes *i*nsipidus *d*iabetes *m*ellitus, *o*ptic nerve *a*trophy, and *d*eafness (DIDMOAD). Diabetes mellitus is typically the first manifestation, usually diagnosed around age 6, and optic nerve atrophy follows around age 11. Diabetes insipidus, sensorineural hearing loss, neurogenic bladder, and obstructive sleep apnea may also develop in the next two decades of life [19].

Patients with Wolfram syndrome type 2 develop cardinal features of Wolfram syndrome type 1, including diabetes mellitus and optic nerve atrophy, but they also tend to develop other symptoms that are not typically seen in patients carrying pathogenic WFS1 variants, such as upper gastrointestinal ulceration and bleeding. Based on clinical and genetic findings, Wolfram syndrome is best characterized as a spectrum of disorders, ranging in clinical severity from mild to severe [20].

27.2.2.1 WFS1-Related Disorders

Some pathogenic variants in the WFS1 gene are associated with a distinct subset of patients who develop only one or a few symptoms seen in Wolfram syndrome. Certain pathogenic variants of the WFS1 gene cause deafness or diabetes alone, while others are associated with deafness together with mild optic nerve atrophy. Another syndrome of neonatal/infancy-onset diabetes, congenital sensorineural deafness, and congenital cataracts has recently been described. All these patients are considered to have WFS1-related disorders, not Wolfram syndrome [21].

27.2.3 Mitochondrial Diabetes (MIDD, MELAS)

Mitochondrial diseases are rare, heterogeneous conditions caused by mutations in either the mitochondrial or nuclear DNA and can present with various clinical symptoms. Mitochondrial mutations are more common and are transmitted through maternal inheritance.

Mitochondrial diabetes most frequently results from the m.3243A>G mutation, responsible for both mitochondrial encephalomyopathy, lactic acidosis, and stroke-like episodes (MELAS) and maternally inherited diabetes and deafness (MIDD).

Clinical features that raise suspicion for mitochondrial diabetes include multi-organ involvement, elevated serum lactate levels, a more rapid progression to insulin therapy, and the earlier onset of diabetes-related complications compared to individuals with type 2 diabetes. Moreover, mitochondrial diabetes should be suspected in patients with clinical features including diabetes and hearing loss on the maternal side.

Diabetes in mitochondrial disease can present insidiously and is usually diagnosed in the fourth decade. This is thought to be primarily due to insulin deficiency secondary to beta-cell dysfunction, although insulin resistance may also occur. Other endocrinopathies reported in patients with mitochondrial disease include hypogonadism, adrenal dysfunction, hypoparathyroidism, and growth hormone deficiency.

MIDD often presents with diabetes in adulthood and bilateral sensorineural hearing loss which is progressive and typically precedes the diagnosis of diabetes. Other clinical features may occur such as macular pattern dystrophy, nephropathy, and neurological symptoms which are more common in rarer forms of mitochondrial diabetes than the classical form. The classic ophthalmic finding in these individuals is pigmentary retinal dystrophy rather than the diabetic retinopathy of type 2 diabetes. Patients also manifest impaired insulin secretion, and insulin treatment is eventually required for most of them [22, 23].

The main clinical characteristics of MELAS are encephalopathy defined by seizures and/or dementia, myopathy with/without red ragged fibers, recurrent headaches and vomiting, and stroke-like episodes below the age of 40 years. Lactic acidosis occurs in up to 94% of MELAS patients due to impaired glucose oxidation with subsequent accumulation of pyruvate and shunting to lactate [24].

27.3 Conclusion

This chapter provides an important insight into the diversity of genetic syndromes with DM. Despite their rarity, genetic syndromes associated with diabetes represent an important group of diseases. The genetic etiologies of these syndromes contribute toward our understanding of the pathophysiology of more common forms of DM, provide potential avenues for future gene identification efforts, promote gene therapy research, and may lead to the development of more personalized medicine treatments. For instance, activating mutations in KCNJ11 and ABCC8 cause a spectrum of diabetes conditions, including isolated neonatal diabetes, childhood diabetes, and adult-onset diabetes. These mutations also cause developmental delay, epilepsy, and neonatal diabetes (DEND) syndrome and are sensitive to sulfonylureas, which target the affected ATP-sensitive potassium channel in pancreatic β cells. Oral sulfonylureas demonstrate superior glycemic control to insulin injections in DEND syndrome, along with improvement of the associated neurological symptoms. As the field of personalized diabetic medicine is expanding, similar approaches are also being developed for the treatment of various symptoms of other diabetic syndromes. In this context valproate acid is being evaluated for its inhibitory effects on endoplasmic reticulum stress-induced apoptosis, which is also the underlying mechanism of the neurological manifestations of WFS.

References

1. American Diabetes A. 2. Classification and diagnosis of diabetes: standards of medical care in diabetes—2020. Diabetes Care. 2020;43(Suppl. 1):S14–31.
2. Yeung RO, Hannah-Shmouni F, Niederhoffer K, Walker MA. Not quite type 1 or type 2, what now? Review of monogenic, mitochondrial, and syndromic diabetes. Rev Endocr Metab Disord. 2018;19(1):35–52.
3. American Diabetes A. Diagnosis and classification of diabetes mellitus. Diabetes Care. 2014;37(Suppl. 1):S81–90.
4. Barrett TG. Differential diagnosis of type 1 diabetes: which genetic syndromes need to be considered? Pediatr Diabetes. 2007;8(Suppl. 6):15–23.
5. Shi D, Motamed M, Mejía-Benítez A, Li L, Lin E, Budhram D, Kaur Y, Meyre D. Genetic syndromes with diabetes: a systematic review. Obes Rev. 2021;22(9):e13303. https://doi.org/10.1111/obr.13303.
6. Hegele RA. Monogenic forms of insulin resistance: apertures that expose the common metabolic syndrome. Trends Endocrinol Metab. 2003;14(8):371–7.
7. Kadowaki H, et al. Four mutant alleles of the insulin receptor gene associated with genetic syndromes of extreme insulin resistance. Biochem Biophys Res Commun. 1997;237(3):516–20.
8. Kirkwood A, et al. Donohue syndrome: a review of literature, case series, and anesthetic considerations. Paediatr Anaesth. 2018;28(1):23–7.
9. Julier C, Nicolino M. Wolcott-Rallison syndrome. Orphanet J Rare Dis. 2010;5:29. https://doi.org/10.1186/1750-1172-5-29.
10. Passone CGB, Vermillac G, Staels W, Besancon A, et al. Mitchell-Riley syndrome: improving clinical outcomes and searching for functional impact of RFX-6 mutations. Front Endocrinol (Lausanne). 2022;13:802351. https://doi.org/10.3389/fendo.2022.802351.
11. Garg A. Clinical review: lipodystrophies: genetic and acquired body fat disorders. J Clin Endocrinol Metab. 2011;96:3313–25.
12. Chan JL, Oral EA. Clinical classification and treatment of congenital and acquired lipodystrophy. Endocr Pract. 2010;16:310–23.
13. Huang Q, Liu X, Zhang Y, Huang J, Li D, Li B. Molecular feature and therapeutic perspectives of immune dysregulation, polyendocrinopathy, enteropathy, X-linked syndrome. J Genet Genomics. 2020;47(1):17–26. https://doi.org/10.1016/j.jgg.2019.11.011.

14. Park JH, Lee KH, Jeon B, Ochs HD, Lee JS, Gee HY, Seo S, Geum D, Piccirillo CA, Eisenhut M, et al. Immune dysregulation, polyendocrinopathy, enteropathy, X-linked (IPEX) syndrome: a systematic review. Autoimmun Rev. 2020;19:102526.
15. Polak M, Shield J. Neonatal diabetes mellitus-genetic aspects. Pediatr Endocrinol Rev. 2004;2:193–8.
16. Khan SA, Parkash A, Ibrahim M. Permanent neonatal diabetes (DEND syndrome). J Coll Physicians Surg Pak. 2016;26(11):114–5.
17. Tahani N, Maffei P, Dollfus H, et al. Consensus clinical management guidelines for Alström syndrome. Orphanet J Rare Dis. 2020;15:253. https://doi.org/10.1186/s13023-020-01468-8.
18. De Franco E, et al. Dominant ER stress-inducing WFS1 mutations underlie a genetic syndrome of neonatal/infancy-onset diabetes, congenital sensorineural deafness, and congenital cataracts. Diabetes. 2017;66(7):2044–53.
19. Rigoli L, Di Bella C. Wolfram syndrome 1 and Wolfram syndrome 2. Curr Opin Pediatr. 2012;24(4):512–7.
20. Urano F. Wolfram syndrome: diagnosis, management, and treatment. Curr Diab Rep. 2016;16(1):6. https://doi.org/10.1007/s11892-015-0702-6.
21. de Muijnck C, Brink JBT, Bergen AA, Boon CJF, van Genderen MM. Delineating Wolfram-like syndrome: a systematic review and discussion of the WFS1-associated disease spectrum. Surv Ophthalmol. 2023;68(4):641–54. https://doi.org/10.1016/j.survophthal.2023.01.012.
22. Takeshima T, Nakashima K. MIDD and MELAS: a clinical spectrum. Intern Med. 2005;44(4):276–7. https://doi.org/10.2169/internalmedicine.44.276.
23. Kyriakidou A, Hadjivassiliou M, Papapostolou A, Picolos MK. Maternally inherited diabetes and deafness (MIDD)—atypical clinical diabetes features leading to the diagnosis. JCEM Case Rep. 2023;1(3):luad047. https://doi.org/10.1210/jcemcr/luad047.
24. El-Hattab AW, Adesina AM, Jones J, Scaglia F. MELAS syndrome: clinical manifestations, pathogenesis, and treatment options. Mol Genet Metab. 2015;116(1–2):4–12. https://doi.org/10.1016/j.ymgme.2015.06.004.

Part IV
Therapy of Diabetes-Related Diseases and Complications

Chapter 28
Dermatologic Treatment with Diabetic Implications

Cristina Bulai Livideanu

Abstract Some drugs, special systemic or topical corticoids, are often used in dermatology. However, they can have a lot of adverse effects, including diabetes mellitus. Often dermatologists are confronted to treat patients with a history of diabetes mellitus, and sometimes these medications can induce de novo type 2 diabetes mellitus.

Other drugs, more recently used by dermatologists can improve type 1 diabetes mellitus, as the baricitinib, an anti-JAK 1 and 2.

In this article we try to abord these three aspects of dermatologic treatments and diabetic implication.

In the practice of dermatology, the clinical practicians can meet three different situations:

1. To treat a patient with a known diabetes mellitus.
2. To discover diabetes mellitus during the treatment of other diseases.
3. Therapies that can avoid the diabetes mellitus.

28.1 Corticosteroids and Known Diabetes Mellitus

Firstly, when we need to treat a patient with known diabetes, we should pay attention to local and oral cortico-therapy. A lot of dermatological diseases need a local or oral cortico-therapy: systemic erythematous lupus (Fig. 28.1), dermatomyositis

C. B. Livideanu (✉)
Dermatology Department, CHU de Toulouse, Toulouse, France
e-mail: livideanu.c@chu-toulouse.fr

K. Fritz, G.-S. Tiplica (eds.), *Cutaneous Manifestations in Diabetes*,
https://doi.org/10.1007/978-3-031-65300-1_28

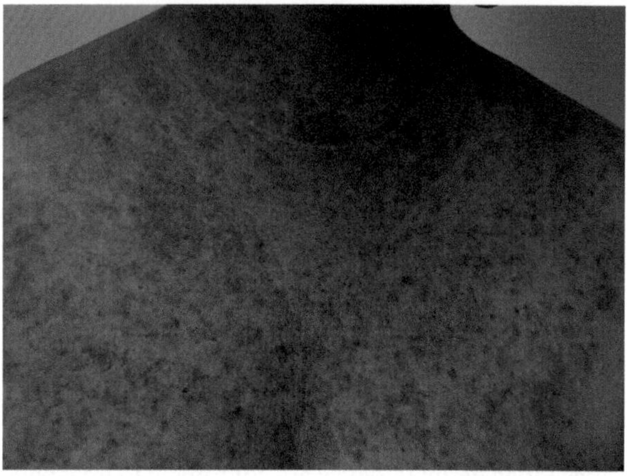

Fig. 28.1 Skin manifestation in systemic erythematosus lupus patient

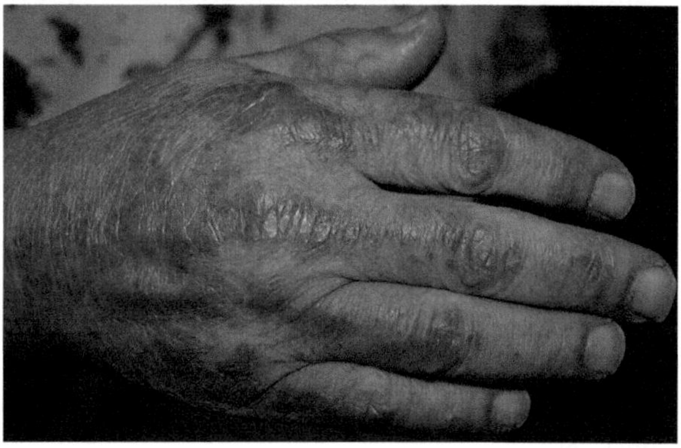

Fig. 28.2 Skin lesions in dermatomyositis patient

(Fig. 28.2), pemphigus (Fig. 28.3), pemphigoid bullous (Fig. 28.4), neutrophilic (Fig. 28.5), eosinophilic dermatosis (Fig. 28.6), mastocytosis (Fig. 28.7), and photodermatosis (Fig. 28.8). Often in these diseases, there is a cortico-dependence at relatively high dosage. If an immunosuppressive treatment is not started at the same time with corticoids, this last aspect (cortico-dependence at relatively high dosage) can induce multiple adverse effects including the worsening of diabetes mellitus.

Actually, as like as we known, there are several adverse effects of oral corticoids, such as perturbation of glycemic level—especially if the restriction of concentrated sweet foods is not avoided—arterial hypertension, cushingoid aspect with adrenal failure, and osteoporosis.

More studies made there several years show the aggravation of diabetes by oral corticoids [1–5].

In some countries as France, the first treatment of bullous pemphigoid is the local cortico-therapy with a very high dosage (40 g of clobetasol propionate cream applied per day, with the amount decreased over 12 months) that is equivalent to an oral cortico-therapy [6].

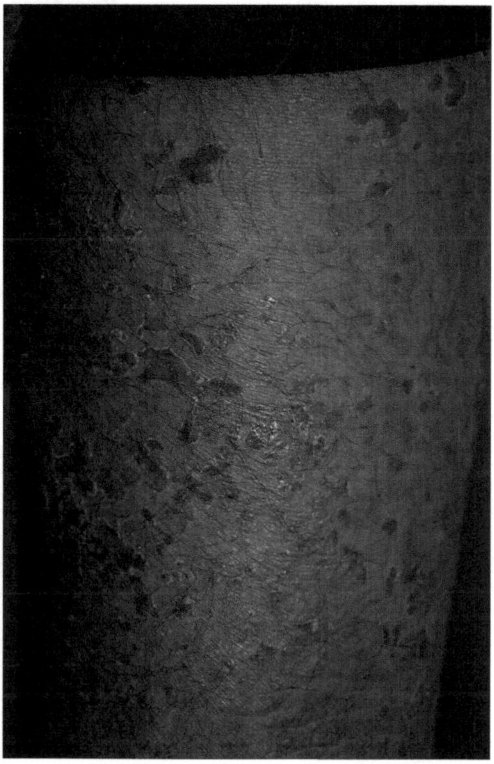

Fig. 28.3 Pemphigus lesions

Over time the atrophic skin (Fig. 28.9) in these patients increased the systemic passage of local cortico-therapy.

So, for the patients with known diabetes mellitus, the use of local or systemic corticoids, whether it is indispensable, has to have careful monitoring and correction of high blood sugar levels with insulin treatment.

28.2 Dapsone and Known Diabetes Mellitus

Dapsone is a treatment often use for neutrophilic diseases or linear bullous IgA disease. However, when we use this treatment to diabetic patients, we should inform her/his patient's diabetologist so that the management of diabetes is done according to the level of glycated hemoglobin A1c [7].

The dapsone has a negative effect on glycated hemoglobin A1c (HbA1c) in diabetic people. Actually, the dapsone dropped significantly the level of HbA1c and does not allow the control of glycemia by this analysis [8]. This adverse event to dapsone is done to interfere with possible hemolysis and/or methemoglobinemia induced by this. The process of methemoglobin formation depletes reduced

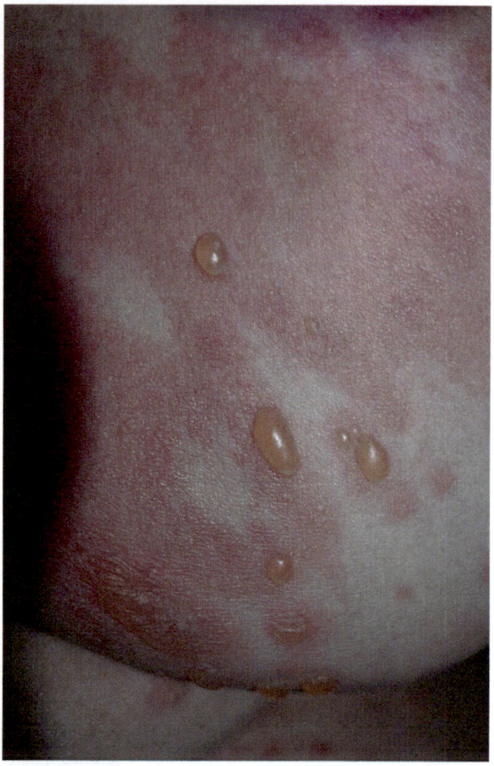

Fig. 28.4 Bullous pemphigoid lesions

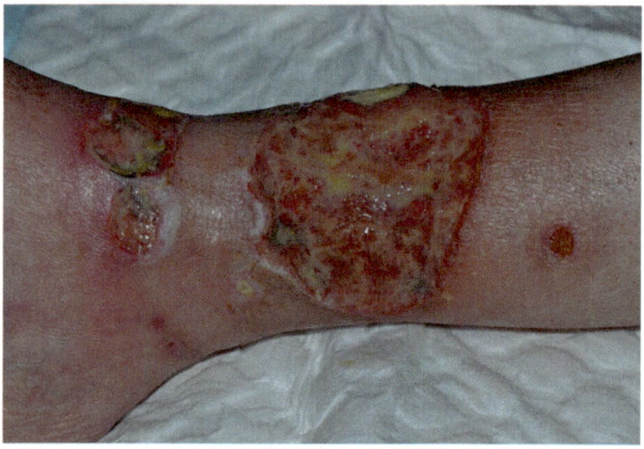

Fig. 28.5 Neutrophilic dermatosis

glutathione and then generates reactive oxygen species and impairs antioxidant defenses [7]. When monitoring diabetes, in the event of a discrepancy between blood sugar and glycated hemoglobin, it is advisable to measure fructosamine.

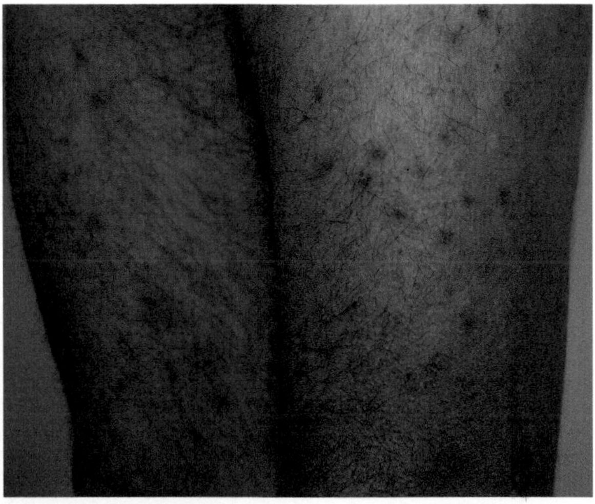

Fig. 28.6 Eosinophilic dermatosis

Fig. 28.7 Skin mastocytosis

28.3 Diabetes Mellitus Induced by Immunosuppressive Drugs

Secondly, some immunosuppressive drugs (ISDs) can induce diabetes mellitus in patients with dermatologic diseases.

Among these drugs corticoids are the main ISD responsible for diabetes mellitus. Actually, corticosteroids increase hepatic glucose production, through gluconeogenesis stimulation, and peripheral insulin resistance has been established for a long time and has deleterious effects on insulin secretion [9].

The predominant factor causing diabetes mellitus by corticosteroids seems to be the aggravation of insulin resistance; however, several studies have displayed deleterious effects on insulin secretion and β cells [10].

Oral corticosteroid users were significantly more likely than pomp proton inhibitor users to develop diabetes mellitus (adjusted rate ratio [aRR], 2.31; 95% confidence interval [95% CI], 2.11–2.54), while the risk of inhaled corticosteroid users was not significantly different from that of PPI users (aRR, 1.03; 95% CI, 0.93–1.14) [11].

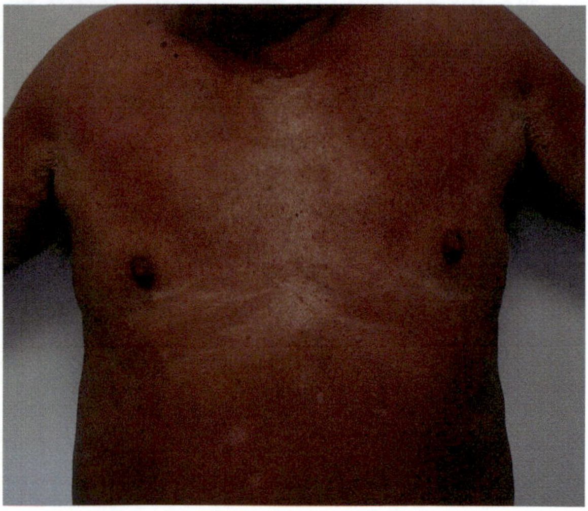

Fig. 28.8 Chronic photodermatosis lesions

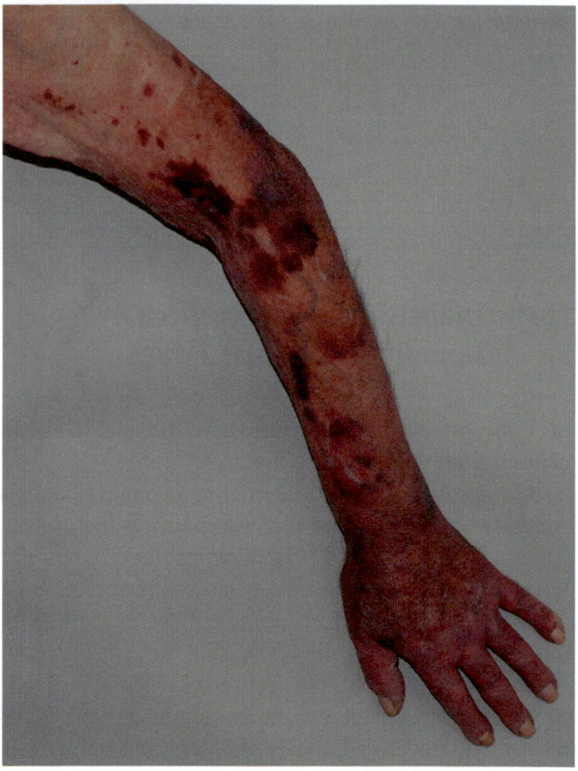

Fig. 28.9 Atrophic skin

Use of corticosteroids beyond 4 weeks has a significant risk of complications. The risks are therefore proportional to the dose and especially to the duration of treatment. Oral, rectal, intramuscular, and intravenous routes of administration have comparable absorption [12].

Local administration is preferable in terms of undesirable effects, but we must not lose sight of the fact that intra-articular, peri-articular, and epidural infiltrations are still absorbed systemically, often in a slow and prolonged manner and therefore have negative effects, so, adverse effects are also possible. Inhaled corticoids are also partially resorbed, and their use should be limited over time [12].

The equivalency of different corticoids, their anti-inflammatory and mineralocorticoid activity, the half-life, and the duration of biological action are shown in Table 28.1 [12].

The analysis of various factors invites us to propose rules of good practice for the prescription of corticosteroid treatments:

- Only initiate treatment with corticosteroids if there is sufficient evidence of objective benefits in this indication.
- Except in an emergency, always prefer a possible alternative treatment, especially if it is more specific (antihistamine, etc.).
- Administer the corticosteroid in sufficient doses and for a sufficient duration to be able to evaluate its effectiveness.
- Evaluate this effectiveness using objective, measurable, and reproducible criteria.
- Administer the corticosteroid at the lowest possible dose which maintains this effectiveness.

Table 28.1 Comparison of the properties of the main synthetic corticoids

	Equivalent dose (mg)	Relative anti-inflammatory activity	Relative mineralocorticoid activity	Half-life (minutes)	Duration of biological action (hours)
Hydrocortisone	20	1	1	80–120	8
Cortisone acetate	25	0.8	0.8	80–120	8
Prednisone	5	4	0.8	200	16–36
Prednisolone	5	4	0.8	120–300	16–36
Methylprednisolone	4	5	0.5	120–300	16–36
Triamcinolone	4	5	0	150–350	16–36
Betamethasone	0.75	25	0	150–350	16–36
Dexamethasone	0.68	30	0	150 to >350	36–72
Fludrocortisone	–	–	200	150 to >350	16–36

Dose equivalence refers to oral or intravenous administration of steroids. The anti-inflammatory and mineralocorticoid activities are expressed in relation to those of cortisol (data obtained from in vitro experiments). Prednisone, prednisolone, and methylprednisolone are strong glucocorticoids and weak mineralocorticoids. Triamcinolone, betamethasone, and dexamethasone do not have mineralocorticoid activity. Fludrocortisone is only used as a mineralocorticoid

- Do not prolong the treatment beyond the duration which is necessary to obtain the desired response.
- Stop treatment if no objective benefit is observed, if serious side effects occur, or if maximum benefit has been achieved.
- Treat associated conditions which increase the risk of corticosteroid toxicity and implement effective prevention measures [12].

Calcineurin inhibitors seemed to induce diabetes mellitus by a number of mechanisms, including decreased insulin secretion and a direct toxic effect on the pancreatic β cells. In vitro studies stress on the increased apoptosis of β cells when exposed to these drugs. In patients developing diabetes mellitus with calcineurin inhibitors, conversion from tacrolimus to cyclosporine could improve or reverse glucose tolerance abnormalities. However, more recent studies show that the risk of developing diabetes mellitus was not increased in comparison with CsA-based therapy [13].

28.4 Therapies That Can Prevent Diabetes Mellitus

Finally, some therapies seem to avoid diabetes mellitus. Type 1 diabetes is an autoimmune disease characterized by rapid destruction of insulin-producing pancreatic β cells by autoreactive T lymphocytes in children. Treatments that block cytokine signaling or target T or B lymphocytes have been successfully evaluated in animal models [14].

Janus kinase (JAK) inhibitors, including baricitinib (an inhibitor of JAK1 and 2), block cytokine signaling and are effective disease-modifying treatments for several autoimmune diseases such as atopic dermatitis, alopecia areata, etc.

A first-in-human international trial, funded by the International Diabetes Research Foundation and published in the New England Journal of Medicine, shows that baricitinib, an orally administered JAK1 and 2 inhibitors, can preserve production insulin by the body and slow the progression of type 1 diabetes in people who started treatment within 100 days of diagnosis.

The randomized double-blind study of Phase 2 human trial testing baricitinib versus placebo-monitored blood sugar and insulin production in 91 young, recently diagnosed type 1 diabetics over a 1-year period. Among these patients, aged 10–30 years at inclusion and suffering from type 1 diabetes diagnosed in the previous 100 days, 60 received baricitinib (4 mg once daily) and 31 a placebo [15].

The primary endpoint was the mean C-peptide level (representative of the quantity of insulin produced endogenously), determined from the area under the concentration time curve, during an insulin tolerance test 2-h mixed meal at week 48. Researchers also monitored participants' total daily insulin dose, blood sugar, and HbA1c levels [15].

Autoreactive CD8+ T cells in type 1 diabetes bind to the self-antigen peptide linked to HLA class I molecules on the surface of β cells and are activated by this peptide, resulting in the release of perforin and granzymes that cause β-cell death. The interaction between CD8+ T cells and HLA class I molecules has been shown to require intracellular signaling molecules associated with Janus kinase (JAK) [15].

Inhibitors of JAK1 and JAK2 isoforms decrease cytokine-induced major histocompatibility complex class I expression in islets and cultured islet cells, decrease CD8+ T-cell activation, and block the formation of immune synapses between β cells and CD8+ T cells to prevent β-cell death.

Furthermore, activating mutations in the signaling molecules STAT 110 (signal transducer and activator of transcription) and STAT311 downstream of JAKs are associated with the development of autoimmune diabetes [15].

In patients with new-onset type 1 diabetes, daily treatment with baricitinib for 48 weeks appears to preserve β-cell function, as estimated by the average C-peptide level stimulated by a mixed meal. In preclinical studies, nonobese diabetic mice that experienced remission of type 1 diabetes with JAK inhibitor treatment also had a progressive relapse after stopping this treatment, and in patients with autoimmune alopecia and juvenile idiopathic arthritis, relapse was observed after discontinuation of JAK inhibitor therapy [15].

It can therefore be assumed that a loss of β-cell function will be observed in study participants after stopping baricitinib. In future trials, researchers may consider giving baricitinib to patients while β-cell function persists or, earlier in the course of type 1 diabetes, at a point where it may still be possible to modify the course progression of autoimmune disease.

It would be more interesting to counter autoimmune dysfunction even earlier in the progressive course of the autoimmune disease. In most autoimmune diseases, there is in fact a very early stage ("window of opportunity") where immunomodulatory treatments really modify the progressive course of the disease, transforming an aggressive disease for the structures of the human body, into a less harmful disease [14].Conflict of InterestNone.

References

1. Conn H, Poynard T. Corticosteroids and peptic ulcer: meta-analysis of adverse events during steroid therapy. J Intern Med. 1994;236:619–32. https://doi.org/10.1111/j.1365-2796.1994.tb00855.x.
2. Dunning T. Corticosteroid medications and diabetes mellitus. Pract Diabetes Int. 1996;13(6):186–8. https://doi.org/10.1002/pdi.1960130610.
3. Lieberman P, Patterson R, Kunske R. Complications of long-term steroid therapy for asthma. J Allergy Clin Immunol. 1972;49:329–36. https://doi.org/10.1016/0091-6749(72)90131-5.
4. Smyllie H, Connolly C. Incidence of serious complications of corticosteroid therapy in respiratory disease. Thorax. 1968;23:571–81. https://doi.org/10.1136/thx.23.6.571.
5. Faul JL, Cormican LJ, Tormey VJ, et al. Deteriorating diabetic control associated with high-dose inhaled budesonide. Eur Respir J. 1999;14:242–3. https://doi.org/10.1183/09031936.99.141.
6. Joly P, Roujeau J-C, Benichou J, et al. A comparison of oral and topical corticosteroids in patients with bullous pemphigoid. N Engl J Med. 2002;346:321–7. https://doi.org/10.1056/NEJMoa011592.

7. Veggi LM, Pretto L, Ochoa EJ, et al. Dapsone induces oxidative stress and impars antioxidant defenses in rat liver. Life Sci. 2008;83:155–63. https://doi.org/10.1016/j.lfs.2008.05.016.
8. Lai Y-C, Wang C-S, Wang Y-C, et al. Falsely decreased HbA1c in a type 2 diabetic patient treated with dapsone. J For Med Ass. 2014;111:109–12.
9. Paty BW, Harmon JS, Marsh CL, et al. Inhibitory effects of immuno suppressive drugs on insulin secretion from HIT-T15 cells and Wis tar rat islets. Transplantation. 2002;73:353. https://doi.org/10.1097/00007890-200202150-00007.
10. McMahon M, Gerich G, Rizza R. Effects of glucocorticoids on car bohydrate metabolism. Diabetes Metab Rev. 1988;4:17. https://doi.org/10.1002/dmr.5610040105.
11. Blackburn D, Hux J, Mamdani M. Quantification of the risk of corticosteroid-induced diabetes mellitus among the elderly. J Gen Intern Med. 2002;17:717–20. https://doi.org/10.1046/j.1525-1497.2002.10649.x.
12. Maiter D. Du bon usage des corticoïdes en dermatologie clinique. In: C Colmant, D. Maiter, B.Vandeleene, M. Baeck, L. de Montjoye, editors. DermatologIe et endocrinologie. Accessed 14 January 2024: https://www.louvainmedical.be/sites/default/files/content/article/pdf/colmant_0.pdf, DOI: https://doi.org/10.1136/bmjopen-2023-077348
13. Penfornis A, Kury-Paulin S. Immunosuppressive drug-induced diabetes. Diabetes Metab. 2006;32:539–46. https://doi.org/10.1016/S1262-3636(06)72809-9.
14. Type 1 diabetes JAK inhibitor preserves insulin-producing pancreatic β cells. Fréquence médicale. Accessed 14 January 2024: requencemedicale.com/generaliste/actualites/11072-Diabete-de-type-1-un-inhibiteur-de-JAK-preserve-les-cellules-pancreatiques-productrices-d-insuline.
15. Waibel M, Wentworth JM, So M, et al. Baricitinib and β-cell function in patients with new-onset type 1 diabetes. N Engl J Med. 2023;389:2140–50. https://doi.org/10.1056/NEJMoa2306691.

Chapter 29
Adverse Skin and Systemic Reactions to Antidiabetic Treatments

Florence Tétart and Krisztian Gaspar

Abstract The different forms of diabetes mellitus affect millions of people worldwide. Depending on the types they suffer, patients are treated by insulins or by different antidiabetic drugs with various actions on glucose metabolism. As a result of recent developments, diabetic patients may be provided with new devices (e.g., glucose sensor, insulin pump) that increase compliance and therapeutic adherence. Just like any drugs, antidiabetics, as well as the supplementary instruments, may be able to provoke the formation of hypersensitivity reactions or other adverse events; however, fortunately such occasions occur rarely. The chapter introduces the most common hypersensitivity reactions to different type of antidiabetic drugs or complementary devices.

29.1 Introduction

The prevalence of diabetes worldwide reaches to 10.5% in the adult population, and it represents a genuine public health issue. While nowadays the disorder affects over half-a-billion people, it is estimated that in 20 years, it will dramatically raise to threat almost 800 million people in the world [1].

Florence Tétar and Krisztian Gaspar contributed equally to this work.

F. Tétart (✉)
Department of Allergology, Centre Erik Satie, CHU Rouen, Rouen, France

Department of Dermatology, CHU Rouen, Rouen, France
e-mail: florence.tetart@chu-rouen.fr

K. Gaspar (✉)
Department of Dermatology, Centre of Excellence, Faculty of Medicine, University of Debrecen, Debrecen, Hungary

HUN-REN-UD Allergology Research Group, Debrecen, Hungary
e-mail: gaspar.krisztian@med.unideb.hu

K. Fritz, G.-S. Tiplica (eds.), *Cutaneous Manifestations in Diabetes*,
https://doi.org/10.1007/978-3-031-65300-1_29

There are several forms of diabetes, such as type 1 diabetes, which is more common in children and adolescents, type 2 diabetes, and other rarer types of diabetes like gestational diabetes and maturity-onset diabetes of the young. The ratio of type 1 and type 2 diabetes is about 1–9. Treatment of type 1 diabetes is mainly based on insulin therapy and therapeutic education of the patient and his family. In type 2 diabetes, the therapeutic target is glycated hemoglobin (Hb) A1C less than or equal to 7% for most diabetic patients, and the therapeutic strategy is based on four axes: hygienic rules, dietary guidelines, the possible use of insulin therapy, and self-glycemic control by the patient. Therapeutic patient education is also fundamental in the management [2].

Besides the obvious insulin replacement in type 1 diabetes, the number of special treatments available in type 2 diabetes has increased significantly in recent years. The oral antidiabetic drugs (OADs) may be prescribed as monotherapy, dual therapy, or triple therapy that act on insulin sensitization, stimulation of beta cells, alpha-glucosidase inhibition, and sodium-glucose-linked transporter 2 inhibition. Available antidiabetic drugs are biguanides, sulfonylureas, glinides, alpha-glucosidases, gliptins (diphosphodiesterase IV inhibitors). Glucagon-like-peptide 1 (GLP-1) analogues are available as subcutaneous (SC) injections [2]. Additionally, glycemic control has been revolutionized by the arrival of continuous glucose recording devices.

Although "allergies" or hypersensitivities (HS) related to diabetes treatments remain rare, allergologists and dermatologists are likely to be confronted with them more often.

29.2 Hypersensitivity Reactions to Biguanides

Metformin is the most preferred biguanide available in the treatment of type 2 diabetes. Its predictable adverse effects are mainly related to gastrointestinal symptoms such as nausea, vomiting, abdominal pain, and diarrhea, while lactic acidosis may occur in case of drug overdose. Compared to the frequency metformin applied in diabetes, HS to metformin is very rare, and only few reports are available in the literature. The explanations behind the development of HS to metformin are scarce and poorly understood. Rapid onset laryngeal angioedema was reported by Atik et al. shortly (within 3 h) after metformin intake [3], while delayed HS had been registered in a form of DRESS [4], fixed-drug eruptions after several reintroductions of the drug [5–7], leukocytoclastic vasculitis [8, 9], erythema multiforme [10] or erythroderma [11].

29.3 Hypersensitivity to Sulfonylureas

Hypoglycemic sulfonamides have been prescribed less frequently since the introduction of new oral antidiabetics. Generally sulfonylureas are well tolerated and HS reactions are infrequent. A case of erythematous toxiderma with erythroderma has been described with gliclazide [12], in which the imputability of the drug was proven by a positive patch test. Stevens-Johnson syndrome (SJS) also occurred in a 31-year-old man after taking glipizide. In this latter case, no allergy testing was performed [13].

29.3.1 Cross-Reactivity with Other Sulfonamides and Paraphenylenediamine (PPD)

The question of cross-reactivity with sulfonamides such as sulfamethoxazole (SMX) or sulfadiazine (SDZ) often arises. The drug contains the chemical structure sulfonamide ($-SO_2NH_4$). There are many drugs that meet this definition, which can be classified into three groups according to Johnson et al. [14]:

- Sulfonylarylamines (sulfonamide chemical group attached to a benzene ring with an amine function (NH2) at the N4 position) in which antibiotics such as SMX and SDZ are mentioned.
- Non-sulfonylarylamines (sulfonamide chemical group attached to the benzene ring or other cyclic structure without the amine group at the N4 position) containing sulfonylureas, carbonic anhydrase-inhibitor diuretics, loop diuretics, thiazide diuretics, cyclooxygenase 2 inhibitors, and protease inhibitors.
- The molecules belonging to the third group have a sulfonamide group not directly bound to the benzene ring, e.g., triptans.

A literature review by Johnson et al. shows that the risk of cross-reactivity between antibiotic sulfonamides and sulfonylureas may not be based on any reliable data. Strom et al. studied reactions in over eight million Britons in a 12-year period. The risk of non-antibacterial sulfonamide HS is six times higher with a history of antibacterial sulfonamide HS (9.9%) compared to subjects with no history of allergic risk. Nevertheless, this risk remains low, less than 10% in the studied population. On the other hand, the same patients had reacted more frequently to penicillin (14%); the association may therefore be more related to a predisposition to HS reactions rather than to cross-reactivity with sulfonamides [15]. A study by Tornero et al. on sulfonamide cross-reactivity in patients with SMX EPF seems to confirm these data: in 28 patients tested by patch test and then reintroduction test, 4 had a positive patch test for SMX and 1 for SDZ. Of the 22 patients who agreed to reintroduction, 6 had cross-reactivity with SDZ, and none had cross-reactivity with other non-antibacterial sulfonamides [16]. Based on these results, it may be concluded that there is no contraindication to treating a patient, who is labeled allergic to SMX, with an antidiabetic product containing sulfonylurea.

Cross-reactivity has also been reported between PPD and drugs with amine para-*function, such* as sulfonamides. The Ottawa team reported 134 patients with PPD contact allergy and cross-reactivity with sulfonamides in 6% of patients. Thus there is no contraindication to use sulfonamides in patients allergic to PPD, and the cross-reactivity does not need to be mentioned on the PPD exclusion sheets provided to the patient [17].

29.4 Hypersensitivity to Gliptins

Gliptins, dipeptidyl peptidase IV (DPP-IV) inhibitors, are a new class of oral antidiabetic drugs indicated for type 2 diabetes in adults, alone or in combination with metformin (Table 29.1). DPP-IV inactivates glucagon-like peptide, GLP-1, and glucose-dependent insulinotropic peptide (GIP). Inhibition of DPP-IV results in a significant increase in the concentration of GLP-1 and GIP which causes an increase in insulin secretion and a decrease in glucagon secretion. Gliptins, in type 2 diabetics, significantly decrease HbA1C, without effect on patients' weight [18].

In preclinical studies vildagliptin caused skin lesions in chimpanzees [19], while after its commercial launch, there were severe toxiderma cases described. An article investigated the side effects of sitagliptin reported between 2006 and 2008 and reported 26 cases of severe toxidermas, including 2 SJS and 2 Lyell's syndromes [20]. Besides angioedemas (AE) and bullous pemphigoids (BPs) are the most frequent cutaneous side effects in daily practice.

29.4.1 Drug-Induced Bradykinin Angioedema and Gliptins

The angiotensin-converting enzyme (ACE) is responsible for the breakdown of bradykinin. When inhibited, there is an accumulation of bradykinin by default degradation; thus AE develops. Its frequency is approximately 0.2% in patients treated with ACE

Table 29.1 The main antidiabetic drugs

Drug class	DCI	Class characteristics
Biguanides	Metformin	Variations of hypersensitivity reactions (EPF, EMP, lichen, etc.)
Sulfamides	Gliclazide Glibenclamide Glimepiride Glipizide	Rare cross-reactivity with other sulfonamides and PPD justifying no contraindication
Gliptins or phosphodiesterase IV inhibitors	Sitagliptin Vildagliptin Saxagliptin	Bradykinin angioedema in association with ACE inhibitors, induced bullous pemphigoids, vildagliptin more often involved
Gliptins or phosphodiesterase IV inhibitors in combination with metformin	Sitagliptin + metformin Vildagliptin + metformin Saxagliptin + metformin	
Glinides	Repaglinide	Some cases of erythematous drug dermatitis
Alpha-glucosidase inhibitors	Acarbose Miglitol	Low digestive absorption Exceptional cases of AGEP
GLP1 analogues (injections)	Dulaglutide Exenatide Liraglutide	Few hypersensitivity reactions

inhibitors [21]. It is interesting to note that ACE inhibitors are frequently prescribed for diabetic patients to treat possible hypertension, for its nephroprotective effect and for cardiac purposes. DPP-IV (inhibited by gliptins) inactivates incretins and influences the degradation of bradykinin; thus IDPP-IV increases the half-life of bradykinins and promotes the occurrence of bradykinin AEs, especially in patients treated with ACE inhibitors [22–24]. A meta-analysis by Brown et al. compares the incidence of AEs in patients treated with vildagliptin and in patients treated with the comparator in phase III randomized clinical trials. Out of 13,921 patients treated in these trials, 55 had AE, including 27 confirmed cases. Of these 27 confirmed cases, 19 patients were in the vildagliptin group. Of these 19 patients, 14 (73%) were treated with ACE inhibitors, 11 of whom had been treated for more than a year. The risk of developing AE was greater in the group treated with 100 mg vildagliptin versus 50 mg, which effect is consistent with the pharmacological mechanism of bradykinin AEs [22]. The occurrence of AE in a patient treated with gliptins without association with an ACE inhibitor seems possible, too [25]. One observation reports the disappearance of AE upon switching from vildagliptin treatment to another gliptin, alogliptin [26]. Gibbs et al. suggest that the degree of inhibition of DPP-IV is different depending on the form of gliptin prescribed, so does the occurrence of AE vary depending on the molecule [27]. Thus, AEs are reported in the meta-analysis of clinical trials of vildagliptin, while no cases are reported in the meta-analysis of sitagliptin [22, 28].

29.4.2 Bullous Pemphigoids and Gliptins

Bullous pemphigoid (BP) is an autoimmune skin disease characterized by the occurrence of subepidermal bullae mainly in the elderly (incidence of 162 cases per million inhabitants in those over 70 years) [29]. Two recent pharmacovigilance studies have confirmed the increased risk of occurrence of BP in a patient treated with gliptins. All gliptins are suspected, which suggests a class effect; however, vildagliptin is overrepresented in these two studies [30, 31]. A study based on data from the Finnish Health Insurance Registry showed a tenfold risk of BP occurrence in patients treated with vildagliptin. This risk was also increased in patients taking a combination of gliptin and metformin, but there was no increased risk when metformin was taken alone [32]. A retrospective French-Swiss case-control study, carried out between 2014 and 2016, highlighted evidence of an increased risk of occurrence of BP when taking gliptin (adjusted odds ratio (OR) = 2.64; CI: 1.19–5.85; $p = 0.02$) with an additional risk when taking vildagliptin (adjusted OR = 3.57; CI: 1.07–11.84; $p = 0.04$) [33]. In this study gliptin cessation along with BP treatment resulted in a complete remission in 95% of cases. A work of the French Society of Dermatology compared the frequency of prescription of gliptins in a population suffering from BP and in the general population (data from the Health Data Institute). After indirect age standardization, 6% of patients with BP took gliptins versus 3.8% in the general population ($p < 0.001$), 2.4% versus 2.5% for sitagliptin, and 3.7% versus 0.8% for vildagliptin ($p < 0.001$) [34]. The possible mechanism of gliptin-induced BP is not elucidated: it may be de novo BP or revelation of BP in patients likely to present one.

Gliptin-induced BP has been described with a specific, rather noninflammatory phenotype (low amounts of circulating and skin-infiltrating eosinophils), with immunoglobulin (Ig)G, IgE, and IgA humoral responses to BP180 and BP230 antigens reduced in frequency and titers compared with those in patients with idiopathic BP; additionally IgG reactivity targets multiple BP180 epitopes other than noncollagenous region 16A [35]. The question in these drug-induced autoimmune diseases is always whether or not to stop the drug responsible. A study compared the evolution of BP after 3 months relative to the continuation or discontinuation of gliptin (interestingly, 67.5% of these patients were taking vildagliptin). 65% of patients achieved complete response of their BP after the discontinuation of gliptin, whereas only 5% of patients achieved complete response when the gliptin was continued. Therefore, stopping the drug seems to allow a complete response within 3–6 months [36].

29.5 Hypersensitivity to Glinides

Glinides (e.g., repaglinide, nateglinide) are a class of insulin-secreting OADs prescribed as monotherapy or in combination with metformin. The known side effects are mainly digestive ones (such as hypoglycemia, nausea, vomiting, diarrhea, dyspepsia), and occasionally headache may occur. Their use from the allergological point of view is safe, HS is unlikely. One case of maculopapular rash after repaglinide use was published. Although allergy tests (0.5 µg/mL repaglinide prick test and 0.05% repaglinide in water and petroleum jelly patch test) were negative, reintroduction tests (repaglinide 0.125 µg; 0.25 µg; 0.5 µg) and consequent histopathology confirmed HS in this case [37]. There are 17 cases mentioned in the French national pharmacovigilance database of HS to glinides.

29.6 Hypersensitivity to Alpha-Glucosidase Inhibitors

Acarbose is the most often used alpha-glucosidase inhibitor in diabetes. One case of erythema multiforme [38] and three cases of acute generalized exanthematous pustulosis (AGEP) [39, 40] related to acarbose have been reported. Acarbose has very low digestive absorption, and low serum levels are still enough to trigger AGEP.

29.7 Hypersensitivity to Glucagon-like Peptide-1 (GLP-1) Analogues

GLP-1 analogues (e.g., exenatide, liraglutide, dulaglutide) increase insulin secretion and inhibit glucagon secretion, slow gastric emptying, and increase feelings of satiety. Side effects are mainly digestive problems (diarrhea, nausea, vomiting), risk of hypoglycemia, and rarely injection site reactions. Allergic reactions to GLP-1 analogues have been described in the literature. Steveling et al. reported the development of type 1 HS reaction (urticaria, pruritus, shortness of breath) after reintroduction of exenatide in a 52-year-old diabetic male patient. Sensitization to the drug was proved by intradermal tests [41]. Perez et al. also reported immediate allergic responses after the reintroduction of exenatide [42] that must make the physician being very cautious prior to restarting of the drug after long drug-holiday period. The development of anaphylactic shock has also been reported after exenatide use [43, 44]. Such alerting accidents had led to the need to develop the desensitization protocol for exenatide allergy patients [45]. Late-type dermal HS reactions have also been reported with liraglutide [46] and with semaglutide [47].

29.8 Hypersensitivity to Insulin

Human insulin is a peptide hormone synthesized by B cells of the islets of Langerhans, consisting of two polypeptide chains and disulfide bridges. In the 1980s, the first commercially available insulins of bovine or porcine origin, which are responsible for many cases of hypersensitivity, were replaced by recombinant human insulins (insulin zinc and insulin neutral protamine hagedorn (NPH)) insulin is an insoluble intermediate-acting insulin preparation, which are less allergenic. Since 1990, advances in genetic engineering have made it possible to commercialize human insulin analogues. Their primary chemical structure differs from human insulin by an amino acid (AA), which makes it possible to mimic physiological insulin secretion after subcutaneous absorption. In 2014, the first biosimilar insulin was introduced. This therapeutic revolution has led to a decrease in the frequency of HS to insulins, about 0.1–3% of users [48]. These hypersensitivity reactions can occur in children, type 2 diabetics, and women with gestational diabetes as well [49–51]. Possible differential diagnoses should be eliminated, such as contact eczema with antiseptics, soaps, latex that may be contained in cartridge caps, allergy to insulin pump cannapul, etc. [52]. The mechanisms of HS to insulins are, in descending order of frequency, (1) type 1-mediated HS reactions responsible for localized injection site reactions and/or generalized reactions, by far the most frequent, (2) delayed type 4 HS responsible for itchy erythematous nodules, (3) HS mediated by type 3 immune complexes responsible for localized reactions or serum disease [53].

The injection technique appears to be important with a case of HS described in a patient who performed his injections intradermally instead of SC [54].

All insulins can be responsible for HS with significant cross-reactivity linked to their identical chemical structure "within one AA." From this different AA comes the name of the analogues: for example, in insulin lispro, a proline is replaced by a lysine, and in insulin glargine, the asparagine is replaced by a glycine. There may also be a possibility to develop a HS reaction with insulin analogues in patients naïve to human insulin treatment [55] and HS to biosimilar insulin glargine [56]. It is therefore essential to carry out allergological tests by prick test and intradermal reactions (up to pure concentration if necessary) under hospital supervision. It is necessary to count the number of units administered to patients during these tests and monitor patients' blood sugar levels during the investigation. In the event of cross-reactivity between all insulins (the most common case), the insulin which reacted the least can be chosen for tolerance induction by SC injections or by continuous SC injection (insulin pump) [57, 58]. SC insulin glargine may be chosen preferentially in the first case. Indeed, insulin glargine forms precipitates under the skin, which means that it is released very gradually and thus mimics a continuous SC injection [59]. Several continuous SC injection desensitization protocols have been published. When allergy tests were performed again after these protocols, they were negative, and the patients could be treated again with SC injections.

29.9 Hypersensitivity to the Glycemic Sensor of Non-needle Glucose Meters and Insulin Pump Adhesives

The FreeStyle® glucose meter has revolutionized the care of people with diabetes, allowing them to measure their blood glucose levels several times a day using a sensor placed on their shoulder for a period of 15 days, thus avoiding repeated spears of the fingers. Skin reactions to these devices—irritation or contact allergy—are the first cause of device abandonment. Collaboration between dermato-allergologists and diabetologists has enabled us to identify new contact allergens and to try to improve the composition of these medical devices. A capillary blood glucose sensor consists of a catheter inserted subcutaneously, connected to a transmitter unit, all held to the skin by an adhesive patch for 10–15 days, depending on the model. The main models are the FreeStyle Libre® from Dexcom® and the Enlite®.

Insulin pumps consist of an insulin reservoir and a needle inserted subcutaneously and held on the skin for 3–5 days by an adhesive patch. Depending on the device, the two parts are connected by tubing (wired pump) or not (patch pump). Such devices are Omnipod®, paradigm MiniMed Quick-set®, and Medtrum®.

When the insulin pump is connected to the capillary glycemia sensor, insulin can be injected directly according to predefined parameters based on capillary glycemia levels. This method is the first step toward an artificial pancreas. In the event of a skin reaction, this is a major challenge for patients, particularly those with type 1 diabetes.

Skin reactions appear to be frequent: according to a recent French study, 29% of insulin pump users and 28% of blood glucose sensor users had skin reactions, and these were the cause of device discontinuation in 2.1% of insulin pump users and 3.2% of blood glucose sensor users [60]. Skin reactions can range from erythema and itching to pain, vesicles, and, more rarely, lipodystrophy, pigmentation disorders (hyper- or hypopigmentation), and hematomas. Eczematous patches can be linked to either irritant dermatitis or allergic contact dermatitis. The clinical appearance does not always allow us to distinguish between the two. In the case of irritant dermatitis, the patient readily describes a burning sensation, and the skin is erythematous, scaly, purpuric without vesicle formation. The dermatitis is limited to the area of contact with the adhesion, and there is no secondary generalization of the eruption. In allergic contact dermatitis, on the other hand, the patient describes severe itching. The skin is highly inflammatory, erythematous, edematous, vesicular, and sometimes even bullous. The eczema often extends beyond the area of contact and may even become generalized.

Skin dryness, exposure to increased humidity (e.g., perspiration), and prolonged contact with the adhesive are all factors that contribute to irritant dermatitis. Irritation then provides the "breeding ground" for allergen sensitization: the skin barrier altered by irritation encourages allergens to penetrate the skin, leading to sensitization and allergic contact dermatitis. In the case of our diabetic patients, sensitization is often triggered by wearing a blood glucose sensor, which is changed only every 10–15 days, followed by contact allergy to it and to the insulin pump, which is changed more frequently.

Allergy prevention involves managing and preventing irritation by simple measures, such as restoring the skin barrier through proper moisturizing, using nonirritating cleansing gels like soap-free surgras and regularly changing the sites where medical devices are applied.

Only allergological investigation and the identification of a contact allergen can confirm that contact dermatitis is allergic to the medical device in question.

Insulin pumps and blood glucose sensors are medical devices. Legislation (EU Regulation 2017/745) was unclear about the labeling of these devices, and collaboration with companies on composition was difficult. Allergen identification then required chemical analyses of the devices by research laboratories. Several learned societies took a stand on the need for better labeling [61]. Legislation has since evolved. Since May 26, 2021, labeling must include the product's serial number, the name of an authorized European representative for manufacturers outside the EU, additional warnings and precautions concerning the device, and a list of all the medical substances it contains derived from tissues and cells, all carcinogenic or mutagenic substances, or all substances toxic for reproduction, as well as a clear symbol indicating that the product is a medical device.

Isobornyl acrylate (IBOA) is contained in several devices for diabetic patients as an identified allergen. It is an acrylate monomer commonly used in many products such as inks, floor coverings, adhesives, plasticizers, and paints. In 2017, when the FreeStyle Libre© sensor was launched, numerous cases of contact eczema occurred, with negative allergological investigations for the usual allergens. The Antwerp team then used chromatographic analysis to identify the presence of IBOA in the sensor. A few cases of contact eczema caused by IBOA in an insulin infusion set had been reported in 1995 [62]. Several patients with contact eczema to FreeStyle® subsequently tested positive for this allergen [63]. Patients allergic to IBOA have been tested with original adhesives not yet attached to the plastic casing, and the tests remained negative, reinforcing this hypothesis of IBOA migration from the plastic casing glue to the adhesive [64]. Since then, the allergen has been removed from the composition of FreeStyle Libre but identified in other devices such as the Enlite® sensor, the Medtrum® A6, a new version of the Dexcom G6, Omnipod® insulin pumps, and the Paradigm MiniMed Quick-Set infusion set [64–66]. The European Chemicals Agency (ECHA) recognizes IBOA as a category 1A skin sensitizer (associated risk phrase H317: may cause an allergic reaction). Current legislation thus obliges manufacturers to indicate the presence of IBOA if its concentration exceeds 0.1% in medical devices in direct contact with the skin. However, IBOA can cause contact allergies at lower concentrations (even <100 ppm). IBOA has even been voted Allergen of the Year 2020 by the American Contact Dermatitis Society [67].

Other molecules have been identified in medical devices. Ethyl cyanoacrylate has been identified in the Platinum G4 Dexcom® sensor. This allergen is used in the nail industry, and patients sensitized by this sensor may subsequently develop allergic contact eczema to gel nails [68]. N-N-dimethylacrylamide (DMAA) has been identified in FreeStyle® Libre and Medtronic® insulin pump kits [65]. DMAA is an allergen often present in association with IBOA in UV-curing adhesives such as Loctite®. Sensitization to DMAA appears to be less frequent than sensitization to IBOA [69]. Other acrylates have been identified more anecdotally: phenoxyethoxy ethylacrylate, 2,2′-methylenebis(6-tert-butyl-4-methylphenol) monoacrylate MBPA, dipropylene glycol diacrylate DPGDA [66].

Colophane, derived from pine gum, is a widespread allergen used for its sticky properties, for example, in violin bows, or modified in shoe varnishes, glues, and other products. Modified rosin and related molecules such as methyl dehydroabietate, abitol, and abietic acid have been used in insulin pumps such as the Omnipod®, the Enlite® blood glucose sensor, and the insulin pump kit of the same brand. An Italian study showed that almost half of diabetic children with skin reactions to their blood glucose meter were sensitized to rosin [70]. Some patients use adhesive barrier wipes to increase the adherence of their device. Rosin has been identified as the allergen responsible for skin reactions to these wipes [71].

Benzoyl peroxide and epoxy resins have also been cited in the literature. When an eczematous patch appears while using blood glucose sensors or insulin pumps, the only way to formally differentiate between irritant dermatitis and allergic contact dermatitis is to carry out a patch test. The principle of patch testing is to apply allergen-containing cups to the patient's back, under occlusion for 48 h. After the removal the response must be read and evaluated at 48 h, 72/96 h, and 1 week. Semi-open tests are also recommended, when pieces of the devices in question are applied to the patient's skin under a nonocclusive dressing. When the test is read, it is also determined whether the patient has a reaction to a particular allergen, and the practitioner then interprets these tests to establish their relevance (presence/absence of sensitization). These tests can be carried out by a dermatologist, or by an allergist, or ideally by a dermato-allergist. It should be noted that, following the outbreak of contact allergies to FreeStyle® libre, IBOA, not previously marketed, is now available from Chemotechnique at a concentration of 0.1% in petroleum. For dermatologists and allergists who do not have access to complementary test materials, a good knowledge of cross-reactivity between allergens in the standard European serial and allergens in medical devices for diabetic patients is essential.

IBOA does not cross-react with other acrylates, notably 2-hydroxyethylmethacrylate (2-HEMA) present in the standard test, but crosses with sesquiterpène lactone mix. This allergen is found in plants of the Compositae and Asteraceae families. Ethyl cyanoacrylate does not cross-react with IBOA but does cross-react with other acrylates, including 2-HEMA. As with any contact allergy, sensitized patients must avoid contact with the allergen in question. Medical devices containing the molecule(s) responsible cannot therefore be offered to the patient in theory. However, it sometimes happens that a patient allergic to a medical device containing IBOA can tolerate a medical device containing it without a skin reaction. The two hypotheses are that the IBOA is present but in lesser quantities and that there is immunity tolerance. It is possible to limit direct exposure by interposing a dressing between the device and the skin. However, this has three limitations. Firstly, the allergen may migrate through the dressing; secondly, the dressing itself may contain allergens such as rosin; and thirdly, the UK Medicines and Healthcare products Regulatory Agency (MHRA) advises against the application of skin barriers or dressings and warns of the risk of device malfunction. Application of a corticosteroid nasal spray (fluticasone propionate, mometasone, clobetasol propionate 0.05% in an alcohol-based solution) under the device may prevent skin irritation [72].

29.10 Conclusion

"Allergies" or HS to antidiabetic drugs are rare, but with the prevalence of diabetes rising sharply, allergists and dermatologists are likely to be increasingly confronted with them. Diabetics are often polymedicated, and drug interactions such as between ACE inhibitors and gliptins can lead to pharmacological side effects such as bradykinic AEs. IgE-mediated allergies, which are potentially serious, are described in particular with insulins of any kind. Medical devices (glycemic sensors, insulin pumps) can be the cause of contact eczema, allowing new allergens such as IBOA to be (re)discovered.

Acknowledgments The work of KG was supported by Hungarian Research Grants (NKFIH K-142348 and NKFIH PD-131689) and Hungarian Research Network (HUN-REN).

FT and KG are representatives of European Reference Network for Rare Skin Diseases (ERN-Skin) ToxiTEN Group.

References

1. Sun H, Saeedi P, Karuranga S, et al. IDF diabetes atlas: global, regional and country-level diabetes prevalence estimates for 2021 and projections for 2045. Diabetes Res Clin Pract. 2022;183:109119.
2. Dahlen AD, Dashi G, Maslov I, et al. Trends in antidiabetic drug discovery: FDA approved drugs, new drugs in clinical trials and global sales. Front Pharmacol. 2022;12:807548.
3. Atik D, Büyükcam F, Yilmaz D, et al. Angioedema after the first dose of metformin. Am J Emerg Med. 2013;31:634–5.
4. Voore P, Odigwe C, Mirrakhimov AE, et al. DRESS syndrome following metformin administration: a case report and review of the literature. Am J Therapeut. 2016;23:1970–3.

5. Steber CJ, Perkins SL, Harris KB. Metformin-induced fixed-drug eruption confirmed by multiple exposures. Am J Case Rep. 2016;17:231–4.
6. Ramırez-Bellver JL, Lopez J, Macias E, et al. Metformin induced generalized fixed drug eruption with cutaneous hemophagocytosis. Am J Dermatopathol. 2017;39(6):471–5.
7. Abtahi-Naeini B, Momen T, Amari R, et al. Metformin-induced generalized bullous fixed-drug eruption with a positive dechallenge-rechallenge test: a case report and literature review. Case Rep Dermatol Med. 2023;2023:6353919.
8. Ben Salem C, Hmouda H, Slim R, et al. Rare case of metformin-induced leukocytoclastic vasculitis. Ann Pharmacother. 2006;40(9):1685–7.
9. Czarnowicki T, Ramot Y, Ingber A, et al. Metformin-induced leukocytoclastic vasculitis: a case report. Am J Clin Dermatol. 2012;13(1):61–3.
10. Burger DE, Goyal S. Erythema multiforme from metformin. Ann Pharmacother. 2004;38:1537.
11. Diaz JM, Brunen JMG, Cameo RB, et al. Erythroderma and chronic lichenification due to metformin. Eu J Case Rep Intern Med. 2019;6:001119.
12. Ozuguz P, Dogruk Kacar S, Ozuguz U, et al. Erythroderma secondary to gliclazide: a case report. Cutan Ocul Toxicol. 2014;33:342–4.
13. Cheng JB, Anderson RC, Cruz PD. Stevens-Johnson syndrome associated with glipizide therapy. Dermatitis. 2006;17:36–8.
14. Johnson KK, Green DL, Rife JP, et al. Sulfonamide cross-reactivity: fact or fiction? Ann Pharmacother. 2005;39:290–1.
15. Strom BL, Schinnar R, Apter AJ, et al. Absence of cross-reactivity between sulphonamide antibiotics and sulphonamide non-antibiotics. N Engl J Med. 2003;349:1628–35.
16. Tornero P, De Barrio M, Baeza L, et al. Cross-reactivity among p-amino group coumpounds in sulfonamide fixed drug eruption: diagnostic value of patch testing. Contact Derm. 2004;51:57–62.
17. Laberge L, Pratt M, Fong B, et al. A 10-year review of p-phenylenediamine allery and related para-amino compounds at the Ottawa patch test clinic. Dermatitis. 2011;22:322–34.
18. Herman GA, Bergman A, Liu F, et al. Pharmacokinetics and pharmacodynamic effects of the oral DPP-4 inhibitor sitagliptin in middle-aged obese subjects. J Clin Pharmacol. 2006;46:876–86.
19. European Medical Agency. EMA monkey study report. http://www.ema.europa.eu/docs/en_GB:document_library/EPAR-hcientific_Discussion/human/000807/WC500030597.pdf. Accesses September 2013.
20. Desai S, Brinker A, Swann J, et al. Sitagliptin-associated drug allergy: review of spontaneaous adverse event reports. Arch Intern Med. 2010;170:1169–71.
21. Brown T, Gonzalez J, Monteleone C. Angiotensin-converting enzyme inhibitor-induced angioedema: a review of the literature. J Clin Hypertens. 2017;19:1377–82.
22. Smolinska S, Antolin-Amerys D, Popescu FD. Bradykinin metabolism and drug induced angioedema. Int J Mol Sci. 2023;24:11649.
23. Hahn J, Trainotti S, Hoffmann TK, et al. Drug-induced inhibition of angiotensin converting enzyme and dipeptidyl peptidase 4 results in nearly therapy resistant bradykinin induced angioedema: a case report. Am J Case Rep. 2017;18:576–9.
24. Faisant C, Armengol G, Bouillet L, et al. Angioedema triggered by medication blocking the renin/angiotensin system: retrospective study using the french national pharmacovigilance database. J Clin Immunol. 2016;36:95–102.
25. Ohyama K, Shindo J, Takahasi T, et al. Pharmacovigilance study of the association between dipeptidyl peptidase-4 inhibitors and angioedema using the FDA adverse event reporting system (FAERS). Sci Rep. 2022;12:13122.
26. Saisho Y, Itoh H. Dipeptidyl peptidase-4 inhibitors and angioedema: a class effect? Diab Med. 2013;30:e149–50.
27. Gibbs JP, Fredrickson J, Barbee T, et al. Quantitative model of the relationship between dipeptidyl peptidase-4 inhibition and response: meta-analysis of alogliptin, saxagliptin, sitagliptin and vildagliptin efficacy results. J Clin Pharmacol. 2012;52:1494–505.

28. Williams-Herman D, Engel SS, Round E, et al. Safety and tolerability of sitagliptin in clinical studies: a pooled analysis of data from 10246 patients with type 2 diabetes. BMC Endocr Disord. 2010;10:7.
29. Joly P, Baricault S, Sparsa A, et al. Incidence and mortality of bullous pemphigoid in France. J Invest Dermatol. 2012;132:1998–2004.
30. Garcia M, Aranburut A, Palacios-Zabalza I, et al. Dipeptidyl peptidase-IV inhibitors induced bullous pemphigoid: a case report and analysis of cases reported in the European pharmacovigilance database. J Clin Pharm Ther. 2016;41:368–70.
31. Bene J, Moulis G, Bennami I, et al. Bullous pemphigoid and dipeptidyl peptidase IV inhibitors: a case-non case study in the French pharmacovigilance database. Br J Dermatol. 2016;175:296–301.
32. Varpuluoma O, Försti AK, Jokelainen J, et al. Vildagliptin significantly increases the risk of bullous pemphigoid: a finish nationwide registry study. J Invest Dermatol. 2018;138:1659–61.
33. Benzaquen M, Borradori L, Berbis P, et al. Dipeptidyl peptidase-IV inhibitors, a risk factor for bullous pemphigoid. Retrospective multicenter case-control study from France and Switzerland. J Am Acad Dermatol. 2018;78:1090–6.
34. Plaquevent M, Tétart F, Fardet L, et al. Higher frequency of dipeptidyl peptidase-4 inhibitor intake in bullous pemphigoid patients than in the French general population. J Invest Dermatol. 2016;136:2201–10.
35. Salemme A, Fania L, Scarabello A, et al. Gliptin-associated bullous shows peculiar features of anti-BP180 and BP230 humoral response: results of a multicentre study. J Am Acad Dermatol. 2022;87:56–63.
36. Prugnit-Rouanet M, Delaumenie S, Couraud A, et al. Gliptin-induced bullous pemphigoid: withdrawal of gliptin allows for faster control of the disease. Eur J Dermatol. 2022;32:368–72.
37. Rojas P, Sanchez L, Santos A, et al. Hypersensitivity to repaglinide. J Investig Allergol Clin Immunol. 2011;21:245–7.
38. Kono T, Hayami M, Kobayashi H, et al. Acarbose-induced generalised erythema multiforme. Lancet. 1999;354:396–7.
39. Poszepczynska-Guigne E, Viguier M, Assier H, et al. Acute generalized exanthematous pustulosis induced by drugs with low-digestive absorption: acarbose and nystatin. Ann Dermatol Venereol. 2003;130:439–42.
40. Wu CS, Chang WY, Lan CCE, et al. Acute generalized exanthematous pustulosis possibly induced by acarbose. Int J Dermatol. 2008;47:1313–5.
41. Steveling EH, Winzeler B, Bircher AJ. Systemic allergic reaction to the GLP-1 receptor agonist exenatide. J Phar Tech. 2014;30(5):182–6.
42. Perez E, Martinez-Tadeo J, Callero A, et al. A case report of allergy to exenatide. J Allergy Clin Immunol Pract. 2014;2(6):822–3.
43. Ornelas C, Caiado J, Lopes A, et al. Anaphylaxis to long-acting release exenatide. J Investig Allergol Clin Immunol. 2018;28(5):332–4.
44. Liu X, Zhai A, Zhang B. A case report of severe adverse reaction of exenatide: anaphylactic shock. Medicine. 2022;101(39):e30805.
45. Yegit OO, Saribeyliler G, Karadag P, et al. The first successful desensitization protocol in exenatide allergy: a case report. Allergy Asthma Clin Immunol. 2023;19(1):2.
46. Carvallo A, Silva C, Gastaminza G, et al. Delayed hypersensitivity reaction to liraglutide: a case report. J Investig Allergol Clin Immunol. 2020;30(5):367–9.
47. Ouellette S, Frias G, Shah R, et al. Dermal hypersensitivity reaction to semaglutide: two case reports. J Drugs Dermatol. 2023;22(4):413–6.
48. Jacquier J, Chik CL, Senior PA. A practical, clinical approach to the assessment and management of suspected insulin allergy. Diabet Med. 2013;30:977–85.
49. Mastrorilli C, Rizzuti L, Cangelosi AM, et al. Long-acting insulin allergy in a diabetic child. Int J Immunopathol Pharmacol. 2017;30(2):174–7.
50. Kim GJ, Bum Kim S, Jo SI, et al. Two cases of allergy to insulin in gestational diabetes. Endocrinol Metab. 2015;30:402–7.

51. Morton A, Laurie J. Allergic reactions to insulin detemir in women with gestational diabetes mellitus. Roy Austr Coll Gen Pract. 2016;45:485–6.
52. Chen YM, Huang H. Allergy to soft cannula of insulin pump in diabetic patient. Pak J Med Scio. 2017;33:245–7.
53. Murray BR, Jewell JR, Jackson KJ, et al. Type III Hypersensitivity reaction to subcutaneous insulin preparations in a type I diabetic. J Gen Intern Med. 2017;32:841–5. https://doi.org/10.1007/s11606-017-4036-7.
54. Chakraborty PP, Biswas SN, Patra S. Faulty injection technique: a preventable but often overlooked factor in insulin allergy. Diabetes Ther. 2016;7:163–7.
55. Bzowyckyj AS, Stahnke AM. Hypersensitivity reactions to human insulin analogs in insulin-naïve patients: a systematic review. Ther Adv Endocrinol Metab. 2018;9(2):53–65.
56. Garcia-Nares H, Leyva-Carmon MI, Perez-Xochipa N, et al. Hypersensitivity reaction to a biosimilar insulin glargine. J Diabetes. 2015;7:155–7.
57. Hasselmann C, Pecquet C, Bismuth E, et al. Continuous subcutaneous insulin infusion allows tolerance induction and diabetes treatment in a type I diabetic child with insulin allergy. Diabet Metab. 2013;39:174–7.
58. Yuan T, Zhao W, Wang L, et al. Continuous subcutaneous insulin infusion as an effective method of desensitization therapy for diabetic patients with insulin allergy: a 4-year single center experience. Clin Therapeut. 2016;38(11):2489–94.
59. Hara M, Izumida Y, Sato N, et al. Successful desensitization by glargine administration in a patient with insulin allergy: a case report. Diabetes Res Clin Pract. 2009;84:48–9.
60. Diedisheim M, Pecquet C, Julla JB, et al. Prevalence and description of the skin reactions associated with adhesives in diabetes technology devices in an adult population: results of the CUTADIAB study. Diabetes Technol Ther. 2023;25(4):279–86.
61. Herman A, Uter W, Rustemeyer T, et al. Position statement: the need for EU legislation to require disclosure and labelling of the composition of medical devices. J Eur Acad Dermatol Venereol. 2021;35:1444–8.
62. Busschots AM, Meuleman V, Poesen N, et al. Contact allergy to components of glue in insulin pump infusion sets. Contact Derm. 1995;33:205–6.
63. Herman A, Aerts O, Baeck M, et al. Allergic contact dermatitis caused by isobornylacrylate in freestyle libre, a newly introduced glucose sensor. Contact Derm. 2017;77(6):367–73.
64. Kamann S, Aerts O, Heinemann L. Further evidence of severe allergic contact dermatitis from isobornyl acrylate while using a continuous glucose monitoring system. J Diabetes Sci Technol. 2018;12:630. https://doi.org/10.1177/1932296818762946.
65. Herman A, Baeck M, De Montjoye L, et al. Allergic contact dermatitis caused by isobornyl-acrylate in the Enlite® glucose sensor and the paradigm® MiniMed quick-set® insulin infusion set. Contact Derm. 2019;81:432–7.
66. Raison-Peyron N, Mowitz M, Bonardel N, et al. Allergic contact dermatitis caused by isobornyl acrylate in Omnipod, an innovative tubeless insulin pump. Contact Derm. 2018;79:76–80.
67. Aerts O, Herman A, Mowitz M, et al. Isobornyl acrylate. Dermatitis. 2020;31:4–12.
68. Peeters C, Herman A, Goossens A, et al. Allergic contact dermatitis caused by 2-ethyl cyanoacrylate contained in glucose sensor sets in two diabetic adults. Contact Derm. 2017;77:426–9.
69. Mowitz M, Herman A, Baeck M, et al. N,N-dimethylacrylamide: a new sensitizer in the FreeStyle Libre glucose sensor. Contact Derm. 2019;81:27–31.
70. Lombardo F, Salzano G, Crisafulli G, et al. Allergic contact dermatitis in pediatric patients with type 1 diabetes: an emerging issue. Diabetes Res Clin Pract. 2020;162:108089.
71. Huang C, DeKoven J. An unexpected source of glucose monitor-associated allergic contact dermatitis. Contact Derm. 2021;85:235.
72. Paret M, Barash G, Rachmiel M. "Out of the box" solution for skin problems due to glucose-monitoring technology in youth with type 1 diabetes: real-life experience with fluticasone spray. Acta Diabetol. 2020;57:419–24.

Chapter 30
The Impact of Diabetes on Aesthetic Procedures

Klaus Fritz, Carmen Salavastru, Seher Eren, and George-Sorin Tiplica

Abstract Diabetes can have several impacts on aesthetic medicine, influencing both the safety and efficacy of various aesthetic procedures. Here are some key aspects of the impact of diabetes on aesthetic medicine:

Dry skin: Individuals with diabetes often experience dry skin, a condition known as xerosis, which may affect the overall texture and appearance of the skin.

Increased suseptibility to infections: Diabetes can compromise the immune system, making individuals more prone to skin infections. Aesthetic procedures involve the introduction of foreign substances, and compromised skin integrity may heighten the risk of infections. This underscores the importance of strict hygiene and post-procedure care to minimize the risk of complications.

Wound healing: Diabetes is associated with delayed wound healing. This can be a significant concern in aesthetic procedures where incisions, injections, or other manipulations are made, as impaired healing may affect the final outcome and increase the risk of complications.

Collagen metabolism: Diabetes can impact collagen metabolism, affecting the elasticity and structural integrity of the skin. This may influence the long-term

K. Fritz (✉)
Carol Davila University of Medicine and Pharmacy, Bucharest, Romania

Dermatology and Laser Consulting, Landau, Germany
e-mail: drklausfritz@drklausfritz.com

C. Salavastru
Carol Davila University of Medicine and Pharmacy, Bucharest, Romania

Colentina Clinical Hospital, Bucharest, Romania

Dermato-Oncology Research Facility, Pediatric Dermatology Discipline, "Colentina" Clinical Hospital, Bucharest, Romania

S. Eren
Hautärzte am Marktplatz, Dr. Bettinger und Kollegen, Karlsruhe, Germany

G.-S. Tiplica
Carol Davila University of Medicine and Pharmacy, Bucharest, Romania

Colentina Clinical Hospital, Bucharest, Romania

K. Fritz, G.-S. Tiplica (eds.), *Cutaneous Manifestations in Diabetes*,
https://doi.org/10.1007/978-3-031-65300-1_30

results of procedures such as dermal fillers, where collagen plays a crucial role in maintaining skin volume and firmness.

Vascular complications: Diabetes is linked to vascular complications, including poor blood circulation. This may have implications for procedures like laser treatments or other interventions that rely on adequate blood supply for optimal results.

As aesthetic interventions gain popularity, understanding the impact of diabetes on procedures is crucial for both clinicians and patients.

This article aims to provide a review of existing medical publications, exploring the relationship between diabetes and the outcomes of aesthetic procedures.

Studies suggest that diabetes may influence the efficacy and safety of procedures like botulinum toxin and hyaluronic acid injections. Factors such as altered collagen metabolism and compromised skin health in diabetes may affect the longevity of results and the overall satisfaction of patients.

Educating patients with diabetes about the potential risks and challenges associated with aesthetic procedures is crucial. Close monitoring during and after procedures is necessary to promptly address any complications and ensure optimal outcomes.

30.1 Aging Skin and Diabetes

Investigating the relationship between glucose metabolism and perceived age, Noordam et al. [1] conducted a study employing facial photographs to assess perceived age in conjunction with the measurement of non-fasted glucose and insulin levels in a cohort of 602 participants. Among nondiabetic subjects, the study revealed a noteworthy increase in perceived age by 0.40 years ($SE = 0.14$, $P = 0.006$) for each 1 mmol/L rise in glucose levels. Consequently, the research establishes a connection between elevated glucose levels and an augmented perceived age, even in individuals without diabetes.

Individuals presenting an older appearance than their chronological age confront an elevated risk of morbidity and mortality, as emphasized by Christensen et al. in 2009 [2]. Numerous intrinsic and extrinsic factors contribute to perceived age, encompassing alterations in facial features like skin wrinkling [3], skin color uniformity [4], lip size, and sagging skin [5]. All these elements have been associated with the perception of age.

The link between skin aging and glucose levels is evident, supported by research indicating that prolonged exposure to hyperglycemic conditions triggers premature cellular senescence in human skin fibroblasts [6, 7]. Diabetic patients, characterized by heightened collagen cross-links, exhibit advanced glycation end products (AGEs) resulting from prolonged exposure to elevated glucose levels [8]. These cross-links impede efficient repair mechanisms, contributing to premature skin aging.

The notion that elevated glucose levels serve as an "aging accelerator" finds support in research spanning lower model organisms and humans. Genetic modifications in the insulin and insulin-like growth factor signaling pathway in lower model organisms significantly extend lifespan [9, 10]. Noordam et al. [1] observed a trend toward a higher perceived age in diabetic subjects compared to their nondiabetic counterparts. Additionally, in nondiabetic individuals, higher glucose levels were independently linked to an elevated perceived age. Cumulatively, these findings suggest that exposure to heightened glucose levels may indeed precipitate premature aging of the skin.

30.2 Alopecia and Diabetes

30.2.1 Male Pattern Hair Loss

Numerous prior investigations have delved into the correlation between metabolic syndrome (MS) and insulin resistance (IR) with androgenetic alopecia (AGA), yielding inconsistent results. In a study by Bakry et al. [11], significant disparities were identified in various parameters, including body weight ($P < 0.001$), height ($P = 0.002$), waist circumference ($P < 0.001$), body mass index ($P < 0.001$), systolic ($P < 0.001$), and diastolic blood pressure ($P < 0.001$), fasting glucose ($P < 0.001$), triglycerides ($P < 0.001$), high-density lipoprotein cholesterol ($P < 0.01$), fasting insulin ($P = 0.02$), and homeostasis model assessment of insulin resistance ($P < 0.001$). Notably, a statistically significant association was observed between androgenetic alopecia and metabolic syndrome ($P = 0.002$), as well as between androgenetic alopecia and insulin resistance ($P < 0.001$).

30.2.2 Female Pattern Hair Loss

In individuals with diabetes, particularly those utilizing insulin for blood sugar control, the risk of developing insulin resistance over time has been linked to androgenetic alopecia (AGA) in both men and women. AGA, known as male pattern baldness or female pattern hair loss, exhibited a noteworthy association with Type 2 diabetes. A study found an increased risk of severe central scalp hair loss in women with Type 2 diabetes, with a multivariable hazard ratio of 1.68 (95% CI, 1.38–2.06) overall, escalating to 2.05 (95% CI, 1.48–2.85) for diabetes duration of ≥10 years [12]. The precise mechanism leading to central hair loss remains elusive, but it is suggested that high glucose levels may damage blood vessels crucial for supplying oxygen and nutrients to hair follicles.

Androgenetic Alopecia in Women: The occurrence of androgenetic alopecia in women is attributed to the impact of the testosterone metabolite dihydrotestosterone on androgen-sensitive hair follicles [13]. There is speculation that vascular impairment resulting from hyperglycemia could adversely affect hair follicles [14], potentially contributing to hair loss. The compromised blood vessels impeding the delivery of oxygen and nutrients to hair follicles may underlie alopecia in patients with diabetes mellitus.

30.2.3 Alopecia Areata

Diabetes also heightens the susceptibility to alopecia areata, a condition associated with autoimmune reactions. Both insulin-dependent diabetes mellitus and alopecia areata universalis are believed to share autoimmune mechanisms and can coexist [15]. Patients with alopecia areata often exhibit signs of insulin resistance [16]. Notably, women with type 1 diabetes are particularly prone to autoimmune conditions, including various forms of alopecia areata (79%), rheumatoid arthritis (73%), and hypothyroidism (69%) [17] (Picture 30.1).

30.2.4 Botulinum Toxin and Diabetes

Botulinum toxin, renowned for its muscle-paralyzing properties, is widely utilized in aesthetic medicine. Minimally invasive procedures such as botulinum toxin injections are generally considered safe for individuals with diabetes. However, there

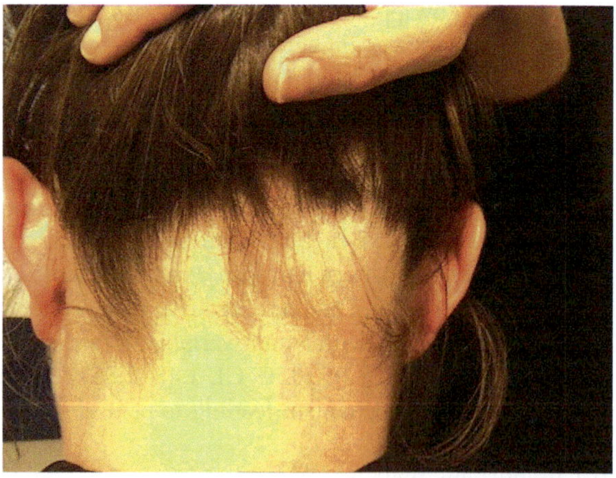

Picture 30.1 Alpoecia areata

exists an elevated risk of infection at the injection site for people with diabetes due to increased skin sensitivity, potentially leading to heightened pain and discomfort during treatment. While no double-blind studies explicitly demonstrate the impact of diabetes on medication metabolism, diabetic patients are advised to discuss any concurrent medications, supplements, or vitamins they may be taking, as these factors could influence their response to botulinum toxin.

30.2.4.1 The Therapeutic Use of Botulinum Toxin a in Diabetes Patients

Botulinum toxin injection into the pylorus has proven to be a safe and symptom-improving approach for patients with diabetic gastroparesis [18]. Despite the existence of a patent for the use of botulinum toxin in treating diabetes (European patent office EP 1250146 B1), this application has not been widely adopted in medical practice. Botulinum toxin type A (BTX-A) has been suggested as a potential treatment for painful diabetic peripheral neuropathy (DPN). In 4 studies involving 231 patients, intradermal BTX-A injection demonstrated effectiveness and safety in alleviating DPN pain. However, larger-scale, well-designed randomized controlled trials are warranted for further validation [19, 20].

30.2.5 Cellulitis and Diabetes

Distinct from cellulite, which characterizes a cobblestone-like appearance on the skin surface of the upper legs, primarily in women, cellulitis is an infection affecting the skin and tissues beneath. Although there is no conclusive evidence indicating increased frequency or severity of cellulitis in diabetic patients, some suggest a potential link between fungal foot infections and the development of lower limb cellulitis [21]. Nevertheless, major case-control studies do not uniformly support this association [22].

Reduced lymphatic drainage may lead to diabetic foot issues or ulcers. Patients with diabetes face a 30-fold higher risk of lower-extremity amputation due to infection compared to those without diabetes [23, 24]. Additionally, diabetes elevates the risk of diabetic foot infections by 12–25%, attributed to neuropathy-related sensory, motor, and/or autonomic disturbances, leading to diminished injury recognition and increased vulnerability to foot ulcerations progressing to infections [25].

Peripheral arterial disease further hampers blood flow, limiting the body's ability to combat infections. Notably, no associations were observed with hypertension, diabetes mellitus, body mass index, and the duration of lymphedema [26].

30.2.6 Chemical Peeling and Diabetes

Chemical peeling entails the application of a chemical agent with defined strength, leading to skin exfoliation and subsequent regrowth, fostering skin rejuvenation. This technique-dependent procedure, while generally safe, can present specific complications in individuals with diabetes, including persistent erythema, irritation, pruritus, and pain shortly after peeling. Additionally, infections or loss of cutaneous barrier and tissue injury may occur due to microvascular damage. Diabetes, particularly in severe cases, poses a relative contraindication for resurfacing procedures, especially medium-deep or deep chemical peels [27, 28]. Microdermabrasion or chemical peels increase the risk of skin injury, emphasizing the need to avoid such procedures if cuts or abrasions are present until fully healed.

Diabetics, with their compromised blood circulation and diminished immune response, may experience delayed wound healing and increased susceptibility to infections, even from minor injuries such as those resulting from chemical peeling (Picture 30.2). The impairment of granulocyte function contributes to a heightened propensity for infections, affecting aspects like adherence, chemotaxis, phagocytosis, and bactericidal effect [29–33].

30.2.7 Collagen and Diabetes

There is no evidence indicating that collagen injections cause specific side effects in diabetic patients compared to healthy individuals. While complications like delayed wound healing and infections may occur after injections or invasive procedures, there is no distinct evidence of increased risks for diabetic patients. In fact, collagen may offer potential benefits for diabetic wounds, as seen in cases where an injectable biomaterial implant improved healing in diabetic ulcers [34].

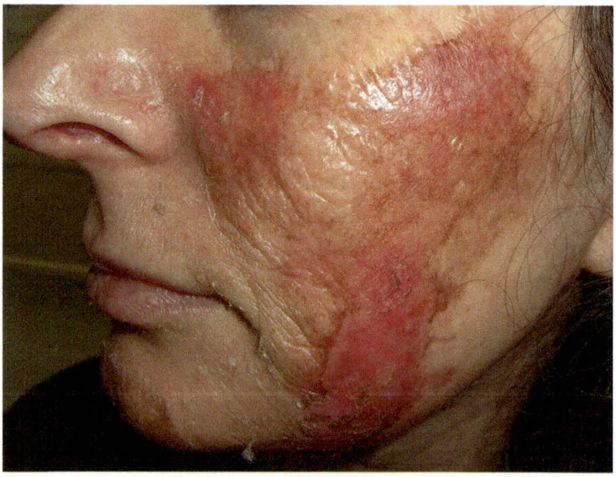

Picture 30.2 Delayed healing after chemical peel

Histopathological analysis revealed positive effects of a radiation-cross-linked bilayer collagen scaffold on skin regeneration and remodeling in diabetic rats. This scaffold not only significantly accelerated diabetic wound healing but also promoted angiogenesis factor (CD31) production, with vascularization observed as early as day 7 [35]. Diabetes-induced changes in collagen metabolism and structure are acknowledged, and collagens may play a role in regulating glucose homeostasis through various mechanisms [36].

Although repeated insulin injections can result in skin thickening and increased collagen fibers, there is no evidence suggesting accelerated collagen degradation in diabetic patients [37]. Appropriate site rotation in insulin injection remains crucial to mitigate adverse effects.

30.2.8 Cryotherapy and Diabetes

Cryotherapy, involving extreme cold exposure, demonstrated blood sugar and cholesterol reduction in a study involving obese patients. However, complications such as nerve damage, frostbite, Raynaud's phenomenon, cold-induced urticaria, and slowed wound healing may arise. In thermotherapy, skin burns may occur, particularly in patients with diabetes mellitus, multiple sclerosis, poor circulation, and spinal cord injuries. While cryolipolysis may offer benefits for obesity patients, caution is warranted, especially considering potential complications in individuals with diabetes.

30.2.9 HIFU and Diabetes

High-intensity focused ultrasound (HIFU) delivers focused energy at depths ranging from 1.1 to 1.6 cm in subcutaneous tissue, elevating local tissue temperature at the focal point. This process induces nearly immediate cell death without harm to surrounding tissues, leading to clinical tissue tightening. The efficacy of HIFU treatment relies on stimulating the body's natural healing responses, making it essential for individuals with immune deficiencies and uncontrolled diabetes to undergo a comprehensive medical evaluation before undergoing treatment. Advanced transducers now allow penetration depths of 6, 9, and 13 mm, making HIFU a noninvasive procedure for localized fat reduction, potentially influencing metabolism similarly to other fat reduction methods [38–42].

In urology and gynecology, HIFU serves as an established therapy for tumor destruction or nerve sensitivity blockage, offering certain patients a noninvasive alternative to surgery with reduced complications and lower costs. HIFU precisely targets the desired area without causing harm to surrounding tissue, with the option for repeated applications if necessary. Notably, high-intensity focused ultrasound has demonstrated safe and reversible suppression of nerve conduction in diabetic rat nerves under appropriate stimulation parameters, suggesting its potential for reversible blockade of sensory nerves and peripheral pain relief [43].

30.2.10 Hyaluronic Acid and Diabetes

Hyaluronic acid injections have become increasingly prevalent in the aesthetic industry for nonsurgical skin rejuvenation, wrinkle reduction, volume enhancement, and improvement of skin texture. As a natural substance in the skin known for its moisturizing properties, hyaluronic acid is generally considered safe for use in individuals with diabetes. The complex sugar in hyaluronic acid fillers is unrelated to the sugar associated with diabetes. However, individuals with diabetes, who may have an elevated susceptibility to infections and delayed wound healing, should consider their risk profile before undergoing aesthetic interventions like hyaluronic acid injections.

Research by Miller et al. [44] underscore the impact of diabetes on collagen metabolism, particularly affecting skin elasticity. Brown et al.'s retrospective analysis emphasizes the importance of individualized treatment plans for diabetic patients undergoing aesthetic procedures, considering their unique risks and side effects [45]. Gupta et al.'s [46] literature review explores current research perspectives on hyaluronic acid application in diabetes, advocating for a nuanced approach. Furthermore, hyaluronic acid can be beneficial for treating diabetic wounds, as evidenced by its increased wound healing rate in diabetic foot ulcerations [47].

30.2.11 Hydroxyl Apatite and Diabetes

Hydroxyl apatite does not pose specific problems for individuals with diabetes. In fact, a study demonstrates that the CS/HA composite material improves diabetes-induced impaired osteointegration of titanium by reactivating the Wnt/β-catenin pathway. This finding suggests a target point for biomaterial modification to enhance clinical performance in diabetic patients [48]. Glucose, as an active chemical agent, influences the degradation of hydroxyapatite nanostructure in a concentration-dependent manner [49].

30.3 Hyperhidrosis and Diabetes

Hyperhidrosis, characterized by excessive sweating, can be either primary (idiopathic) or secondary to medication or underlying health conditions. Diabetes, as a systemic disorder, can impact the body in various ways, including overstimulating the sweat glands. This can lead to challenges in maintaining a consistent internal body temperature. Fluctuations in blood sugar levels, especially extreme ones, can influence perspiration, resulting in either hyperhidrosis (excessive sweating) or anhidrosis (lack of sweating). Automatic neuropathy, which is nerve damage affecting organ control, can be a consequence of prolonged and untreated high blood glucose levels (National Institute of Diabetes and Digestive and Kidney Diseases).

Automatic neuropathy extends its effects to the sweat glands, causing variable responses depending on the severity of nerve damage. In some areas of the body, the sweat glands may cease functioning, while in others, they may become overly active. Sweating induced by automatic neuropathy is particularly noticeable at night or during meals.

Gustatory sweating (GS) is a specific form characterized by profuse sweating during or immediately after eating and is recognized as a complication of diabetes mellitus. In a hospital-based cohort of patients with both type 1 and type 2 diabetes, the prevalence of gustatory sweating was documented at 11%, twice as high as in nondiabetic control individuals. Associations between GS and known diabetes complications were observed specifically in type 2 diabetes. Higher odds for GS were found in people with diabetes over the age of 45 compared to a control group without diabetes [50]. The link between neuropathy and gustatory sweating was postulated, and a strong association was proposed between gustatory sweating and thermoregulatory sweating in the context of diabetic neuropathy [51].

In the assessment of pathological loss of sweating, various patterns were identified, including distal loss in 65%, segmental loss in 25%, and isolated dermatomal loss in 25%. Global anhidrosis, affecting the entire body surface, was noted in 16% of patients with profound autonomic neuropathy. The degree of clinical dysautonomia correlated with the percentage of body surface anhidrosis. Additionally, discrete zones of anhidrosis on the thorax and abdomen were observed in patients with painful diabetic radiculopathy, correlating with muscle fibrillation potentials. Distal loss of sweating consistently correlated with abnormal neuropathic indicators, pointing to a distal axonal neuropathy [52].

30.4 Keloids and Scars

Hypertrophic scars emerge immediately after wound healing and confine themselves to the injury site, whereas keloids take longer to manifest and can extend beyond the original injury area. Hypertrophic scars typically resolve over time, with or without intervention, while keloids may persist long-term despite treatment efforts. Diabetes is believed to influence keloid formation, progression, and infection due to heightened NLRP3 inflammasome activity in diabetic wounds, a factor considered crucial in keloid fibrosis [53, 54]. Despite the increased susceptibility to infection in diabetes mellitus, it is not identified as a risk factor for keloid infection in this study, although a higher proportion of diabetic individuals was observed in patients with suppurative keloids [55] (Pictures 30.3 and 30.4).

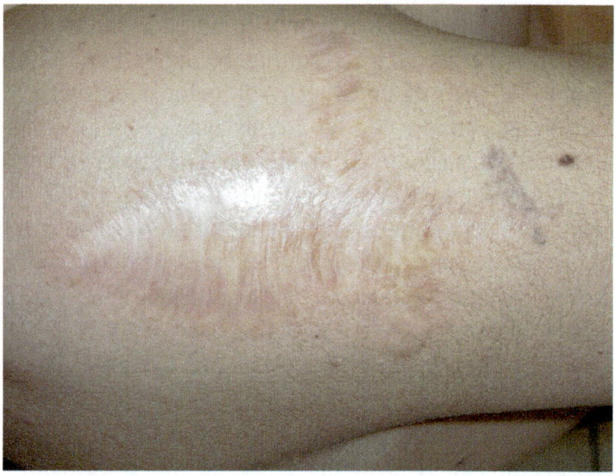

Picture 30.3 Wide scar post poor healing

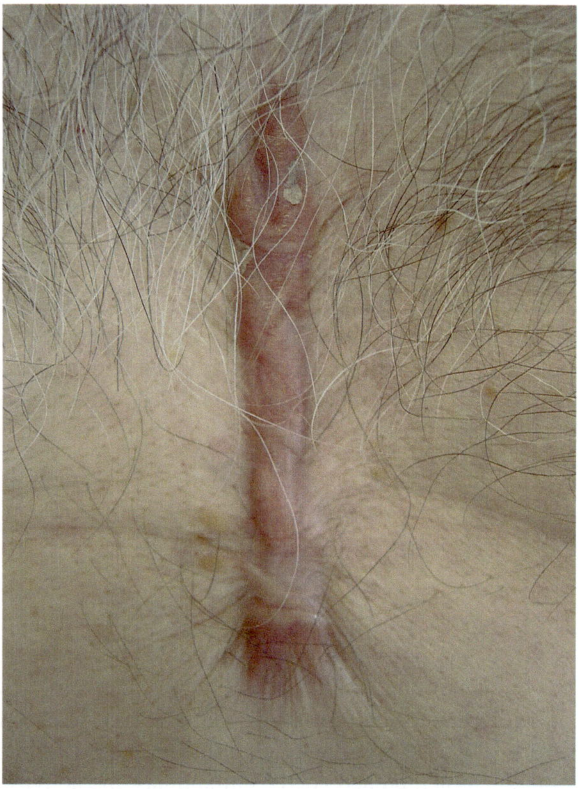

Picture 30.4 Keloid

30.4.1 Lasers and Diabetes

Laser therapy holds potential benefits for individuals with diabetes, particularly in addressing specific complications:

30.4.1.1 Diabetic Peripheral Neuropathy (DPN)

Low-level laser therapy (LLLT) has been explored as a potential treatment for DPN, a chronic complication of diabetes affecting nerve function. Clinical studies suggest that LLLT may alleviate symptoms and enhance nerve function in DPN patients, providing a non-pharmacological avenue for improving quality of life.

Ongoing systematic reviews and meta-analyses aim to evaluate the effectiveness and safety of LLLT for DPN.

Case reports have shown improvements, especially in dermopathy with numbness, pain, or paresthesia after low-level light therapy, although standardized protocols are lacking.

Energy density and wavelength are critical factors influencing LLLT effects, with the potential for combining laser and magnetic field therapy for enhanced outcomes [56].

30.4.1.2 Effects on Glycemia

Some laser exposure parameters have been associated with effects on glycemia and diabetes management, particularly nonsurgical lasers and low-level light therapy. Hypoglycemic effects of nonsurgical lasers have been reported in diabetes types 1 and 2, involving different laser types and combinations with magnetic fields and electricity [57].

Low-level laser therapy (LLLT) has also been found to reduce glycemia on DM type 1 patients. A gradual reduction of glycemia was noted during the course of treatment. In long-term controls, a reduction in HbA1c was reported. Results confirm previous observations and need for further research on large cohorts [58].

30.4.1.3 Diabetic Retinopathy

Laser treatment is a common approach for diabetic retinopathy, mitigating the risk of severe vision loss and blindness in advanced cases.

However, it is crucial to note that laser therapy does not cure diabetic retinopathy, restore lost vision, or prevent future vision loss without proper diabetes and blood pressure management.

30.4.1.4 LASIK (Laser-Assisted in Situ Keratomileusis)

Individuals with type 1 or type 2 diabetes can undergo LASIK surgery for vision correction, although eligibility is determined based on various clinical factors.

Effective diabetes management is essential to prioritize overall health and prevent complications related to LASIK surgery.

30.5 Lipolysis (Cryo-, Injection-), Liposuction, and Diabetes

Cryolipolysis causes no reported problems for individuals with diabetes, although there might be a slight increase in numbness due to diabetic predisposition to nerve issues. Both type 1 and type 2 diabetic patients have experienced excellent results with cryolipolysis, offering a nonsurgical option preferred by many. In contrast, mesenteric fat cryolipolysis has shown a safe reduction in mesenteric fat volume, resulting in improved glycemic control, insulin sensitivity, and blood pressure compared to sham controls [59] (Picture 30.5).

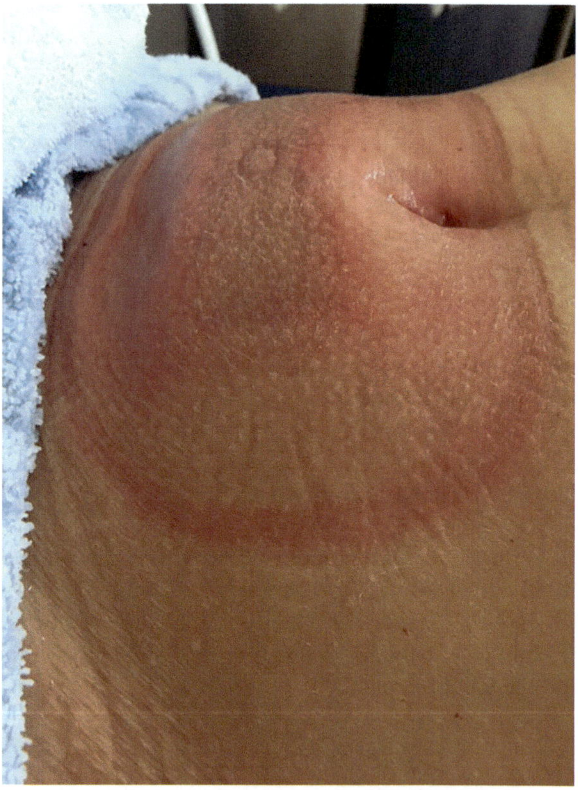

Picture 30.5 Cryolipolysis

While fat-dissolving procedures, including injections, are generally suitable for healthy patients, they are not recommended for lipodystrophy or immunocompromised individuals, including those with type 1 diabetes. Liposuction has demonstrated effectiveness in combating diabetes, particularly in patients who have gained weight rapidly, such as during pregnancy, stress, or post-injury. However, nonsurgical fat removal lacks similar metabolic benefits compared to surgical interventions, and evidence supporting its metabolic advantages is currently inconclusive [60].

30.5.1 Pigmentation of the Skin and Diabetes

Diabetes can impact various skin pigmentation disorders, including diabetic dermopathy, acanthosis nigricans (AN), necrobiosis lipoidica diabeticorum, diabetic blisters, eruptive xanthomatosis, and psoriasis, which are more prevalent in individuals with type 2 diabetes. Acanthosis nigricans (AN) is often associated with insulin resistance (see separate chapters).

30.5.2 Plastic Surgery and Diabetes

Diabetes is an independent risk factor for major complications, especially infection, after aesthetic surgical procedures [61]. The complexity of the procedure and the extent of tissue removal or reconstruction can influence the risk of complications in people with diabetes [62]. While eyelid procedures may not exhibit the same association between A1c levels and delayed wound healing, more complex surgeries like tummy tuck or breast reduction may pose a higher risk for diabetics. Diabetic wounds have an extended inflammatory phase during wound healing, which may lead to chronic wounds [63, 64] and increased complications in surgical procedures.

In the beginning macrophages arrive (M1) during the inflammation phase of wound healing. They are phagocytic and proinflammatory. They are eventually replaced by M2 macrophages that are anti-inflammatory, synthesize extracellular matrix (ECM), and promote angiogenesis [65]. In diabetic wounds, macrophages produce excessive proinflammatory cytokines [66]. Additionally, the inflammatory macrophage does not readily transition to the anti-inflammatory macrophage in diabetic wounds [65].

Neutrophils play a role in promoting inflammation through the release of cytotoxic enzymes, inflammatory mediators, and free radicals, exacerbating oxidative stress. This oxidative stress, in turn, leads to additional tissue damage and impedes the proper healing of diabetic wounds. In diabetic wound environments, there is an increased production of neutrophil extracellular traps (NETs), which heightens the inflammatory response, thereby hindering the healing process. Furthermore, molecular alterations such as changes in micro-ribonucleic acid (miRNA) levels also contribute to the dysregulated inflammation in diabetic wounds. Although the miRNA associated with healing initially shows similar levels in uninjured diabetic and non-diabetic skin, their expression differs upon injury, indicating a role in contributing to the disrupted inflammatory response [65]. The dysregulation of these molecular mechanisms further adds to the pathological inflammation observed in diabetic wounds.

Research findings from both diabetic and human models consistently highlight that persistent inflammation is a key factor in the impaired healing observed in diabetic wounds. This prolonged inflammatory state significantly delays the healing trajectory, thereby elevating the risk of chronic wounds.

It is also associated with diabetic mice models, reducing inflammation by inducing the transition from M1 to M2 macrophages, increased levels of several prohealing growth factors, thereby improving wound healing [67]. Thus, curbing inflammation during the healing process is crucial to minimize scarring in diabetic patients [68–71].

Managing inflammation during the healing process is crucial to minimize scarring in diabetic patients.

Benefits of plastic surgery for diabetics include improvements in physical appearance and medical conditions related to diabetes, such as alleviating back pain or reducing the risk of skin infections. Cosmetic procedures can boost self-confidence and improve mental health, positively impacting overall well-being.

30.5.3 Varicose Veins, Spider Veins, Telangiectasia, and Diabetes

Diabetes itself doesn't directly cause varicose veins or spider veins, but it can influence their development and severity. Individuals with diabetes are more susceptible to venous disorders due to risk factors like poor circulation, obesity, high blood pressure, and peripheral arterial disease. Proper blood sugar management is crucial to prevent or mitigate skin and nerve damage caused by venous stasis ulcers. While diabetes doesn't directly cause spider veins, it contributes to poor circulation, especially in the feet and legs. **Type 1 diabetes** can contribute to varicose veins due to **hyperglycemia**, which leads to weight gain—one of the major causes of varicose veins. Pregnant women with **gestational diabetes** may experience impaired circulation in the extremities, further increasing the risk of varicose veins. Elevated blood sugar levels weaken blood vessels, making the vascular system more susceptible to infections like **leg ulcers**. Proper blood sugar management is essential to prevent or mitigate skin and nerve damage caused by venous stasis ulcers. **Spider veins** are smaller, dilated blood vessels visible near the skin's surface. While diabetes itself doesn't directly cause spider veins, it contributes to poor circulation, especially in the feet and legs.

30.5.4 Wrinkles and Diabetes

Diabetes can indeed have an impact on the skin, including the development of wrinkles on the face. Let's explore this further.

Glycation and Collagen: **Glycation** is a process where sugar molecules bind to proteins (including collagen and elastin) in the skin. This can interfere with the skin's natural regeneration process. Once the sugar-protein bond forms, collagen and elastin become less efficient at repairing themselves. As a result, fine lines and wrinkles may become more noticeable.

Ozempic Face: Some patients using the type 2 diabetes medication semaglutide (Ozempic) have reported sagging and aging of facial skin. Rapid weight loss associated with Ozempic use may contribute to this phenomenon (see also antiaging).

References

1. Noordam R, Gunn DA, Tomlin CC, Maier AB, Mooijaart SP, Slagboom PE, Westendorp RG, de Craen AJ, van Heemst D, Leiden Longevity Study Group. High serum glucose levels are associated with a higher perceived age. Age (Dordr). 2013;35(1):189–95. https://doi.org/10.1007/s11357-011-9339-9.
2. Christensen K, Thinggaard M, McGue M, Rexbye H, Hjelmborg JV, Aviv A, Gunn D, van der Ouderaa F, Vaupel JW. Perceived age as clinically useful biomarker of ageing: cohort study. BMJ. 2009;339:b5262. https://doi.org/10.1136/bmj.b5262.
3. Gunn DA, Rexbye H, Griffiths CE, Murray PG, Fereday A, Catt SD, Tomlin CC, Strongitharm BH, Perrett DI, Catt M, Mayes AE, Messenger AG, Green MR, van der Ouderaa F, Vaupel JW, Christensen K. Why some women look young for their age. PLoS One. 2009;4(12):e8021. https://doi.org/10.1371/journal.pone.0008021.
4. Matts PJ, Fink B, Grammer K, Burquest M. Color homogeneity and visual perception of age, health, and attractiveness of female facial skin. J Am Acad Dermatol. 2007;57(6):977–84. https://doi.org/10.1016/j.jaad.2007.07.040.
5. Ozdemir R, Kilinc H, Unlu RE, Uysal AC, Sensoz O, Baran CN. Anatomicohistologic study of the retaining ligaments of the face and use in face lift: retaining ligament correction and SMAS plication. Plast Reconstr Surg. 2002;110(4):1134–47. https://doi.org/10.1097/00006534-200209150-00019.
6. Blazer S, Khankin E, Segev Y, Ofir R, Yalon-Hacohen M, Kra-Oz Z, Gottfried Y, Larisch S, Skorecki KL. High glucose-induced replicative senescence: point of no return and effect of telomerase. Biochem Biophys Res Commun. 2002;296(1):93–101. https://doi.org/10.1016/S0006-291X(02)00818-5.
7. Dekker P, Maier AB, van Heemst D, de Koning-Treurniet C, Blom J, Dirks RW, Tanke HJ, Westendorp RG. Stress-induced responses of human skin fibroblasts in vitro reflect human longevity. Aging Cell. 2009;8(5):595–603. https://doi.org/10.1111/j.1474-9726.2009.00506.x.
8. Paul RG, Bailey AJ. Glycation of collagen: the basis of its central role in the late complications of ageing and diabetes. Int J Biochem Cell Biol. 1996;28(12):1297–310. https://doi.org/10.1016/S1357-2725(96)00079-9.
9. Bartke A. Impact of reduced insulin-like growth factor-1/insulin signaling on aging in mammals: novel findings. Aging Cell. 2008;7(3):285–90. https://doi.org/10.1111/j.1474-9726.2008.00387.x.
10. Lakowski B, Hekimi S. Determination of life-span in Caenorhabditis elegans by four clock genes. Science. 1996;272(5264):1010–3. https://doi.org/10.1126/science.272.5264.1010.

11. Bakry OA, Shoeib MA, El Shafiee MK, Hassan A. Androgenetic alopecia, metabolic syndrome, and insulin resistance: is there any association? A case-control study. Indian Dermatol Online J. 2014;5(3):276–81. https://doi.org/10.4103/2229-5178.137776.
12. Coogan PF, Bethea TN, Cozier YC, Bertrand KA, Palmer JR, Rosenberg L, Lenzy Y. Association of type 2 diabetes with central-scalp hair loss in a large cohort study of African American women. Int J Womens Dermatol. 2019;5(4):261–6. https://doi.org/10.1016/j.ijwd.2019.05.010.
13. Piraccini BM, Alessandrini A. Androgenetic alopecia. G Ital Dermatol Venereol. 2014;149:15–24.
14. Miranda JJ, Taype-Rondan A, Tapia JC, Gastanadui-Gonzalez MG, Roman-Carpio R. Hair follicle characteristics as early marker of type 2 diabetes. Med Hypotheses. 2016;95:39–44.
15. Taniyama M, Kushima K, Ban Y, Kaihara M, Nagakura H, Sekita S, Katagiri T, Sueki H. Simultaneous development of insulin dependent diabetes mellitus and alopecia areata universalis. Am J Med Sci. 1991;301(4):269–71. https://doi.org/10.1097/00000441-199104000-00009.
16. Shahidi-Dadras M, Bahraini N, Rajabi F, Younespour S. Patients with alopecia areata show signs of insulin resistance. Arch Dermatol Res. 2019;311(7):529–33. https://doi.org/10.1007/s00403-019-01929-6.
17. Narang M, Prasad S, Mahavar S, Jain A, Kumar R, Gupta B. Diabetes type-1 with alopecia areata. J Indian Acad Clin Med. 2012;13(3):261–2.
18. Lacy BE, Crowell MD, Schettler-Duncan A, Mathis C, Pasricha PJ. The treatment of diabetic gastroparesis with botulinum toxin injection of the pylorus. Diabetes Care. 2004;27(10):2341–7. https://doi.org/10.2337/diacare.27.10.2341.
19. Salehi H, Moussaei M, Kamiab Z, Vakilian A. The effects of botulinum toxin type a injection on pain symptoms, quality of life, and sleep quality of patients with diabetic neuropathy: a randomized double-blind clinical trial. Iran J Neurol. 2019;18(3):99. https://doi.org/10.18502/ijnl.v18i3.1632.
20. Wang C, Zhang Q, Wang R, Xu L. Botulinum toxin type a for diabetic peripheral neuropathy pain: a systematic review and meta-analysis. J Pain Res. 2021;14:3855–63. https://doi.org/10.2147/JPR.S340390.
21. Bristow IR, Spruce M. C fungal foot infection, cellulitis and diabetes: a review. Diabet Med. 2009;26(5):548–51. https://doi.org/10.1111/j.1464-5491.2009.02722.x.
22. Halpern JS. Fungal infection, not diabetes, is risk factor for cellulitis. Br Med J London Bd. 2012;345 https://doi.org/10.1136/bmj.e5877.
23. Atkins RC, Zimmet P. Diabetic kidney disease: act now or pay later. Saudi J Kidney Dis Transpl. 2010;21:217–21.
24. Geerlings SE, Hoepelman AI. Immune dysfunction in patients with diabetes mellitus (DM). FEMS Immunol Med Microbiol. 2011;26:256–65.
25. Muller LM, Gorter KJ, Hak E, Goudzwaard WL, Schellevis FG, Hoepelman AI, et al. Increased risk of common infections in patients with type 1 and type 2 diabetes mellitus. Clin Infect Dis. 2005;41:281–8.
26. Teerachaisakul M, Ekataksin W, Durongwatana S, Taneepanichskul S. Risk factors for cellulitis in patients with lymphedema: a case-controlled study. Lymphology. 2013;46(3):150–6.
27. Brody HJ. Complications of chemical peeling. J Dermatol Surg Oncol. 1989;15(09):1010–9.
28. Nikalji N, Godse K, Sakhiya J, Patil S, Nadkarni N. Complications of medium depth and deep chemical peels. J Cutan Aesthet Surg. 2012;5(04):254–60.
29. Wheat LJ. Infection and diabetes mellitus. Diabetes Care. 1980;3:187.
30. Halprin KM, et al. Glucose and glycogen metabolism in the human epidermia. J Invest Dermatol. 1966;46:43.
31. Urbach E, et al. Carbohydrate metabolism and the skin. Syphilology. 1945;52:301.
32. Aagenaaes O, et al. Light and electron-microscopic study of skin-capillaries of diabetics. Diabetes. 1961;10:253.
33. Handlesman MB, et al. Skin-vascular alterations in diabetes mellitus. Arch Intern Med. 1962;110:70.

34. Skorman SE. Use of injectable collagen to treat chronic diabetic foot ulcers. J Foot Surg. 1987;26(6):511–5.
35. Li H, Chen X, Ren K, et al. Qualitative study on diabetic cutaneous wound healing with radiation crosslinked bilayer collagen scaffold in rat model. Sci Rep. 2023;13:6399. https://doi.org/10.1038/s41598-023-33372-z.
36. Bondarenko LB. Diabetes and collagen: interrelations. Avicenna J Med Biochem. 2019;7(2):64–71. https://doi.org/10.34172/ajmb.2019.12.
37. Murao S, Murao K, Nagata T, Shimizu M, Miyai Y. Repeated insulin injection without site rotation affects skin thickness—ultrasonographic and histological evaluation. J Diabetes Invest. 2022;13(6):997–1003. https://doi.org/10.1111/jdi.13753.
38. Fonseca VM, Campos PS, Certo TF, de-Faria LT, Juliano PB, Cintra DE, Liebano RE, da Silva C, Guidi RM, Sant'Ana E. Efficacy and safety of noninvasive focused ultrasound for treatment of subcutaneous adiposity in healthy women. J Cosmet Laser Ther. 2018;20(6):341–50.
39. Fatemi A, Kane MAC. High-intensity focused ultrasound effectively reduces waist circumference by ablating adipose tissue from the abdomen and flanks: a retrospective case series. Aesth Plast Surg. 2010;34:577–82.
40. Mazzoni D, Lin MJ, Dubin DP, Khorasani H. Review of non-invasive body contouring devices for fat reduction, skin tightening and muscle definition. Austr J Dermatol. 2019;60(4):278–83.
41. Shek SY, Yeung CK, Chan JC, Chan HH. Efficacy of high-intensity focused ultrasonography for noninvasive body sculpting in Chinese patients. Lasers Surg Med. 2014;46(4):263–9.
42. Halachmi S, Lapidoth M. Safety and tolerability of a focused ultrasound device for treatment of adipose tissue in subjects undergoing abdominoplasty, a placebo control pilot study. Dermatologic Surg. 2013;39:752–4.
43. Lee YF, Lin CC, Cheng JS, Chen GS. Nerve conduction block in diabetic rats using high-intensity focused ultrasound for analgesic applications. Br J Anaesth. 2015;114(5):840–6. https://doi.org/10.1093/bja/aeu443.
44. Miller C, et al. Diabetes and collagen metabolism: impacts on skin elasticity. Diabet Res Pract. 2020;30(3):145–57.
45. Brown R, et al. Risks and side effects of aesthetic procedures in diabetic patients: a retrospective analysis. J Dermatol Complic. 2021;40(1):55–6.
46. Gupta M, et al. Current research perspectives on hyaluronic acid application in diabetes: a literature review. Dermatol Diabetes. 2022;15(4):210–25.
47. Chen CP, Hung W, Lin SH. Effectiveness of hyaluronic acid for treating diabetic foot: a systematic review and meta-analysis. Dermatol Ther. 2014;27(6):331–6. https://doi.org/10.1111/dth.12153.
48. Ma XY, Feng YF, Ma ZS, Li X, Wang J, Wang L, Lei W. The promotion of osteointegration under diabetic conditions using chitosan/hydroxyapatite composite coating on porous titanium surfaces. Biomaterials. 2014;35(26):7259–70. https://doi.org/10.1016/j.biomaterials.2014.05.028.
49. Martins ML, Iessi IL, Quintino MP, Damasceno DC, Rodrigues CG. Glucose is an active chemical agent on degradation of hydroxyapatite nanostructure. Mater Chem Phys. 2020;240:122166. https://doi.org/10.1016/j.matchemphys.2019.122166.
50. Klarskov CK, von Rohden E, Thorsteinsson B, Tarnow L, Lommer KP. Gustatory sweating in people with type 1 and type 2 diabetes mellitus: prevalence and risk factors. Endocrinol Diabetes Metab. 2021;4(4):e00290. https://doi.org/10.1002/edm2.290.
51. Shaw JE, Parker R, Hollis S, Gokal R, Boulton AJM. Gustatory sweating in diabetes mellitus. Diabet Med. 1996;13(12):1033–7. https://doi.org/10.1002/(SICI)1096-9136(199612)13:12<1033:AID-DIA280>3.0.CO;2-B.
52. Fealey RD, Low PA, Thomas JE. Thermoregulatory sweating abnormalities in diabetes mellitus. Mayo Clin Proc. 1989;64(6):617–28. https://doi.org/10.1016/S0025-6196(12)65338-5.
53. Louiselle AE, Niemiec SM, Zgheib C, Liechty KW. Macrophage polarization and diabetic wound healing. Transl Res. 2021;236:109–16.

54. Huang C, Ogawa R. Role of Inflammasomes in keloids and hypertrophic scars-lessons learned from chronic diabetic wounds and skin fibrosis. Int J Mol Sci. 2022;23(12):6820.
55. Liang Z, Zhang M, Hao Y, et al. Risk factors associated with keloid infections: a five-year retrospective study. Int Wound J. 2023;20(6):2215–23. https://doi.org/10.1111/iwj.14099.
56. Lin L, Li J, Lin J, et al. Effectiveness and safety of low-level laser therapy in diabetic peripheral neuropathy: a protocol for a systematic review and meta-analysis. Syst Rev. 2021;10:96. https://doi.org/10.1186/s13643-021-01656-y.
57. Longo L. Non surgical laser and light in the treatment of chronic diseases: a review based on personal experiences. Laser Phys Lett. 2010;7:771. https://doi.org/10.1002/lapl.201010056.
58. Abdelhalim NM, Abdelbasset WK, Alqahtani BA, Samhan AF. Low-level laser therapy for diabetic dermopathy in patients with type 2 diabetes: a placebo-controlled pilot study. J Lasers Med Sci. 2020;11(4):481–5. https://doi.org/10.34172/jlms.2020.75.
59. Mazor R, Babkin A, Littrup PJ, Alloush M, Sturek M, Byrd JP, Hernandez E, Bays H, Grunvald E, Mattar SG. Mesenteric fat cryolipolysis attenuates insulin resistance in the Ossabaw swine model of the metabolic syndrome. Surg Obes Relat Dis. 2023;19(4):374–83. https://doi.org/10.1016/j.soard.2022.10.023.
60. Badran S, Doi SA, Iskeirjeh S, Aljassem G, Jafarian N, Clark J, Habib AM, Glass GE. Metabolic changes after nonsurgical fat removal: a dose response meta-analysis. J Plast Reconstr Aesthet Surg. 2023;77:68–77. https://doi.org/10.1016/j.bjps.2022.10.054.
61. Bamba R, Gupta V, Shack RB, Grotting JC, Higdon KK. Evaluation of diabetes mellitus as a risk factor for major complications in patients undergoing aesthetic surgery. Aesthet Surg J. 2016;36(5):598–608. https://doi.org/10.1093/asj/sjv241.
62. Sardar N, Akin J, Williams K. Diabetes and eyelid surgery: a 12 year analysis of surgical complications. Invest Ophthalmol Vis Sci. 2020;61(7):3972.
63. Dasari N, Jiang A, Skochdopole A, Chung J, Reece EM, Vorstenbosch J, Winocour S. Updates in diabetic wound healing, inflammation, and scarring. Semin Plast Surg. 2021;35(3):153–8. https://doi.org/10.1055/s-0041-1731460.
64. Zhao R, Liang H, Clarke E, Jackson C, Xue M. Inflammation in chronic wounds. Int J Mol Sci. 2016;17(12):E2085.
65. Davis FM, Kimball A, Boniakowski A, Gallagher K. Dysfunctional wound healing in diabetic foot ulcers: new crossroads. Curr Diab Rep. 2018;18(01):2.
66. Boniakowski AE, Kimball AS, Jacobs BN, Kunkel SL, Gallagher KA. Macrophage-mediated inflammation in normal and diabetic wound healing. J Immunol. 2017;199(1):17–24. https://doi.org/10.4049/jimmunol.1700223.
67. Mirza RE, Fang MM, Weinheimer-Haus EM, Ennis WJ, Koh TJ. Sustained inflammasome activity in macrophages impairs wound healing in type 2 diabetic humans and mice. Diabetes. 2014;63(03):1103–14.
68. Rosique RG, Rosique MJ, Farina Junior JA. Curbing inflammation in skin wound healing: a review. Int J Inflamm. 2015;2015(1):316235.
69. Dekker den A, Davis FM, Kunkel SL, Gallagher KA. Targeting epigenetic mechanisms in diabetic wound healing. Transl Res. 2019;204:39–50.
70. Mahdavian Delavary B, van der Veer WM, van Egmond M, Niessen FB, Beelen RHJ. Macrophages in skin injury and repair. Immunobiology. 2011;216(07):753–62.
71. Boyce DE, Ciampolini J, Ruge F, Murison MS, Harding KG. Inflammatory-cell subpopulations in keloid scars. Br J Plast Surg. 2001;54(06):511–6.

Index

K. Fritz, G.-S. Tiplica (eds.), *Cutaneous Manifestations in Diabetes*,
https://doi.org/10.1007/978-3-031-65300-1

GPSR Compliance

The European Union's (EU) General Product Safety Regulation (GPSR) is a set of rules that requires consumer products to be safe and our obligations to ensure this.

If you have any concerns about our products, you can contact us on ProductSafety@springernature.com

In case Publisher is established outside the EU, the EU authorized representative is:

Springer Nature Customer Service Center GmbH
Europaplatz 3
69115 Heidelberg, Germany

Batch number: 10726058

Printed by Printforce, the Netherlands